TAKES THE GUESSWORK
OUT OF DIETING

From abalone to zwiebach, from Burger King to Wendy's, whether you are dining in or eating out, whether you want to lose five pounds or fifty, *Calories and Carbohydrates* will help you achieve your dieting goals. This is the key to ensuring that you eat a healthy, well-balanced diet while getting sufficient vitamins, minerals, and other nutrients. Organized in an easy-to-use, A-to-Z fashion, this book provides the most accurate and dependable calorie and carbohydrate counts for almost everything you eat and drink, allowing you to diet with ease—and to lose as never before.

CALORIES
AND
CARBOHYDRATES

Barbara Kraus

CALORIES AND CARBOHYDRATES

NEW REVISED EDITION

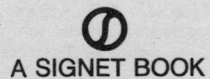

A SIGNET BOOK

SIGNET
Published by the Penguin Group
Penguin Putnam Inc., 375 Hudson Street,
New York, New York 10014, U.S.A.
Penguin Books Ltd, 27 Wrights Lane,
London W8 5TZ, England
Penguin Books Australia Ltd, Ringwood,
Victoria, Australia
Penguin Books Canada Ltd, 10 Alcorn Avenue,
Toronto, Ontario, Canada M4V 3B2
Penguin Books (N.Z.) Ltd, 182–190 Wairau Road,
Auckland 10, New Zealand

Penguin Books Ltd, Registered Offices:
Harmondsworth, Middlesex, England

Published by Signet, an imprint of Dutton NAL, a member of
Penguin Putnam Inc.

First Signet Printing, August, 1973
Second Revised Edition (Seventh Printing), July, 1975
Third Revised Edition (Fourteenth Printing), March, 1979
Fourth Revised Edition (Nineteenth Printing), May, 1981
Fifth Revised Edition (Twenty-fourth Printing), May, 1983
Sixth Revised Edition (Twenty-seventh Printing), June, 1985
Seventh Revised Edition (Thirty-fourth Printing), April, 1987
Eighth Revised Edition (Thirty-seventh Printing), March, 1989
Ninth Revised Edition (Forty-second Printing), March, 1991
Tenth Revised Edition (Forty-third Printing), March, 1993
Eleventh Revised Edition (Forty-fifth Printing), May, 1995
Twelfth Revised Edition (Forty-sixth Printing), January, 1997
Thirteenth Revised Edition, February, 1999
10 9 8 7 6 5 4 3

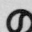 REGISTERED TRADEMARK—MARCA REGISTRADA

Printed in the United States of America

For Audra Thompson

Contents

Introduction ix

Abbreviations and Symbols, Equivalents xv

Dictionary of Brand Names
and Basic Foods 1

Introduction

This dictionary of foods lists several thousand brand-name products and basic foods with their caloric and carbohydrate content. The calorie yield of your diet versus the amount of energy you expend is the key to whether you maintain your ideal weight, gain too many pounds or lose weight.

Because of the relationship of weight to health, many individuals are "counting calories" at every meal. Interest has also been directed to the carbohydrate content of the diet in relation to weight control. Comprehensive information on these values in basic foods and brand-name products is not readily available in any one source. Nor is the information regularly supplied in single-serving portions. (For example, the United States Department of Agriculture supplies counts primarily in bulk-sized portions.) To compound the problem, hundreds of new food items appear in our stores every year.

Analyses of foods to provide information on nutritive values are extremely expensive to conduct. Many small companies have not been able to afford to have their products analyzed and thus were unable to provide data for this book or were able to provide only the calories or only the carbohydrates. Other companies have simply never gotten around to having the analyses done. Other companies simply refuse to supply nutritional information. New requirements for labeling nutritive values of products may provide information on additional items in the future. Therefore, wherever data for carbohydrates were unavailable, blank spaces were left which may be filled in by the reader at a later time.

Arrangement of This Book

Foods are listed alphabetically by brand name or by the name of the food. The singular form is used for most entries—e.g., Blackberry instead of Blackberries. Most items are listed individually though a few are grouped under the general food category. For example, all candies are listed together so that if you are looking for *Mars* bar, you look first under Candy, Commercial, then under *M* in alphabetical order; but, if you are looking for a breakfast food such as oatmeal, you will find it under *O* in the main alphabet. Other foods that are grouped include Baby Food, Gravy, Ice Cream, Marinade Mix, Pie, Sauce, Soft Drinks, Soup, and "Vegetarian Foods." Many cross references are included to assist in finding items called by different names.

Under the main headings, it was often not possible or even desirable to follow an alphabetical arrangement. For basic foods such as apricots, for example, the first entries are for the fresh product weighed with seeds as it is purchased in the store, then the fruit in small portions as they may be eaten or measured. These entries are followed by the processed products, canned (although it may actually be a bottle or jar), dehydrated, dried and frozen. This basic plan, with adaptations where necessary, was followed for fruits, vegetables and meats.

In almost all entries where data were available the U.S. Department of Agriculture figures are shown first. The Department values represent averages from several manufacturers and are shown for comparison with the values from individual companies or for use where particular brands are not available.

All brand-name products have been italicized and company names appear in parentheses.

Portions Used

The portion column is a most important one to read and note. Common household measures are used insofar as possible. For some items, the amounts given are those commonly purchased in the store, such as 1 pound of meat. These quantities can be divided into the number of servings used in the home, and the nutritive values available to each person served can then be readily determined. Of course, any ingredients added when preparing such products must also be taken into account.

The smaller portions given are for foods as served or measured in moderate amounts, such as ½ cup of juice reconstituted, or 4 ounces of meat. Be sure to adjust the calories and carbohydrates to the actual portions you use. For example, if you serve 1 cup of juice instead of ½ cup, multiply the calories and carbohydrates shown for the smaller amount by 2.

Don't fool yourself about the size of portions you use. If you are serious about controlling the calories and carbohydrates in your diet, weigh your foods until you can accurately gauge the weight visually. Remember, the calories and carbohydrates go up with any increase in the weight of foods. Remember, too, that 4 ounces by weight may be very different from 4 fluid ounces or ½ cup. Ounces in the table are always ounces by weight unless specified as fluid ounces, or fractions of a cup or other volumetric measure. Foods that are fluffy in texture, such as flaked coconut and bean sprouts, vary greatly in weight per cup depending on how tightly they are packed into the cup. Such foods as canned green beans also vary when weighed with or without liquid; for example, canned green beans with liquid weigh 4.2 ounces for ½ cup, but drained beans weigh 2.5 ounces for the same ½ cup. Check the weights of your serving portions regularly. Bear in mind that you can cut calories and carbohydrates by cutting the serving size.

It was impossible to convert all the portions to a uniform basis. Some sources were only able to report data in terms of weights with no information on cup or other volumetric measures. I have shown small portions in quantities that might reasonably be expected to be served or measured in the home. Package sizes are useful to show the composition of products as they are purchased and may be divided into the number of serving portions prepared from the entire product, taking into account any added ingredients.

You will find in the portion column the phrases "weighed with bone," or "weighed with skin and seeds" or other inedible parts. These descriptions apply to the products as you purchase them in the markets, but the caloric values and the carbohydrate content as shown are for the amount of edible food after you discard the bone, skin, seed or other inedible part. The weight given in the "measure or quantity" column is to the nearest gram or fraction of an ounce.

Data on the composition of foods are constantly changing for many reasons. Better sampling and analytical methods, improvements in marketing procedures and changes in formulas of mixed products, all may alter values for carbohydrates and other nutrients as well as caloric values. Weights of packaged foods are frequently changed. It is essential to read label information to be informed about these matters and to make intelligent use of food tables.

This book, along with the individual calorie annual guide (*The Barbara Kraus 1996 Calorie Guide to Brand Names and Basic Foods*), is constantly revised and updated to help keep you as up-to-date as possible.

Calories

What is a calorie? It is not a nutrient nor is it a good guide to the nutritive value of food. It is more like a yardstick to measure the energy that a food will yield in the body. You need energy for your body functions as well as for exercise. If your diet contains more calories than your body uses for these purposes, the extra "energy" will be stored as fat.

If your plan is to cut down on calories, the easiest way to do so is to consult the calorie column of this counter and keep an accurate count of your total intake of food and beverages for a period of seven days. If you have not gained or lost weight during that week divide that number by seven and you'll have your maintenance diet expressed in calories. To lose weight, you must reduce your daily or weekly intake of calories below this maintenance level. (To gain, increase the intake.)

One pound of fat is equal to 3,500 calories. Add this number of calories to those you need to balance your energy requirements and you will gain one pound; subtract it, and you will lose a pound.

Carbohydrates

The carbohydrate column shows the amount of this nutrient in grams for the quantities of foods indicated in the portion column. Some dietitians are giving special attention to this nutrient at present in connection with weight control. Carbohydrates include sugars, starches, some acids and other nutrients.

Other Nutrients

Do not forget that other nutrients are extremely important in diet planning—protein, fat, minerals and vitamins. Calories yielded by alcohol must also be taken into consideration. From a nutrition viewpoint, perhaps the best advice that can be given to the dieter is to eat a varied diet with all classes of foods represented. Meat, fish, chicken, fats and oils, milk, vegetables, fruits and grain products are all important sources of essential nutrients and some foods from each of these classes of foods should be included in the diet every day. With the great abundance and variety of foods on the grocer's shelves, there is no reason why the dieter should not enjoy a tasty, nutritious and attractive diet. Just eat in moderation and there is no need to eliminate any one food altogether, except in special conditions under a doctor's directions. Choose wisely and eat well.

Sources of Data

Values in this dictionary are based on publications issued by the U.S. Department of Agriculture and on data submitted by manufacturers and processors. The U.S. Department of Agriculture issues basic tables on food composition for use in the United States. The commercial products from USDA publications represent average values obtained on products of more than one company. The figures designated "home recipe" are based on recipes on file with the Department of Agriculture. Data on commercial products listed by brand name in this publication are based on values supplied by manufacturers and processors for their own individual products. Very few supermarket brand names, such as Safeway or private labels, were included in this book because they are not usually analyzed under these trade names. Every care has been taken to interpret the data and the descriptions supplied by the companies as fully and accurately as possible. Many values have been recalculated to different portions from those submitted in order to bring about greater uniformity among similar items.

Calories in these different sources are not always on a strictly uniform basis. In the Department of Agriculture, calories are calculated using specific factors, which make allowances for losses in digestion and metabolism. The technical explanation of these factors is given in Handbook 74 of the USDA. Most manufacturers use average factors of 4, 9 and 4 for calories yielded by each gram of protein, fat and carbohydrate respectively; a factor of 7 is used as an average value to calculate the calories from one gram of alcohol. These differences in procedure will give somewhat different results for products of similar composition. Some manufacturers have adopted the values from U.S. Department of Agriculture publications as representative of their own products. In these cases, it will be apparent in the table that the data from the companies match exactly those from USDA publications.

Bear in mind that small differences in calorie values on similar products of the same weight are not important in diet planning. They may be due to different methods of calculating the calories or to small differences in the nutritive values of the samples analyzed because no two foods ever have exactly the same composition. Some differences may also be due to the way the food was measured, as noted in the case of green beans earlier.

Carbohydrates in this book are usually total carbohydrates by difference. A few manufacturers reported only "available carbohydrates." These values were omitted.

Abbreviations and Symbols

(USDA) = United States Department
    of Agriculture
(HHS/FAO) = Health and Human
    Services/Food
    and Agriculture
    Organization
* = prepared as package directs[1]
< = less than
& = and
" = inch
canned = bottles or jars
    as well as cans
dia. = diameter

fl. = fluid
liq. = liquid
lb. = pound
med. = medium
oz. = ounce
pkg. = package
pt. = pint
qt. = quart
sq. = square
T. = tablespoon
Tr. = trace
tsp. = teaspoon
wt. = weight

Italics or name in parentheses = registered trademark,®
The letters DNA indicate that data are not available.

Equivalents

By Weight
1 pound = 16 ounces
1 ounce = 28.35 grams
3.52 ounces = 100 grams

By Volume
1 quart = 4 cups
1 cup = 8 fluid ounces
1 cup = ½ pint
1 cup = 16 tablespoons
2 tablespoons = 1 fluid ounce
1 tablespoon = 3 teaspoons

[1]If the package directions call for whole or skim milk, the data given here are for whole milk, unless otherwise stated.

Food	Measure	Cals.	Carbs.

A

ABALONE (USDA):
Raw, meat only	4 oz.	111	3.9
Canned	4 oz.	91	2.6

AC'CENT ¼ tsp. 3 0.0

ACEROLA, fresh fruit
	¼ lb. (weighed with seeds)	52	12.6

ACEROLA JUICE 1 fl. oz. 6 1.5

AGNOLETTI
Fresh, refrigerated
  (See **PASTA, DRY OR FRESH, REFRIGERATED**)
  Frozen (Buitoni):
Cheese filled	2-oz. serving	196	33.4
Meat filled	2-oz. serving	206	31.7

ALBACORE, raw, meat only (USDA) 4 oz. 201 0.0

ALCOHOL (See **DISTILLED LIQUOR**)

ALE (See **BEER & ALE**)

ALFALFA SEEDS (USDA)
Sprouted	1 cup	10	1.0

ALFALFA SPROUTS
canned (Jonathan's):
Plain	1 cup	25	3.0
With garlic	1 cup	27	4.0
With onion	1 cup	25	3.0

ALLSPICE (French's) 1 tsp. 6 1.3

Food	Measure	Cals.	Carbs.
ALMOND:			
Fresh (USDA):			
In shell	10 nuts	60	2.0
Shelled, raw, natural, with skins	1 oz.	170	5.5
Roasted:			
Dry (Planters)	1 oz.	170	6.0
Honey roast (Eagle)	1 oz.	150	10.0
Oil:			
(Fisher)	1 oz.	178	5.5
(Tom's)	1 oz.	180	6.0
ALMOND BUTTER (Hain):			
Raw, natural	1 T.	95	1.5
Toasted, blanched	1 T.	105	1.5
ALMOND DELIGHT, cereal (Ralston/Purina)	¾ cup (1 oz.)	110	23.0
ALMOND EXTRACT (Virginia Dare) pure	1 tsp.	10	0.
ALMOND PASTE (USDA)	1 oz.	127	12.4
ALOE VERA JUICE (Sunburst) 100%	1 oz.	2	.5
ALPHA-BITS, cereal (Post)	1 cup (1 oz.)	113	24.6
AMARANTH, raw, trimmed (USDA)	4 oz.	41	7.4
AMARETTO DI SARONNO **LIQUEUR,** 28% alcohol	1 fl. oz.	83	9.0
AMBROSIA JUICE, canned (Knudson & Sons)	8 fl. oz.	110	27.0
ANCHOVY, PICKLED, canned:			
(USDA) flat or rolled, not heavily salted, drained	2-oz. can	79	.1
(Granadaisor)	2-oz. can	80	Tr.
ANGEL HAIR PASTA (See **PASTA, DRY OR FRESH, REFRIGERATED**)			
ANISE EXTRACT (Virginia Dare) 76% alcohol	1 tsp.	22	0.

Food	Measure	Cals.	Carbs.
ANISE SEEDS (USDA)	1 T.	21	3.0
ANISETTE:			
(DeKuyper)	1 fl. oz.	95	11.4
(Mr. Boston)	1 fl. oz.	87	10.8
APPLE:			
Fresh (USDA):			
Eaten with skin	2½" dia. (4.1 oz.)	61	15.3
Eaten without skin	2½" dia. (4.1 oz.)	53	13.9
Canned:			
(Comstock):			
Rings, drained	1 ring (1.1 oz.)	30	7.0
Sliced	⅙ of 21-oz. can	45	10.0
(Lucky Leaf):			
Chipped	4 oz.	50	12.0
Rings, spiced, green or red	4 oz.	100	24.0
Sliced:			
Regular, dessert	4 oz.	70	16.0
Sweetened:			
In syrup	4 oz.	50	13.0
In water	4 oz.	50	12.0
Whole, baked	1 apple	110	28.0
(White House):			
Rings, spiced	.7-oz. ring	11	8.0
Sliced	½ cup (4 oz.)	54	14.0
Dried:			
(Del Monte) uncooked, sliced	1 oz.	70	18.5
(Sun-Maid/Sunsweet) chunks	2-oz. serving	150	42.0
(Town House)	2-oz. serving	150	40.0
(Weight Watchers):			
Chips	¾-oz. pkg.	70	19.0
Snacks	.5-oz. pkg.	50	13.0
Frozen (USDA), sweetened, slices	10-oz. pkg.	264	68.9
*APPLE, CANDY			
*(Concord) microwaveable:			
Candy	1 apple	50	14.0
Caramel	1 apple	150	27.0
APPLE, ESCALLOPED:			
Canned (White House)	½ cup (4.5 oz.)	163	39.0
Frozen (Stouffer's)	4-oz. serving	130	27.0

Food	Measure	Cals.	Carbs.
APPLE, GLAZED, frozen (Budget Gourmet) in raspberry sauce	5-oz. serving	110	22.0
APPLE-APRICOT JUICE, canned (Knudson & Sons)	8 fl. oz.	120	29.0
APPLE-BANANA JUICE, canned (Knudson & Sons)	8 fl. oz.	120	29.0
APPLE-BLACKBERRY JUICE, canned:			
(Knudson & Sons)	8 fl. oz.	100	24.0
(Santa Cruz) natural, organic	8 fl. oz.	120	29.0
APPLE-BLUEBERRY JUICE DRINK, canned (Boku)	6 fl. oz.	90	22.0
APPLE-BOYSENBERRY JUICE, canned:			
(Knudson & Sons)	8 fl. oz.	110	28.0
(Santa Cruz) natural, organic	8 fl. oz.	120	29.0
APPLE BROWN BETTY, home recipe (USDA)	1 cup	325	63.9
APPLE BUTTER:			
(Empress) regular or spiced	1 T.	37	9.0
(Home Brands)	1 T.	51	13.5
(Piedmont)	1 T.	37	7.5
(White House)	1 T.	38	9.0
APPLE CHERRY BERRY DRINK, canned:			
(Lincoln)	6 fl. oz.	90	23.0
(Veryfine)	6 fl. oz.	97	24.7
APPLE-CHERRY CIDER, canned:			
(McCain) junior	4.2-fl.-oz. container	50	13.0
(Red Creek)	6 fl. oz.	113	28.0
APPLE-CHERRY JUICE COCKTAIL, canned: *Musselman's*	8 fl. oz.	110	28.0

Food	Measure	Cals.	Carbs.
(Red Cheek)	6 fl. oz.	113	28.0
APPLE CIDER:			
Canned:			
(Johanna Farms)	½ cup	56	14.5
(Mott's) sweet	½ cup	59	14.6
(S. Martinelli) sparkling	6 fl. oz.	100	25.0
(Town House)	6 fl. oz.	90	23.0
(Tree Top)	6 fl. oz.	90	22.0
*Frozen (Tree Top)	6 fl. oz.	90	22.0
*Mix:			
Country Time	8 fl. oz.	98	24.5
(Hi-C)	6 fl. oz.	72	18.0
APPLE-CRANBERRY CIDER,			
canned (Indian Summer)	6 fl. oz.	100	24.0
APPLE-CRANBERRY DRINK,			
canned:			
(Mott's)	8 fl. oz.	141	35.2
(Tropicana):			
Regular	8 fl. oz.	147	36.0
Single Serve	8 fl. oz.	140	34.4
APPLE-CRANBERRY JUICE:			
Canned:			
(Knudson & Sons)	6 fl. oz.	82	21.0
(Mott's):			
Regular	6 fl. oz.	83	24.0
Box	8.45-fl.-oz. container	136	34.0
(Santa Cruz) organic	6 fl. oz.	86	21.0
(Tree Top)	6 fl. oz.	100	25.0
(Veryfine) cocktail	6 fl. oz.	97	24.7
*Frozen (Tree Top)	6 fl. oz.	100	25.0
APPLE CRISP, frozen:			
(Pepperidge Farm)	4-oz. serving	240	41.0
(Weight Watchers) *Sweet Celebrations*	3½-oz. serving	190	40.0
APPLE DRINK, canned:			
Capri Sun, natural	6¾ fl. oz.	90	22.7
(Hi-C)	6 fl. oz.	92	23.0
(Johanna Farms) *Ssips*	8.45-fl.-oz. container	130	32.0

Food	Measure	Cals.	Carbs.
APPLE DUMPLINGS, frozen (Pepperidge Farm)	1 dumpling (3.1 oz.)	260	33.0
APPLE-GRAPE-CHERRY JUICE, canned (Welch's) *Orchard Cocktail*	8.45-fl.-oz. container	150	38.0
APPLE-GRAPE JUICE:			
Canned:			
(Juicy Juice)	6 fl. oz.	90	10.0
(Juicy Juice)	8.45-fl.-oz. container	120	29.0
(Mott's)	8.45-fl.-oz. container	128	32.0
(Mott's)	9½-fl.-oz. can	139	37.0
(Red Cheek)	6 fl. oz.	109	27.0
(Tree Top)	6 fl. oz.	100	25.0
*Frozen (Tree Top)	6 fl. oz.	100	25.0
APPLE JACKS, cereal (Kellogg's)	1 cup (1 oz.)	110	26.0
APPLE JAM (Smucker's)	1 T.	53	13.5
APPLE JELLY:			
Sweetened:			
(Kraft)	1 T.	51	12.0
(Polaner)	1 T.	53	13.5
(Smucker's) regular, cinnamon or mint	1 T.	54	12.0
Dietetic:			
(Estee)	1 T. (.6 oz.)	6	0.0
(Featherweight)	1 T.	12	3.0
Slenderella	1 T.	21	6.0
APPLE JUICE:			
Canned:			
(Ardmore Farms)	6 fl. oz.	90	22.2
(Borden) *Sippin' Pak*	8.45-fl.-oz. container	110	28.0
(Indian Summer)	6 fl. oz.	90	21.0
(Juicy Juice)	6 fl. oz.	90	21.0
(Knudson & Sons) gravenstein	6 fl. oz.	82	21.0
(Land O' Lakes)	6 fl. oz.	90	22.0
(McCain) junior	4.2-fl.-oz.		

Food	Measure	Cals.	Carbs.
	container	50	13.0
(Minute Maid)	8.45-fl.-oz.		
	container	128	31.9
(Mott's)	6 fl. oz.	88	22.0
(Ocean Spray)	6 fl. oz.	90	23.0
(Red Cheek)	6 fl. oz.	97	24.0
(S. Martinelli) sparkling	6 fl. oz.	100	25.0
(Snapple) Apple Crisp	6 fl. oz.	105	27.0
(Town House)	6 fl. oz.	90	23.0
(Tree Top) any type	6 fl. oz.	90	22.0
(Very Fine) 100% juice	6 fl. oz.	80	20.2
(White House)	6 fl. oz.	87	22.0
Chilled (Minute Maid):			
Regular	6 fl. oz.	91	22.7
On the Go	10-fl.-oz. bottle	140	35.0
*Frozen:			
(Minute Maid)	6 fl. oz.	91	22.7
(Sunkist)	6 fl. oz.	59	14.5
(Tree Top)	6 fl. oz.	90	22.0
APPLE JUICE DRINK, canned:			
Squeezit (General Mills)	6¾-fl.-oz. bottle	110	27.0
(Sunkist)	8.45 fl. oz.	140	34.0
APPLE NECTAR, canned			
(Libby's)	6 fl. oz.	100	25.0
APPLE-ORANGE-PINEAPPLE COCKTAIL canned (Welch's) *Orchard Tropical Cocktail*:			
Regular	6 fl. oz.	100	25.0
Individual container	8.45-fl.-oz.		
	container	140	35.0
APPLE-PEACH JUICE, canned			
(Knudson & Sons)	6 fl. oz.	105	25.5
APPLE-PEAR JUICE, canned or *frozen			
(Tree Top)	6 fl. oz.	90	22.0
APPLE PIE (See **PIE**, Apple)			
APPLE PUNCH DRINK, canned (Red Cheek)	6 fl. oz.	113	28.0

Food	Measure	Cals.	Carbs.
APPLE RAISIN CRISP, cereal			
(Kellogg's)	⅔ cup (1 oz.)	130	32.0
APPLE-RASPBERRY DRINK,	10-fl.-oz.		
canned (Mott's)	container	158	40.0
APPLE-RASPBERRY JUICE:			
Canned, regular pack:			
(Knudson & Sons)	6 fl. oz.	82	21.0
(Mott's)	8.45-fl.-oz.		
	container	124	31.0
(Mott's)	9½-fl.-oz.		
	container	134	35.0
(Red Cheek)	6 fl. oz.	113	28.0
(Santa Cruz) natural, organic	6 fl. oz.	90	21.8
(Tree Top)	6 fl. oz.	80	21.0
(Very Fine) cocktail	6 fl. oz.	82	20.2
*Frozen (Tree Top)	6 fl. oz.	80	21.0
APPLE SAUCE, canned:			
Regular:			
(Hunt's) *Snack Pack*:			
Regular	4¼ oz.	80	19.0
Natural	4¼ oz.	50	12.0
Raspberry	4¼ oz.	80	21.0
Strawberry	4¼ oz.	80	20.0
(Mott's):			
Regular, jarred:			
Plain	6 oz.	150	36.0
Chunky	6 oz.	132	31.2
Cinnamon	6 oz.	144	34.8
Single-serve cups:			
Regular	4 oz.	100	24.0
Cherry	3¾ oz.	72	17.0
Cinnamon	4 oz.	101	24.0
Peach	3¾ oz.	75	18.0
Pineapple	3¾ oz.	86	21.0
Strawberry	3¾ oz.	76	18.0
(Town House)	½ cup	85	23.5
(Tree Top) Cinnamon or			
original	½ cup	80	22.0
(White House) regular	½ cup (5 oz.)	80	22.0
Dietetic or natural:			
(Country Pure)	4 oz.	50	12.0
(Del Monte lite	4 oz.	50	13.0
(Featherweight)	4 oz.	50	12.0

Food	Measure	Cals.	Carbs.
(Mott's):			
Regular	4 oz.	53	13.3
Single-serve cup	4 oz.	53	13.0
(S&W) *Nutradiet*	4 oz.	55	14.0
(Tree Top) natural	4 oz.	60	14.0
(White House):			
Natural	½ cup (4.7 oz.)	50	12.0
Apple juice added	½ cup (4.7 oz.)	50	13.0
APRICOT:			
Fresh (USDA):			
Whole	1 lb. (weighed with pits)	217	54.6
Whole	3 apricots (about 12 per lb.)	55	13.7
Halves	1 cup (5½ oz.)	79	19.8
Canned, regular pack, solids & liq.:			
(USDA):			
Juice pack	4 oz.	61	15.4
Extra heavy syrup	4 oz.	115	29.5
(Stokely-Van Camp)	½ cup (4.6 oz.)	110	27.0
(S&W) in heavy syrup:			
Peeled, whole	½ cup	100	26.0
Unpeeled, halves	½ cup	110	28.0
(Town House) unpeeled, halves	½ cup	110	28.0
Canned, dietetic, solids & liq.:			
(Country Pure) halves	½ cup	60	15.0
(Diet Delight):			
Juice pack	½ cup (4.4 oz.)	60	15.0
Water pack	½ cup (4.3 oz.)	35	9.0
(Featherweight):			
Juice pack	½ cup	50	12.0
Water pack	½ cup	35	9.0
(Libby's) Lite	½ cup (4.4 oz.)	60	15.0
(S&W) *Nutradiet,* in water:			
Peeled, whole	½ cup	28	7.0
Unpeeled, halves	½ cup	35	9.0
Dried (Town House)	2-oz. serving	140	35.0
APRICOT, CANDIED (USDA)	1 oz.	96	24.5
APRICOT, STRAINED, canned (Larsen) no salt added	½ cup	55	14.5

Food	Measure	Cals.	Carbs.
APRICOT LIQUEUR			
(DeKuyper) 60 proof	1 fl. oz.	82	8.3
APRICOT NECTAR, canned:			
(Ardmore Farms)	6 fl. oz.	94	24.2
(Knudson & Sons)	6 fl. oz.	79	18.0
(S&W)	6 fl. oz.	100	26.0
(Town House)	6 fl. oz.	100	26.0
APRICOT-PINEAPPLE			
NECTAR, canned, dietetic			
(S&W) *Nutradiet*, blue label	6 oz.	52	18.0
APRICOT & PINEAPPLE			
PRESERVE OR JAM:			
Sweetened (Smucker's)	1 T. (.7 oz.)	53	13.5
Dietetic:			
(Featherweight)	1 T.	6	1.0
(Tillie Lewis) *Tasti Diet*	1 T.	12	3.0
APRICOT PRESERVE, dietetic:			
(Estee)	1 T.	6	0.0
(Smucker's) low sugar	1 T.	24.0	6.0
ARBY'S:			
Biscuit:			
Plain	2.9-oz. piece	280	34.0
Bacon	3.1-oz. piece	318	35.0
Ham	4.4-oz. piece	323	34.0
Sausage	4.2-oz. piece	460	35.0
Cakes	3-oz. serving	204	20.0
Cake, Cheese	3-oz. serving	320	23.0
Cheddar fries	5-oz. serving	333	40.0
Chicken fingers	2 pieces	290	20.0
Condiments:			
Croutons	.5-oz. serving	59	8.0
Ketchup	.5-oz. serving	16	4.0
Mustard	.5 oz.	11	Tr.
Cookie, chocolate chip	1-oz. cookie	125	16.0
Croissant:			
Plain	1-piece serving	220	25.0
Bacon & egg	4.3-oz. serving	430	29.0
Ham & cheese	4.2-oz. serving	345	29.0
Mushroom & cheese	5.2-oz. serving	493	34.0
Sausage & egg	5-oz. serving	519	29.0
Curly fries	3.5-oz. serving	337	43.0
Danish, cinnamon nut	3½-oz. piece	360	60.0

Food	Measure	Cals.	Carbs.
French fries	2½-oz. serving	246	30.0
French Toastix	6 pieces	430	52.0
Ham	1 serving	45	0.0
Hot chocolate	8 fl. oz.	110	23.0
Muffin, blueberry	2.7-oz. piece	230	45.0
Orange juice	6 fl. oz.	82	20.0
Platters:			
Bacon	7.8-oz. serving	593	51.0
Egg	7.1-oz. serving	460	45.0
Ham	9.1-oz. serving	518	45.0
Sausage	8.4-oz. serving	640	46.0
Polar Swirl:			
Butterfinger	11.6-oz. serving	457	62.0
Heath	11.6-oz. serving	543	76.0
Oreo	11.6-oz. serving	482	66.0
Peanut butter cup	11.6-oz. serving	517	61.0
Snickers	11.6-oz. serving	511	73.0
Potato, baked:			
Plain	11.5-oz. serving	355	82.0
Broccoli & cheddar	1 serving	445	89.0
Butter & sour cream	1 serving	578	85.0
Deluxe	1 serving	736	86.0
Salad:			
Garden	1 serving	60	12.0
Roast chicken	1 serving	149	12.0
Side	5.3-oz. serving	25	4.0
Salad dressing:			
Regular:			
Blue cheese	2-oz. serving	290	2.0
Honey french	2-oz. serving	280	18.0
Thousand Island	2-oz. serving	260	7.0
Dietetic Italian, light	2-oz. serving	20	3.0
Sandwich, chicken:			
Breast fillet	7.2-oz. serving	445	42.0
Club, roast	8.4-oz. serving	545	37.0
Cordon bleu	8-oz. serving	623	45.0
Grilled:			
Barbeque	7.1-oz. serving	386	47.0
Deluxe	8.1-oz. serving	430	42.0
Sandwich, fish fillet	1 serving	530	50.0
Sandwich, ham & cheese melt	1 serving	330	34.0
Sandwich, roast beef:			
Plain:			
Regular	1 serving	388	33.0
Giant	1 serving	555	43.0
Junior	1 serving	325	35.0
Light, deluxe	1 serving	295	33.0

Food	Measure	Cals.	Carbs.
Super	1 serving	523	50.0
Arby's Melt, with cheddar cheese	1 serving	365	36.0
Arby Q	1 serving	430	48.0
Bac'N Cheddar, deluxe	1 serving	538	38.0
Beef 'N Cheddar	1 serving	485	40.0
Sandwich, roast turkey, deluxe, light	1 serving	260	33.0
Sandwich on sub roll:			
French dip	1 serving	475	40.0
Italian	1 serving	675	46.0
Sauce:			
Arby's	.5-oz. serving	15	3.0
Horsey	.5-oz. serving	60	2.0
Sausage	1 serving	163	0.0
Shake:			
Chocolate	12 fl. oz.	451	76.0
Jamocha	11½ fl. oz.	384	62.0
Vanilla	11 fl. oz.	360	50.0
Soft drink:			
Sweetened:			
Cola:			
Coca Cola Classic	12 fl. oz.	140	38.0
R.C.	12 fl. oz.	170	43.0
Orange (Nehi)	12 fl. oz.	190	47.4
Root beer, *R.C.*	12 fl. oz.	173	42.9
Upper Ten	12 fl. oz.	169	42.3
Dietetic:			
Coca Cola	12 fl. oz.	1	0.0
7 Up	12 fl. oz.	4	0.0
Soup:			
Broccoli, cream of	8 fl. oz.	160	15.0
Chicken noodle, old fashioned	8 fl. oz.	80	11.0
Chowder, clam, Boston	8 fl. oz.	190	18.0
Potato, with bacon	8 fl. oz.	170	23.0
Vegetable, Lumberjack, mixed	8 fl. oz.	89	13.0
Syrup, maple	1.5-oz.	100	25.0
Turnover, Apple	3-oz. serving	303	28.0
ARTHUR TREACHER'S RESTAURANTS:			
Chicken patty	2 patties (4.8 oz.)	369	16.5
Chicken sandwich	5½-oz. serving	413	44.0
Cod fillet, tail shape, *Bake 'n Broil*	5-oz. serving	245	9.7
Coleslaw	3-oz. serving	123	11.0

Food	Measure	Cals.	Carbs.
Fish	5.2-oz. serving	355	19.2
Fish sandwich	5½-oz. serving	440	39.4
French fries, *Chips*	4-oz. serving	275	34.9
Hushpuppy, *Krunch Pup*	1 piece (2 oz.)	203	12.0
Lemon Luv	3-oz. serving	275	35.1
Shrimp	4.1-oz. serving (7 pieces)	381	27.2
ARTICHOKE:			
Fresh (USDA):			
Raw, whole	1 lb. (weighed untrimmed)	85	19.2
Boiled, without salt, drained	15-oz. artichoke	187	42.1
Canned (Cara Mia) marinated, drained	6-oz. jar	175	12.6
Frozen (Birds Eye) hearts, deluxe	⅓ pkg. (3 oz.)	33	6.6
ARUGULA (USDA) raw	1 leaf	1	tr.
ASPARAGUS:			
Fresh (USDA):			
Raw, spears	1 lb. (weighed untrimmed)	66	12.7
Boiled, without salt, drained	1 spear (½" dia. at base)	3	.5
Canned, regular pack, solids & liq.:			
(Del Monte) whole	½ cup	20	3.0
(Green Giant) cuts or spears	½ cup (4 oz.)	20	3.0
(Le Sueur) green spears	½ of 8-oz. can	30	4.0
(S&W) fancy:			
Regular	½ cup	18	3.0
Colossal	½ cup	20	4.0
(Town House) cut or spears	½ cup	20	3.0
Canned, dietetic pack (USDA) drained solids, cut	1 cup (8.3 oz.)	47	7.3
Canned, dietetic pack, solids & liq.:			
(Diet Delight)	½ cup	16	2.0
(S&W) *Nutradiet*	½ cup	17	3.0
Frozen:			
(USDA) cuts & tips, boiled, drained	1 cup (6.3 oz.)	40	6.3
(Birds Eye):			
Cuts	⅓ pkg. (3.3 oz.)	25	3.8
Spears	⅓ pkg. (3.3 oz.)	25	3.9

Food	Measure	Cals.	Carbs.
(Frosty Acres)	3.3-oz. serving	25	4.0
ASPARAGUS PILAF, frozen (Green Giant) microwave *Garden Gourmet*	9½-oz. pkg.	190	37.0
ASPARAGUS PUREE, canned (Larsen) no salt added	½ cup (4.4 oz.)	22	3.5
AU BON PAIN **RESTAURANT**:			
Bagel:			
Plain	1 bagel	380	79.0
Cinnamon	1 bagel	396	86.0
Onion	1 bagel	390	81.0
Sesame	1 bagel	425	81.0
Bread:			
Baguette	1 loaf	810	166.0
Cheese	1 loaf	1670	269.0
Four grain	1 loaf	1420	262.0
Onion herb	1 loaf	1430	263.0
Pita pocket	1 slice	40	9.0
Ponsienne	1 loaf	1490	166.0
Sandwich:			
Multigrain	1 slice	145	38.0
Rye	1 slice	187	36.5
Cheese:			
Boursin	1 serving on a sandwich	290	2.0
Brie	1 serving on a sandwich	300	3.0
Cheddar	1 serving on a sandwich	110	1.0
Provolone	1 serving on a sandwich	155	<1.0
Swiss	1 serving on a sandwich	330	3.0
Chicken pot pie	1 serving	440	46.0
Chicken sandwich:			
Cracked pepper:			
On a French roll	1 sandwich	440	66.0
On a hearth roll	1 sandwich	490	70.0
On a soft roll	1 sandwich	430	51.0
Grilled:			
On a French roll	1 sandwich	450	66.0
On a hearth roll	1 sandwich	550	70.0
On a soft roll	1 sandwich	440	51.0

Food	Measure	Cals.	Carbs.
Tarragon:			
On a French roll	1 sandwich	590	68.0
On a hearth roll	1 sandwich	640	72.0
On a soft roll	1 sandwich	580	53.0
Chili, vegetarian:			
Bowl	1 serving	208	27.0
Cup	1 serving	139	24.0
Cookie, gourmet:			
Chocolate chip	1 piece	280	37.0
Chocolate chunk pecan:			
Regular	1 piece	290	37.0
White	1 piece	300	37.0
Oatmeal raisin	1 piece	250	41.0
Peanut butter	1 piece	290	33.0
Shortbread	1 piece	425	46.0
Croissant:			
Plain	1 croissant	220	29.0
Almond	1 croissant	420	41.0
Apple	1 croissant	250	38.0
Blueberry cheese	1 croissant	380	44.0
Chocolate	1 croissant	400	46.0
Cinnamon raisin	1 croissant	390	60.0
Coconut pecan	1 croissant	440	51.0
Hazelnut chocolate	1 croissant	480	56.0
Raspberry cheese	1 croissant	400	49.0
Strawberry cheese	1 croissant	400	49.0
Sweet cheese	1 croissant	420	45.0
Croissant, hot, filled:			
With ham & cheese	1 serving	370	38.0
With spinach & cheese	1 serving	290	29.0
With turkey & cheddar	1 serving	410	38.0
With turkey and havarti	1 serving	410	38.0
Danish:			
Cheese	1 piece	390	43.0
Cherry	1 piece	335	42.0
Cherry dumpling	1 piece	360	59.0
Raspberry	1 piece	335	43.0
Ham sandwich, country:			
On a French roll	1 sandwich	470	68.0
On a hearth roll	1 sandwich	520	72.0
On a soft roll	1 sandwich	460	53.0
Muffin, gourmet:			
Blueberry	1 muffin	390	66.0
Bran	1 muffin	390	73.0
Carrot	1 muffin	450	48.0
Corn	1 muffin	460	71.0
Cranberry walnut	1 muffin	350	53.0

Food	Measure	Cals.	Carbs.
Oat bran apple	1 muffin	400	71.0
Pumpkin	1 muffin	410	63.0
Whole grain	1 muffin	440	68.0
Roast beef sandwich:			
On a French roll	1 sandwich	500	66.0
On a hearth roll	1 sandwich	550	70.0
On a soft roll	1 sandwich	490	51.0
Roll:			
Alpine	1 roll	220	43.0
Country seed	1 roll	220	37.0
Hearth	1 roll	250	42.0
Petit Pan	1 roll	220	44.0
Sandwich:			
Braided	1 roll	387	64.0
Croissant	1 roll	300	38.0
French	1 roll	320	65.0
Hearth	1 roll	320	65.0
Soft	1 roll	310	50.0
Three-seed raisin	1 roll	250	46.0
Vegetable	1 roll	230	40.0
Salad:			
Chicken tarragon	1 serving	310	24.0
Cracked pepper chicken	1 serving	100	14.0
Garden:			
Large	1 serving	40	8.0
Small	1 serving	20	5.0
Grilled chicken	1 serving	110	9.0
Italian, low calorie	1 serving	68	3.0
Shrimp	1 serving	102	8.0
Tuna	1 serving	350	11.0
Turkey sandwich, smoked:			
On a French roll	1 sandwich	420	65.0
On a hearth roll	1 sandwich	470	69.0
On a soft roll	1 sandwich	410	50.0
Soup:			
Beef barley:			
Bowl	1 serving	112	15.0
Cup	1 serving	75	10.0
Broccoli, cream of:			
Bowl	1 serving	302	18.0
Cup	1 serving	200	12.0
Chicken noodle:			
Bowl	1 serving	119	14.0
Cup	1 serving	79	9.0
Chowder, clam:			
Bowl	1 serving	433	36.0
Cup	1 serving	139	24.0

Food	Measure	Cals.	Carbs.
Minestrone, cup	1 serving	105	20.0
Split pea:			
Bowl	1 serving	264	45.0
Cup	1 serving	176	30.0
Tomato, Florentine:			
Bowl	1 serving	92	15.0
Cup	1 serving	61	10.0
Vegetarian, garden:			
Bowl	1 serving	44	9.0
Cup	1 serving	29	6.0

AUNT JEMIMA SYRUP (See
SYRUP)

AVOCADO, all varieties
(USDA):

Whole	1 fruit (10.7 oz.)	378	14.3
Cubed	1 cup (5.3 oz.)	251	9.5

AVOCADO PUREE

(Calavo)	½ cup (8.1 oz.)	411	15.9

*****AWAKE** (Birds Eye)	6 fl. oz. (6.5 oz.)	84	20.5

B

BABY FOOD:

Apple (Earth's Best)	4½-oz. jar	60	14.0
Apple & apricot (Earth's Best)	4½-oz. jar	70	15.0
Apple-apricot juice (Heinz)			
strained	3½ fl. oz.	47	11.2
Apple & banana:			
(Earth's Best)	4½-oz. jar	60	14.0
(Gerber) *Second Foods*	4-oz. jar	80	19.0
Apple-banana juice:			
(Earth's Best)	4.2 fl. oz.	60	14.0
(Gerber) *Graduates*	6 fl. oz.	135	34.5
Apple & blueberry:			
(Earth's Best)	4½-oz. jar	60	14.0
(Gerber):			
Junior	6-oz. jar	80	19.0

Food	Measure	Cals.	Carbs.
Second Foods	7 T.	51	12.1
Strained	4½-oz. jar	60	14.0
Apple-carrot juice (Gerber)			
Third Foods	4 fl. oz.	50	12.0
Apple-cherry juice:			
(Beech-Nut) *Stages 2*	4 fl. oz.	60	14.0
(Gerber):			
Graduates	6 fl. oz.	80	21.0
Second Foods	4 fl. oz.	60	14.0
(Heinz) strained	3½ fl. oz.	45	10.7
Apple & cranberry with tapioca			
(Heinz) strained	3½-oz. jar	66	15.9
Apple dessert, Dutch:			
(Beech-Nut) *Stages 2*	4½-oz. jar	100	24.0
(Gerber):			
Second Foods	1 T.	11	2.3
Third Foods	1 T.	11	2.4
(Heinz):			
Junior	3½-oz. jar	69	16.3
Strained	3½-oz. jar	69	16.3
Apple-grape juice:			
(Beech-Nut) *Stages 2*	3½ fl. oz.	47	11.3
(Earth's Best)	4.2 fl. oz.	60	14.0
(Gerber):			
Graduates	6 fl. oz.	90	22.0
Second Foods	3.2 fl. oz.	48	11.7
Apple juice:			
(Beech-Nut) *Stages 1*	4.2 fl. oz.	60	15.0
(Earth's Best)	4.2 fl. oz.	60	14.0
(Gerber):			
First Foods, strained	4 fl. oz.	60	14.0
Graduates	3.2 fl. oz.	48	11.7
(Heinz) strained:			
Regular	3½ fl. oz.	48	11.7
Saver size	4.2 fl. oz.	70	17.0
Apple juice dessert (Gerber)			
Second Foods, with yogurt	4-oz. jar	100	18.0
Apple juice with yogurt			
(Gerber) *Second Foods*	3.2 fl. oz.	73	14.2
Apple-peach juice:			
(Gerber) *Second Foods*	4 fl. oz.	60	14.0
(Heinz) strained	3½ fl. oz.	44	10.4
Apple, peach & strawberry			
(Beech-Nut) *Stages 2*	4½-oz. jar	100	24.0
Apple, pear & banana (Beech-Nut) *Stages 2*			

Food	Measure	Cals.	Carbs.
	4½-oz. jar	100	24.0
Apple-pineapple juice (Heinz)			
strained	3½ fl. oz.	47	11.1
Apple & Plum (Earth's Best)	4½-oz. jar	70	16.0
Apples & chicken dinner			
(Gerber) *Second Foods,*			
Simple Recipe	1 T.	9	.1
Apples & ham dinner (Gerber)			
Second Foods, Simple			
Recipe	1 T.	9	1.7
Apples & turkey dinner			
(Gerber) *Second Foods,*			
Simple Recipe	4 oz.	80	13.0
Applesauce:			
(Beech-Nut):			
Baby's First, golden			
delicious	2½-oz. jar	50	11.0
Stages 1, golden delicious	4½-oz. jar	70	17.0
Stages 3	6-oz. jar	90	22.0
(Gerber):			
First Foods	2½-oz. jar	35	9.0
Junior	6-oz. jar	90	20.0
Second Foods	7 T.	52	12.3
Strained	4½-oz. jar	60	14.0
Third Foods	7 T.	51	12.1
(Heinz):			
Beginner Foods	3½-oz. jar	73	18.0
Junior	3½-oz. jar	53	12.4
Strained	3½-oz. jar	53	12.4
Applesauce & apricot:			
(Beech-Nut) *Stages 2*	5½-oz. jar	80	19.0
(Gerber):			
Second Foods	7 T.	53	12.5
Strained	4½-oz. jar	70	15.0
Applesauce & banana (Beech-Nut):			
Stages 2	4½-oz. jar	80	18.0
Stages 3	6-oz. jar	100	25.0
Apricot with pear (Beech-Nut)			
Stages 3	6-oz. jar	120	27.0
Apricot with tapioca:			
(Gerber):			
Junior	6-oz. jar	130	29.0
Second Foods	7 T.	67	16.2
Strained	4½-oz. jar	90	10.0
Third Foods	7 T.	71	17.1
(Heinz):			
Junior	3½-oz. jar	66	15.9

Food	Measure	Cals.	Carbs.
Strained	3½-oz. jar	64	15.3
Banana:			
(Beech-Nut) *Chiquita*:			
Baby First	2½-oz. jar	70	16.0
Stages 1	4½-oz. jar	110	26.0
(Earth's Best)	4½-oz. jar	100	22.0
(Gerber) *First Foods*	2½-oz. jar	70	17.0
Banana & apple (Gerber) strained	4½-oz. jar	90	20.0
Banana-apple dessert (Gerber) *Second Foods*	1 T.	10	2.3
Banana juice with yogurt (Gerber) *Second Foods*	4 fl. oz.	110	21.0
Banana & pineapple (Beech-Nut) *Stages 2*	4½-oz. jar	110	27.0
Banana-pineapple dessert (Beech-Nut) *Stages 2*	4½-oz. jar	110	27.0
Banana & pineapple with tapioca:			
(Beech-Nut) *Stages 2*	4½-oz. jar	110	27.0
(Gerber):			
Junior	6-oz. jar	90	20.0
Strained	4½-oz. jar	60	15.0
(Heinz)	3½-oz. jar	64	15.3
Banana-vanilla dessert (Gerber) *Tropical Foods*	1 T.	12	2.7
Bean dinner, green, with turkey (Gerber) *Second Foods, Simple Recipe*	1 T.	8	1.0
Bean, green:			
(Beech-Nut):			
Stages 1	4½-oz. jar	35	8.0
Stages 3	6-oz. jar	45	10.0
(Gerber) *First Foods*	7 T.	32	6.2
(Heinz):			
Beginner Foods	3½-oz. jar	30	5.9
Strained	3½-oz. jar	25	4.9
Beans & rice dinner:			
(Earth's Best) with green beans	4½-oz. jar	70	14.0
(Gerber) *Tropical Foods*	1 T.	7	1.1
Beef (Gerber):			
Second Foods	7 T.	100	0.1
Third Foods	7 T.	103	0.2
Beef with broth:			
(Beech-Nut) *Stages 1*	2½-oz. jar	80	0.0
(Heinz):			
Junior	3½-oz. jar	123	0.3

Food	Measure	Cals.	Carbs.
Strained	3½-oz. jar	123	0.3
Beef dinner:			
(Beech-Nut):			
Stages 1	2.8-oz. jar	90	0.0
Stages 2, supreme	4½-oz. jar	120	13.0
Stages 3	6-oz. jar	150	14.0
(Gerber):			
Junior:			
Plain	2½-oz. jar	80	1.0
With vegetables, lean meat	4½-oz. jar	100	10.0
Strained, with vegetables,			
lean meat	4½-oz. jar	90	9.0
Third Foods	1 T.	15	Tr.
Beef & egg noodle dinner:			
(Gerber):			
Second Foods	1 T.	9	1.2
Third Foods	1 T.	9	1.3
(Heinz) strained	3½-oz. jar	49	6.3
Beef with egg yolks (Gerber)			
strained	2½-oz. jar	80	0.0
Beef stew (Beech-Nut) *Stages*			
Table Time	6-oz. jar	150	16.0
Beef vegetable entree (Beech-Nut):			
Stages 2	4½-oz. jar	90	10.0
Stages 3	6-oz. jar	160	16.0
Beet:			
(Gerber):			
Second Foods	7 T.	39	8.1
Strained	4½-oz. jar	60	11.0
(Heinz) strained	3½-oz. jar	40	8.3
Broccoli, carrot & cheese			
(Gerber) *Third Foods*	7 T.	44	7.2
Broccoli-chicken dinner			
(Gerber) *Second Foods,*			
Simple Recipe	1 T.	6	.5
Carrot:			
(Beech-Nut):			
Regular, *Stages 3*	6-oz. jar	60	13.0
Regal *Imperial:*			
Baby's First	2½-oz. jar	25	6.0
Stages 1	4½-oz. jar	40	9.0
(Earth's Best)	4½-oz. jar	40	7.0
(Gerber):			
First Foods	2½-oz. jar	25	5.0
Graduates, diced	3.2-oz. jar	22	4.7
Junior	6-oz. jar	80	16.0

Food	Measure	Cals.	Carbs.
Second Foods	7 T.	30	6.1
Strained	4½-oz. jar	35	8.0
Third Foods	7 T.	29	6.0
(Heinz):			
Beginner Foods	3½-oz. jar	30	6.1
Junior	3½-oz. jar	23	4.9
Strained	3½-oz. jar	23	4.9
Carrot & beef dinner (Gerber)			
Second Foods, Simple			
Recipe	1 T.	8	1.2
Carrot & Parsnip (Earth's Best)	4½-oz. jar	60	14.0
Chicken:			
(Beech-Nut) *Stages 1*	2.8-oz. jar	80	0.0
(Gerber):			
Second Foods	7 T.	128	0.0
Third Foods	7 T.	132	0.2
Chicken with broth:			
(Beech-Nut) *Stages 1*	2½-oz. jar	70	0.0
(Heinz) strained	3½-oz. jar	143	0.7
Chicken dinner (Gerber):			
Junior	2½-oz. jar	110	1.0
Third Foods	1 T.	19	Tr.
Chicken noodle dinner			
(Gerber):			
Second Foods	1 T.	8	1.2
Third Foods	1 T.	8	1.2
Chicken rice dinner:			
(Beech-Nut) *Stages 2*	4½-oz. jar	80	11.0
(Gerber) *Tropical Foods*	1 T.	7	1.0
Chicken soup (See Soup,			
Chicken)			
Chicken sticks (Gerber)			
Graduates	1 piece	14	1.5
Cereal:			
Barley, dry, instant:			
(Beech-Nut) *Stages 1*	.5 oz.	60	10.0
(Gerber) *First Foods*	.5 oz.	60	11.0
Corn, dry (Gerber) *Tropical*			
Foods	.5 oz.	60	12.0
Mixed:			
Plain, dry:			
(Beech-Nut) *Stages 2*	.5 oz.	60	12.0
(Earth's Best)	.5 oz.	60	11.0
(Gerber) *Second Foods*	.5 oz.	60	11.0
(Heinz)	.5 oz.	53	10.3
With apples & bananas:			
(Beech-Nut) *Stages 2*	4½-oz. jar	90	19.0

Food	Measure	Cals.	Carbs.
(Heinz) strained	3½-oz. jar	70	15.7
With applesauce & bananas (Gerber) *Third Foods*	1 T.	12	2.6
With bananas (Gerber) *Second Foods,* instant, dry	.5 oz.	60	11.0
Oatmeal:			
Plain, dry (Beech-Nut) *Stages 1*	.5 oz.	60	10.0
Mixed:			
With apples & bananas:			
(Beech-Nut) *Stages 2*	4½-oz. jar	90	17.0
(Heinz) strained	3½-oz. jar	76	16.0
With apples & cinnamon (Gerber) *Third Foods,* instant, dry	1 packet	90	16.0
With applesauce & bananas (Gerber):			
Second Foods	4-oz. jar	90	20.0
Third Foods	1 T.	11	2.4
With bananas (Gerber) *Third Foods,* dry, instant	1 packet	90	16.0
Rice:			
Plain, dry:			
(Beech-Nut) *Stages 1,* instant	.5 oz.	60	12.0
(Earth's Best)	.5 oz.	60	12.0
(Gerber) *First Foods*	.5 oz.	60	11.0
(Heinz) instant	.5 oz.	54	11.0
Mixed:			
With apples (Beech-Nut) *Stages 2,* instant, dry	.5 oz.	60	13.0
With apples & bananas:			
(Beech-Nut) *Stages 2*	4½-oz. jar	100	24.0
(Heinz) strained	3½-oz. jar	70	16.2
With banana:			
(Beech-Nut) *Stages 2,* dry, instant	.5 oz.	60	13.0
(Gerber) *Second Foods,* dry, instant	.5 oz.	60	11.0
With mango (Gerber) *Tropical Foods,* dry, instant	.5 oz.	55	12.0

Food	Measure	Cals.	Carbs.
With mixed fruit (Gerber):			
Junior	6-oz. jar	140	31.0
Third Foods	1 T.	11	2.6
Cereal snack (Gerber)			
Graduates, finger snack:			
Apple-banana	3.2-oz.	405	82.5
Apple-cinnamon	3.2-oz.	407	82.5
Cheese, cottage (Beech-Nut)			
with pineapple:			
Stages 2	4½-oz. serving	130	26.0
Stages 3	6-oz. serving	170	36.0
Custard:			
Chocolate (Heinz) junior	3½-oz. jar	75	14.0
Vanilla:			
(Beech Nut):			
Stages 2	4½-oz. jar	140	24.0
Stages 3	6-oz. jar	180	30.0
(Gerber):			
Junior	6-oz. jar	150	31.0
Second Foods	1 T.	13	2.6
Strained	4½-oz. jar	100	22.0
(Heinz) strained	3½-oz. jar	75	14.0
Cookie:			
Animal-shaped (Gerber):			
Baked, chunky	3½-oz. serving	443	74.8
Cinnamon, *Graduates*	3½-oz. serving	449	78.7
Arrowroot (Gerber)			
Graduates	3½-oz. serving	452	70.3
Corn, creamed:			
(Beech-Nut) *Stages 2*	4½-oz. jar	100	20.0
(Gerber):			
Second Foods	7 T.	62	12.7
Strained	4½-oz. jar	80	16.0
(Heinz) strained	3½-oz. jar	63	14.0
Egg yolk (Gerber) *Second Foods*	7 T.	193	1.0
Formula, infant:			
Canned:			
(Carnation) iron fortified:			
Follow-Up	5 fl. oz.	100	13.2
Good Start	5 fl. oz.	100	11.0
(Enfamil):			
With iron	5 fl. oz.	100	10.3
Low iron	5 fl. oz.	100	10.3
(Gerber):			
With iron	5 fl. oz.	100	10.7
Low iron	5 fl. oz.	100	10.0

Food	Measure	Cals.	Carbs.
Soy, milk-free, iron fortified	5 fl. oz.	100	10.0
(Isomil) soy, milk-free, with iron	5 fl. oz.	100	10.3
(Similac):			
With iron	5 fl. oz.	100	10.7
Low iron	5 fl. oz.	100	10.7
*Mix:			
Liquid:			
(Carnation) iron fortified:			
Follow-Up	5 fl. oz.	100	13.2
Good Start	5 fl. oz.	100	11.0
(Enfamil):			
With iron	5 fl. oz.	100	10.3
Low iron	5 fl. oz.	100	10.3
(Gerber):			
With iron	5 fl. oz.	100	10.7
Low iron	5 fl. oz.	100	10.0
Soy, milk-free, iron fortified	5 fl. oz.	100	10.0
(Isomil) soy, milk-free, with iron	5 fl. oz.	100	10.3
(Similac):			
With iron	5 fl. oz.	100	10.7
Low iron	5 fl. oz.	100	10.7
Powder:			
(Carnation):			
Follow-Up	5 fl. oz.	100	13.2
Good Start	5 fl. oz.	100	11.0
(Enfamil):			
With iron	5 fl. oz.	100	10.3
Low iron	5 fl. oz.	100	10.3
(Gerber):			
With iron	5 fl. oz.	100	10.7
Low iron	5 fl. oz.	100	10.0
Soy, milk-free, iron fortified	5 fl. oz.	100	10.0
(Isomil) soy, milk-free with iron	5 fl. oz.	100	10.3
(Gerber):			
With iron	5 fl. oz.	100	10.3
Low iron	5 fl. oz.	100	10.0
(Isomil) soy, milk-free, with iron	5 fl. oz.	100	10.3
(Similac):			
With iron	5 fl. oz.	100	10.7

Food	Measure	Cals.	Carbs.
Low iron	5 fl. oz.	100	10.7
Fruit dessert:			
(Beech-Nut):			
Stages 2	4½-oz. jar	80	20.0
Stages 3	6-oz. jar	120	28.0
(Gerber):			
Junior	6-oz. jar	130	30.0
Second Foods	7 T.	82	19.7
Strained	4½-oz. jar	100	24.0
Third Foods	7 T.	73	17.6
(Heinz):			
Junior	3½-oz. jar	65	15.7
Strained	3½-oz. jar	66	15.8
Fruit juice, mixed:			
(Beech-Nut) *Stages 2*	4 fl. oz.	70	16.0
(Gerber) *Second Foods*	4 fl. oz.	60	14.0
(Heinz) strained	3½ fl. oz.	50	11.7
Grape juice:			
(Beech-Nut):			
Juice Plus, Stages 2	4 fl. oz.	90	22.0
White, *Stages 1*	4.2 fl. oz.	80	20.0
(Gerber) *First Foods*:			
Red	4 fl. oz.	80	20.0
White	3.2 fl. oz.	65	15.6
(Heinz) white, strained	3½ fl. oz.	58	13.8
Guava dessert (Gerber)			
Tropical Foods, with tapioca	7 T.	69	16.8
Guava juice with mixed fruit			
(Gerber) *Tropical Foods*	3.2 fl. oz.	58	13.8
Guava with tapioca:			
(Beech-Nut) *Stages 2*	4½-oz. jar	100	24.0
(Gerber)	4½-oz. jar	90	20.0
Ham (Gerber):			
Junior	2½-oz. jar	90	0.0
Second Foods	7 T.	120	0.2
Third Foods	7 T.	123	0.1
Ham & vegetables:			
(Beech-Nut) *Stages 2* entree	4½-oz. jar	80	12.0
(Gerber) lean meat dinner:			
Junior	4½-oz. dinner	110	11.0
Strained	4½-oz. dinner	100	10.0
Hawaiian dessert (Gerber):			
Junior	6-oz. jar	150	33.0
Second Foods	7 T.	86	19.7
Third Foods	7 T.	87	20.2
Strained	4½-oz. jar	120	25.0

Food	Measure	Cals.	Carbs.
Lamb:			
(Beech-Nut) *Stages 1*	2.8-oz. jar	70	0.0
(Gerber) *Second Foods*	7 T.	104	0.0
Lamb with broth:			
(Beech-Nut) *Stages 1*	2½-oz. jar	60	0.0
(Heinz) strained	3½-oz. jar	129	0.2
Lamb & vegetable entree			
(Beech-Nut) *Stages 2*	4½-oz. jar	90	13.0
Liver with liver broth (Heinz)			
strained	3½-oz. jar	100	3.6
Macaroni with beef:			
(Beech-Nut) dinner:			
Stages 2	4½-oz. jar	90	13.0
Stages 3	6-oz. jar	160	17.0
(Gerber) *Graduates,* in			
sauce	3.2-oz. jar	78	11.1
Macaroni with cheese dinner			
(Gerber) *Second Foods*	1 T.	9	1.1
Macaroni, tomato & beef dinner:			
(Gerber):			
Second Foods	1 T.	8	1.3
Third Foods	1 T.	9	1.5
(Heinz) junior	3½-oz. jar	52	8.2
Mango-banana dessert			
(Gerber) *Tropical Foods,*			
with passion fruit	7 T.	73	17.7
Mango & banana with passion			
fruit & tapioca (Gerber)			
strained	4½-oz. jar	100	25.0
Mango dessert (Gerber)			
Tropical Foods, with tapioca	7 T.	75	18.2
Mango juice with mixed fruit			
(Gerber) *Tropical Foods*	3.2 fl. oz.	59	14.2
Mango nectar with grape and			
pear juice (Beech-Nut)			
Stages 2	4 fl. oz.	80	19.0
Noodle with beef (Gerber)			
Homestyle, chunky	1 T.	13	1.4
Orange-apple juice (Heinz)			
strained	3½ fl. oz.	50	11.4
Orange juice:			
(Beech-Nut) *Stages 3*	4 fl. oz.	60	14.0
(Gerber) *Second Foods*	4 fl. oz.	60	13.0
(Heinz) strained	3½ fl. oz.	48	10.7
Papaya (Beech-Nut) *Stages 2*	4½-oz. jar	100	24.0
Papaya dessert (Gerber)			
Tropical Foods, with tapioca	7 T.	62	15.1

Food	Measure	Cals.	Carbs.
Papaya-pineapple dessert			
(Gerber) *Tropical Foods*	7 T.	76	18.6
Papaya with tapioca			
(Gerber) strained	4½-oz. jar	80	9.0
Pasta dinner (Earth's Best)	4½-oz. jar	90	13.0
Peach:			
(Beech-Nut):			
Regular, *Stages 3*	6-oz. jar	90	22.0
Yellow cling:			
Baby's First	2½-oz. jar	45	10.0
Stages 1	4½-oz. jar	70	15.0
(Gerber):			
First Foods	2½-oz. jar	20	7.0
Junior	6-oz. jar	110	25.0
Second Foods	7 T.	66	15.3
Strained	4½-oz. jar	90	19.0
(Heinz):			
Beginner Foods	3½-oz. jar	80	18.3
Junior	3½-oz. jar	68	15.4
Strained	3½-oz. jar	68	15.4
Peach with oatmeal & banana			
(Earth's Best)	4½-oz. jar	70	15.0
Peach cobbler:			
(Gerber):			
Second Foods	7 T.	77	18.2
Third Foods	7 T.	77	18.4
(Heinz) strained	3½-oz. jar	72	16.9
Peach nectar with pear & grape			
juice (Beech-Nut) *Stages 2*	4 fl. oz.	70	17.0
Pear:			
(Beech-Nut) Bartlett:			
Baby's First	2½-oz. jar	50	12.0
Stages 1	4½-oz. jar	70	18.0
Stages 3	6-oz. jar	100	24.0
(Earth's Best)	4½-oz. jar	60	14.0
(Gerber):			
First Foods	2½-oz. jar	40	11.0
Junior	6-oz. jar	100	21.0
Second Foods	7 T.	55	12.9
Strained	4½-oz. jar	80	16.0
(Heinz):			
Beginner Foods	3½-oz. jar	76	18.0
Junior	3½-oz. jar	60	14.1
Strained	3½-oz. jar	60	14.1
Pear with applesauce (Beech-Nut) *Stages 2*	4½-oz. jar	80	20.0
Pear-grape juice (Heinz) strained	3½ fl. oz.	43	10.5

Food	Measure	Cals.	Carbs.
Pear juice:			
(Beech-Nut) *Stages 1*	4 fl. oz.	60	15.0
(Earth's Best)	4.2 fl. oz.	60	15.0
(Gerber) strained *First Foods*	4 fl. oz.	60	14.0
(Heinz) strained, saver size	4.2 fl. oz.	70	15.0
Pear & pineapple (Gerber):			
Junior	6-oz. jar	100	21.0
Strained	4½-oz. jar	80	16.0
Third Foods	7 T.	54	12.7
Pear & raspberries (Earth's Best)	4½-oz. jar	60	15.0
Peas:			
(Beech-Nut) tender, sweet:			
Plain, *Baby's First*	2½-oz. jar	40	7.0
Buttered, *Stages 1*	4½-oz. jar	60	10.0
(Gerber):			
Graduates, diced	3.2-oz. jar	44	8.4
Junior	7 T.	47	7.7
(Heinz) *Beginner Foods*	3½-oz. jar	55	9.5
Peas & brown rice (Earth's Best)	4½-oz. jar	80	16.0
Peas & carrots (Beech-Nut)			
Stages 2	4½-oz. jar	60	11.0
Plum with banana & rice			
(Earth's Best)	4½-oz. jar	90	19.0
Plum with rice (Beech-Nut)			
Stages 2	4½-oz. jar	150	34.0
Plum with tapioca:			
(Gerber):			
Second Foods	7 T.	74	17.7
Strained	4½-oz. jar	90	22.0
(Heinz)	3½-oz. jar	67	16.2
Prune (Gerber) *First Foods*	2½-oz. jar	70	17.0
Prune with tapioca:			
(Gerber):			
Second Foods	7 T.	77	18.1
Strained	4½-oz. jar	100	22.0
(Heinz) strained	3½-oz. jar	90	21.5
Potato dinner, with green beans			
(Earth's Best)	4½-oz. jar	100	13.0
Pretzel (Gerber) *Graduates*	3½-oz. serving	403	83.0
Pudding:			
Banana:			
(Beech-Nut) *Stages 2*	4½-oz. jar	100	25.0
(Heinz) strained	3½-oz. jar	74	16.8
Cherry vanilla (Gerber)			
Second Foods	1 T.	10	2.4

Food	Measure	Cals.	Carbs.
Ravioli:			
(Earth's Best) rice and lentil			
dinner	4½-oz. jar	80	13.0
(Gerber):			
Beef with tomato sauce,			
Graduates:			
Regular	3.2-oz. jar	97	16.3
Micro cup	6-oz. serving	170	28.0
Cheese with tomato sauce,			
Graduates:			
Regular	3.2-oz. jar	99	16.3
Micro cup	6-oz. serving	170	28.0
Rice with beef & tomato sauce			
(Gerber) chunky	1 T.	11	1.7
Rice, saucy, with chicken			
(Gerber) chunky	1 T.	11	1.7
Soup:			
Broccoli, cream of (Gerber)			
Third Foods	3.2 oz.	26	2.7
Chicken:			
(Beech-Nut) *Stages Table*			
Time, hearty, with stars	6 oz.	100	15.0
(Gerber) strained	3½ oz.	70	10.0
Potato, cream of (Gerber)			
Third Foods	3.2 oz.	33	5.2
Tomato, cream of (Gerber)			
Third Foods	3.2 oz.	41	7.3
Vegetable, cream of			
(Gerber) *Third Foods*	3.2 oz.	29	4.4
Spaghetti with beef (Beech-Nut) *Stages 3*	6-oz. dinner	170	17.0
Spaghetti with meatballs, mini, and sauce (Gerber)			
Graduates	6-oz. jar	160	21.0
Spaghetti with tomato sauce & beef (Gerber):			
Chunky	1 T.	12	1.8
Junior	6-oz. jar	120	19.0
Third Foods	7 T.	64	10.6
Spaghetti with tomato sauce & meat (Heinz) junior	3½-oz. jar	58	9.6
Spinach, creamed (Gerber) strained	4½-oz. jar	60	9.0
Spinach & potato (Earth's Best)	4½-oz. jar	60	8.0
Squash:			
(Beech-Nut) butternut:			
Baby's First	2½-oz. jar	30	7.0

Food	Measure	Cals.	Carbs.
Stages 1	4½-oz. jar	50	11.0
(Earth's Best) winter	4½-oz. jar	50	12.0
(Gerber):			
First Foods	2½-oz. jar	25	5.0
Junior	6-oz. jar	60	11.0
Strained	4½-oz. jar	35	8.0
Sweet potato:			
(Beech-Nut) *Baby's First*	2½-oz. jar	50	11.0
(Gerber) *Third Foods*	7 T.	33	6.8
(Heinz) strained	3½-oz. jar	32	6.6
Sweet potato dinner with chicken (Earth's Best)	4½-oz. jar	90	13.0
Turkey:			
(Beech-Nut) *Stages 1*	2.8-oz. jar	100	0.0
Turkey with broth:			
(Beech-Nut) *Stages 1*	2½-oz. jar	90	0.0
(Heinz) strained	3½-oz. jar	137	0.4
Turkey dinner:			
(Beech-Nut) *Stages 2,* supreme	4½-oz. jar	120	11.0
(Gerber) junior	2½-oz. jar	100	1.0
Turkey with egg yolks (Gerber) strained	2½-oz. jar	100	1.0
Turkey rice dinner:			
(Beech-Nut):			
Stages 2	4½-oz. jar	70	12.0
Stages 3	6-oz. jar	110	14.0
(Gerber):			
Junior	6-oz. jar	110	14.0
Second Foods	7 T.	55	7.5
Strained	4½-oz. jar	80	10.0
Third Foods	7 T.	55	7.8
Turkey rice dinner with vegetables (Heinz):			
Junior	3½-oz. jar	42	7.9
Strained	3½-oz. jar	47	8.2
Turkey stew with rice (Gerber) *Graduates*	3.2-oz. jar	59	7.6
Turkey sticks (Gerber) *Graduates*	1 stick	14	.1
Turkey vegetable dinner (Gerber) lean meat:			
Junior	4½-oz. jar	100	10.0
Strained	4½-oz. dinner	100	9.0
Tutti frutti dessert (Heinz) junior	3½-oz. jar	67	15.7

Food	Measure	Cals.	Carbs.
Veal:			
(Beech-Nut) *Stages 1*	2.8-oz. jar	60	0.0
(Gerber) junior	2½-oz. jar	80	0.0
Veal with broth (Heinz) strained	3½-oz. jar	130	15.1
Veal & turkey (Gerber) junior	6-oz. jar	100	15.0
Vegetable-bacon dinner (Gerber):			
Second Foods	7 T.	73	8.8
Third Foods	7 T.	77	9.3
Vegetable-beef dinner:			
(Earth's Best)	4½-oz. jar	90	11.0
(Gerber):			
Second Foods	7 T.	65	8.5
Third Foods	7 T.	62	9.2
Vegetable-chicken dinner (Gerber) *Third Foods*	7 T.	51	8.1
Vegetable dinner, summer (Earth's Best)	4½-oz. jar	90	12.0
Vegetable dumpling dinner (Heinz) with beef:			
Junior	3½-oz. jar	47	7.2
Strained	3½-oz. jar	49	8.6
Vegetable-noodle with chicken dinner (Heinz):			
Junior	3½-oz. jar	57	8.7
Strained	3½-oz. jar	54	7.5
Vegetable stew with beef (Gerber) *Graduates*:			
Regular	3.2-oz. jar	71	8.8
Micro cup	6-oz. serving	130	15.0
Vegetable-turkey dinner:			
(Earth's Best)	4½-oz. jar	60	11.0
(Gerber) *Third Foods*	7 T.	49	7.5
Vegetables, garden:			
(Beech-Nut) *Stages 2*	4½-oz. jar	60	11.0
(Earth's Best)	4½-oz. jar	70	15.0
(Gerber) *Second Foods*	7 T.	39	6.4
Vegetables, mixed:			
(Beech-Nut) *Stages 2*	4½-oz. jar	50	12.0
(Gerber):			
Junior	6-oz. jar	70	14.0
Second Foods	7 T.	42	8.4
Strained	3½-oz. jar	60	11.0
(Heinz) strained	3½-oz. jar	44	8.8
Water (Beech-Nut) sodium free, with fluoride	4 fl. oz.	0	0.0

Food	Measure	Cals.	Carbs.
Yogurt:			
Apple:			
(Beech-Nut) *Stages 2,*			
dessert	4½-oz. jar	120	25.0
(Earth's Best) breakfast	4½-oz. jar	100	17.0
Banana:			
(Beech-Nut) *Stages 2*	4½-oz. jar	120	26.0
(Gerber) *Second Foods*	1 T.	11	2.3
(Heinz) strained	3½-oz. jar	83	18.7
Blueberry (Earth's Best)			
breakfast	4½-oz. jar	100	16.0
Fruit, mixed (Gerber) *Second*			
Foods	7 T.	79	18.0
Peach:			
(Beech-Nut) *Stages 2*	4½-oz. jar	120	25.0
(Gerber) *Second Foods*	7 T.	76	17.2
Pear:			
(Beech-Nut) *Stages 2*	4½-oz. jar	130	29.0
(Gerber) *Tropical Foods,*			
with pineapple & banana	7 T.	79	19.3
(Heinz) strained	3½-oz. jar	80	18.1
Tropical (Earth's Best)			
breakfast	4½-oz. serving	110	19.0
BACON, broiled:			
(USDA):			
Medium slice	1 slice		
	(7½ grams)	43	.1
Thick slice	1 slice		
	(12 grams)	64	.2
Thin slice	1 slice (5 grams)	30	.2
(Hormel):			
Black Label	1 slice	30	0.0
Range Brand	1 slice	55	0.0
(Oscar Mayer):			
Center cut	1 slice (4 grams)	25	.1
Lower salt	1 slice	32	.1
Regular slice	6-gram slice	35	.1
Thick slice	1 slice		
	(11 grams)	50	.2
(Shannon) Irish	1-oz. serving	70	0.0
BACON, CANADIAN,			
unheated:			
(USDA)	1 oz.	61	Tr.
(Eckrich)	1-oz. slice	35	1.0
(Hormel):			
Regular	1 oz	45	0.0

Food	Measure	Cals.	Carbs.
Light & Lean	1 slice	17	0.0
(Oscar Mayer):			
Thin	.7-oz. slice	30	0.0
Thick	1-oz. slice	35	.1
BACON, SIMULATED,			
cooked:			
(Louis Rich) turkey	1 slice	32	Tr.
(Oscar Mayer) *Lean 'N Tasty:*			
Beef	1 slice (.4 oz.)	48	.2
Pork	1 slice (.4 oz.)	54	.1
(Swift's) *Sizzlean:*			
Beef	1 strip (4 oz.)	35	Tr.
Pork	1 strip	45	0.0
BACON BITS:			
Bac*Os (Betty Crocker)	1 tsp.	12	1.0
(French's) imitation	1 tsp.	6	Tr.
(McCormick) imitation	1 tsp.	9	.7
(Oscar Mayer) real	1 tsp.	8	.1
BAGEL:			
(USDA):			
Egg	3"-dia. bagel, 1.9 oz.	162	28.3
Water	3"-dia. bagel, (1.9 oz.)	163	30.5
Non-frozen (Thomas') (See also *Dunkin' Donuts*):			
Plain	1 bagel	170	34.0
Cinnamon raisin	1 bagel	160	36.0
Onion	1 bagel	180	35.0
Frozen:			
(Lender's)			
Plain:			
Regular	1 bagel (2 oz.)	150	30.0
Bagelette	.9-oz. bagel	70	14.0
Big 'N Crusty	1 bagel	240	45.0
Soft	2½-oz. bagel	210	36.0
Blueberry	1 bagel (2 oz.)	190	38.0
Cinnamon-raisin,			
Big 'N Crusty	3⅛-oz. bagel	250	49.0
Egg:			
Regular	2-oz. bagel	150	30.0
Big 'N Crusty	1 bagel	250	46.0
Garlic:			
Regular	2-oz. bagel	160	32.0

Food	Measure	Cals.	Carbs.
Big 'N Crusty	3⅛-oz. bagel	250	50.0
Oat bran	2½-oz. bagel	170	36.0
Onion:			
Regular	1 bagel	160	30.0
Big 'N Crusty	1 bagel	230	46.0
Poppy	1 bagel (2 oz.)	160	30.0
Pumpernickel	2-oz. bagel	160	31.0
Raisin-honey	2½-oz. bagel	200	40.0
Rye	2-oz. bagel	150	30.0
Sesame	1 bagel (2 oz.)	160	31.0
(Sara Lee):			
Cinnamon raisin	2½-oz. bagel	200	39.0
Cinnamon raisin	3-oz. bagel	240	48.0
Egg	2½-oz. bagel	200	38.0
Egg	3-oz. bagel	250	48.0
Oat bran	2½-oz. bagel	180	38.0
Oat bran	3-oz. bagel	220	47.0
Onion	2½-oz. bagel	190	37.0
Onion	3-oz. bagel	230	45.0
Plain	2½-oz. bagel	190	38.0
Plain	3-oz. bagel	230	46.0
Poppy seed	2½-oz. bagel	450	37.0
Poppy seed	3-oz. bagel	560	46.0
Sesame seed	2½-oz. bagel	440	37.0
Sesame seed	3-oz. bagel	550	46.0
BAGEL CHIPS (Pepperidge Farm):			
Cheese	.5-oz. serving	70	10.0
Garlic or toasted onion	.5-oz. serving	60	10.0
BAKING POWDER:			
(USDA):			
Phosphate	1 tsp. (3.8 grams)	5	1.1
SAS	1 tsp. (3 grams)	4	.9
Tartrate	1 tsp. (2.8 grams)	2	.5
(Calumet)	1 tsp. (3.6 grams)	2	1.0
(Davis)	1 tsp. (3 grams)	7	1.7
(Featherweight) low sodium, cereal free	1 tsp.	8	2.0
BAKING SODA (Arm & Hammer)	½ tsp.	0	0.0

Food	Measure	Cals.	Carbs.
BALSAMPEAR, fresh (HEW/FAO):			
Whole	1 lb. (weighed with cavity contents)	69	16.3
Flesh only	4 oz.	22	5.1
BAMBOO SHOOTS:			
Raw, trimmed (USDA)	4 oz.	31	5.9
Canned, drained:			
(Chun King)	8½-oz. can	65	12.5
(La Choy)	¼ cup	6	1.0
BANANA (USDA):			
Common yellow:			
Fresh:			
Whole	1 lb. (weighed with skin)	262	68.5
Small size	5.9-oz. banana (7¾" × 1¹¹⁄₃₂")	81	21.1
Medium size	6.3-oz. banana (8¾" × 1¹³⁄₃₂")	101	26.4
Large size	7-oz. banana (9¾" × 1⁷⁄₁₆")	116	30.2
Mashed	1 cup (about 2 med.)	191	50.0
Sliced	1 cup (about 1¼ med.)	128	33.3
Dehydrated flakes	½ cup (1.8 oz.)	170	44.3
Red, fresh, whole	1 lb. (weighed with skin)	278	72.2
BANANA EXTRACT (Durkee) imitation	1 tsp.	15	DNA
BANANA NECTAR, canned (Libby's)	6 fl. oz.	99	24.5
BANANA PIE (See **PIE,** Banana)			
BARBECUE SAUCE (See **SAUCE,** Barbecue)			
BARBECUE SEASONING (French's)	1 tsp. (.1 oz.)	6	1.0

Food	Measure	Cals.	Carbs.
BARBERA WINE:			
(Colony)	3 fl. oz.	68	2.6
(Louis M. Martini) 12½% alcohol	3 fl. oz.	65	.2
BARDOLINO WINE (Antinori)			
12% alcohol	3 fl. oz.	84	6.3
BARLEY, pearl, dry:			
Light (USDA)	¼ cup (1.8 oz.)	174	39.4
Pot or Scotch:			
(USDA)	2 oz.	197	43.8
(Quaker) Scotch	¼ cup (1.7 oz.)	172	36.3
***BARLEY PILAF MIX** (Near East)	1 cup	220	41.0
BASIL:			
Fresh (HEW/FAO) sweet, leaves	½ oz.	6	1.0
Dried (French's)	1 tsp.	3	.7
BASS (USDA):			
Black Sea:			
Raw, whole	1 lb. (weighed whole)	165	0.0
Baked, stuffed, home recipe	4 oz.	294	12.9
Smallmouth & largemouth, raw:			
Whole	1 lb. (weighed whole)	146	0.0
Meat only	4 oz.	118	0.0
Striped:			
Raw, whole	1 lb. (weighed whole)	205	0.0
Raw, meat only	4 oz.	119	0.0
Oven-fried	4 oz.	222	7.6
White, raw, meat only	4 oz.	111	0.0
BATMAN, cereal (Ralston Purina)	1 cup (1 oz.)	110	25.0
BATTER MIX (Golden Dipt):			
Beer, corn dog or original	1 oz.	100	22.0
Fish & chips	1¼ oz.	120	27.0
Tempura	1 oz.	100	22.0
BAY LEAF (French's)	1 tsp.	5	1.0

Food	Measure	Cals.	Carbs.
B & B LIQUEUR, 86 proof	1 fl. oz.	94	5.7
B.B.Q. SAUCE & BEEF, frozen (Banquet) *Cookin' Bag,* sliced	4-oz. pkg.	100	11.0
BEAN, BAKED:			
(USDA):			
With pork & molasses sauce	1 cup (9 oz.)	382	53.8
With pork & tomato sauce	1 cup (9 oz.)	311	48.5
With tomato sauce	1 cup (9 oz.)	306	58.7
Canned:			
(Allen's) *Wagon Master*	1 cup	340	48.0
(B&M) *Brick Oven:*			
Barbecue style	8 oz.	260	48.0
Maple	8 oz.	240	52.0
Pea bean with pork in brown sugar sauce	8 oz.	270	50.0
Red kidney or yellow eye bean in brown sugar sauce	8 oz.	290	42.0
Vegetarian	8 oz.	230	50.0
(Bush's):			
Regular	½ cup (4.6 oz.)	150	29.0
Homestyle	½ cup (4.6 oz.)	160	28.0
With onions	½ cup (4.6 oz.)	150	26.0
Vegetarian	½ cup (4.6 oz.)	140	24.0
(Campbell's):			
Barbecue	7⅞-oz. can	210	43.0
Home style	8-oz. can	220	48.0
With pork & tomato sauce	8-oz. can	270	49.0
Old fashioned, in molasses & brown sugar sauce	8-oz. can	230	49.0
& pork, in tomato sauce	8-oz. can	200	43.0
Vegetarian	7¾-oz. can	170	40.0
(Furman's) & pork, in tomato sauce	8-oz. serving	245	46.4
(Grandma Brown's) home baked	8-oz. serving	300	54.0
(Health Valley):			
Boston, regular or no added salt	8 oz.	202	43.7
Vegetarian, with miso	8 oz.	180	38.0
(Hormel) *Micro-Cup,* with pork	7½ oz.	254	41.0
(Hunt's) & pork	8-oz. serving	270	52.0

Food	Measure	Cals.	Carbs.
(Pathmark) in tomato sauce:			
Regular	1 cup	300	46.0
No Frills	1 cup	320	56.0
(Town House) & pork	1 cup	260	48.0
BEAN, BLACK OR BROWN:			
Dry (USDA)	1 cup	678	122.4
Canned (Goya)	1 cup	250	42.0
*Mix (Fantastic Foods)	½ cup	207	28.0
BEAN, CANNELLINI, canned (Progresso)	1 cup	160	38.0
BEAN, FAVA, canned (Progresso)	4-oz. serving	90	15.5
BEAN, GARBANZO (See **CHICK-PEAS OR GARBANZOS**)			
BEAN, GREEN:			
Fresh (USDA):			
Whole	1 lb. (weighed untrimmed)	128	28.3
French style	½ cup (1.4 oz.)	13	2.8
Boiled (USDA):			
Whole, drained	½ cup (2.2 oz.)	16	3.3
Boiled, 1½" to 2" pieces, drained	½ cup (2.4 oz.)	17	3.7
Canned, regular pack:			
(USDA):			
Whole, solids & liq.	½ cup (4.2 oz.)	22	5.0
Whole, drained solids	4 oz.	27	5.9
Cut, drained solids	½ cup (2.5 oz.)	17	3.6
Drained liquid only	4 oz.	11	2.7
(Allen's) solids & liq:			
Whole	½ cup (4.2 oz.)	21	4.0
Cut	½ cup (4 oz.)	20	4.0
French	½ cup (4.1 oz.)	20	4.0
(Green Giant):			
Cut:			
Regular or kitchen sliced	½ cup	16	4.0
Pantry Express	½ cup	12	3.0
French	½ cup	16	4.0
Whole, almandine	½ cup	45	5.0
(Larsen) *Freshlike*, solids & liq., french or whole	½ cup	20	4.0

Food	Measure	Cals.	Carbs.
(Pathmark):			
Regular or Blue Lake, whole, cut or french cut	½ cup	20	4.0
No frills, cut or french style	½ cup	17	4.0
(S&W):			
Whole:			
Stringless or *Vertical Pak*	½ cup	20	4.0
Dilled	½ cup	60	15.0
Cut or french style, Premium Blue Lake or stringless	½ cup	20	4.0
Cut, Premium Gold	½ cup	20	5.0
(Town House) cut or french style	½ cup	20	4.0
Canned, dietetic or low calorie:			
(USDA):			
Solids & liq.	4 oz.	18	4.1
Drained solids	4 oz.	25	5.4
(Diet Delight) solids & liq.	½ cup (4.2 oz.)	20	3.0
(Featherweight) solids & liq.	½ cup (4 oz.)	25	5.0
(Larsen) *Fresh-Lite*, water pack	½ cup (4.2 oz.)	20	4.0
(Pathmark) no salt added	½ cup	20	5.0
(S&W) *Nutradiet*, cut	½ cup	20	4.0
Freeze-dried (Mountain House)	⅔ cup	25	5.0
Frozen:			
(Bel-Air):			
Cut or whole	3 oz.	25	6.0
French style:			
Plain	3 oz.	25	6.0
With toasted almonds	3 oz.	45	10.0
Italian	3 oz.	35	7.0
(Birds Eye):			
Cut, regular or portion pack	3-oz. serving	25	6.0
French:			
Regular	3-oz. serving	25	6.0
Combination, with almonds	3-oz. serving	50	8.0
Whole:			
Bavarian style, with spaetzle	⅓ of 10-oz. pkg.	100	11.0
Deluxe	⅓ of 9-oz. pkg.	25	5.0

Food	Measure	Cals.	Carbs.
Farm Fresh	4-oz. serving	30	7.0
Petite, deluxe	⅓ of 8-oz. pkg.	20	5.0
	5-oz. serving	70	9.4
(Frosty Acres)	3-oz. serving	25	6.0
(Green Giant):			
Cut or french, with butter sauce	½ cup	30	4.0
Cut, *Harvest Fresh*	½ cup	16	4.0
With mushroom in cream sauce	½ cup	80	10.0
Polybag	½ cup	14	4.0
(Larsen)	3 oz.	25	6.0

BEAN, GREEN, & MUSHROOM CASSEROLE, frozen (Stouffer's)

	Measure	Cals.	Carbs.
	½ of 9½-oz. pkg.	160	13.0

BEAN, GREEN, PUREE, canned (Larsen) no salt added

	Measure	Cals.	Carbs.
	½ cup (4.4 oz.)	35	7.5

BEAN, ITALIAN:

Food	Measure	Cals.	Carbs.
Canned (Del Monte) cut, solids & liq.	4 oz.	25	6.0
Frozen:			
(Birds Eye)	⅓ of pkg. (3 oz.)	31	7.2
(Frosty Acres)	3-oz. serving	30	7.0
(Larsen)	3 oz.	30	7.0

BEAN, KIDNEY OR RED:

Food	Measure	Cals.	Carbs.
(USDA):			
Dry	½ cup (3.3 oz.)	319	57.6
Cooked	½ cup (3.3 oz.)	109	19.8
Canned, regular pack, solids & liq.:			
(Allen's)	½ cup (4.1 oz.)	110	20.0
(Furman's) red, fancy, light	½ cup (4½ oz.)	121	21.2
(Goya):			
Red	½ cup	115	20.0
White	½ cup	100	18.5
(Hunt's):			
Regular	½ cup (3.5 oz.)	80	16.0
Small red	4 oz.	120	21.0
(Pathmark):			
Regular	½ cup	110	20.0
Red, dark	½ cup	110	18.0
White	½ cup	100	18.0
(Progresso) red	½ cup	100	21.0

Food	Measure	Cals.	Carbs.
(Town House) dark or light	½ cup	110	20.0
Canned, dietetic (S&W) *Nutradiet*, low sodium, green label	½ cup	90	16.0
BEAN, LIMA:			
Raw (USDA):			
Young, whole	1 lb. (weighed in pod)	223	40.1
Mature, dry	½ cup (3.4 oz.)	331	61.4
Young, without shell	1 lb. (weighed shelled)	558	100.2
Boiled (USDA) drained	½ cup	94	16.8
Canned, regular pack:			
(USDA):			
Solids & liq.	4 oz.	81	15.2
Drained solids	4 oz.	109	20.8
(Allen's):			
Regular	½ cup	60	9.0
Butter, large	½ cup	105	19.0
(Furman's)	½ cup	92	16.7
(Larsen) *Freshlike*, solids & liq.	½ cup (4 oz.)	80	16.0
(Town House) butter	½ cup	100	18.0
Canned, dietetic, solids & liq.:			
(Featherweight)	½ cup	80	16.0
(Larsen) *Fresh-Lite*, water pack, no salt added	½ cup (4.4 oz.)	80	16.0
Frozen:			
(Birds Eye):			
Baby	⅓ of 10-oz. pkg.	126	24.1
Fordhook	⅓ of 10-oz. pkg.	99	18.5
(Frosty Acres):			
Baby	3.3 oz.	130	24.0
Butter	3.3 oz.	140	26.0
Fordhook	3.3 oz.	100	19.0
(Green Giant):			
In butter sauce	½ cup	83	20.4
Harvest Fresh, or polybag	½ cup	60	15.0
(Health Valley)	½ cup	94	18.0
(Larsen) baby	3.3 oz.	130	24.0
BEAN, MUNG (USDA) dry	½ cup (3.7 oz.)	357	63.3
BEAN, PINK, canned (Goya) solids & liq.	½ cup	115	20.5

Food	Measure	Cals.	Carbs.
BEAN, PINTO:			
Dry (USDA)	4 oz.	396	72.2
Canned:			
(Gebhardt)	½ of 15-oz. can	370	67.0
(Goya):			
Regular	½ cup (4 oz.)	100	18.0
Butter	½ cup	105	17.5
(Green Giant)	½ cup	100	21.0
(Old El Paso)	½ cup	100	19.0
(Progresso)	½ cup (4 oz.)	82	16.5
(Town House)	½ cup	105	18.5
Frozen (McKenzie)	3.2-oz. serving	160	29.0
BEAN, REFRIED, canned:			
(Gebhardt):			
Regular	4 oz.	130	20.0
Jalapeño	4 oz.	110	18.0
Little Pancho (Borden) &			
green chili	½ cup	80	15.0
(Old El Paso):			
Plain	½ cup	110	16.0
With bacon	½ cup	208	24.0
With cheese	½ cup	72	8.0
With green chili	½ cup	98	16.0
With jalapeños	½ cup	62	8.0
With sausage	½ cup	360	16.0
Spicy	½ cup	70	10.0
Vegetarian	½ cup	140	30.0
(Rosarita):			
Regular	4 oz.	130	20.0
Bacon	4 oz.	132	19.6
With beans & onion	4 oz.	125	20.0
With green chilis	4 oz.	116	18.5
With nacho cheese & onion	4 oz.	135	21.1
Spicy	4 oz.	120	18.7
Vegetarian	4 oz.	120	18.7
BEAN, ROMAN, canned, solids & liq:			
(Goya)	½ cup (2.3 oz.)	81	15.0
(Progresso)	½ cup	110	18.0
BEAN, YELLOW OR WAX:			
Raw, whole (USDA)	1 lb. (weighed untrimmed)	108	24.0
Boiled (USDA) 1" pieces, drained	½ cup (2.9 oz.)	18	3.7

Food	Measure	Cals.	Carbs.
Canned, regular pack, solids & liq.:			
(Comstock)	½ cup (4.2 oz.)	20	4.0
(Larsen) *Freshlike*, cut, solids & liq.	½ cup (4.2 oz.)	25	5.0
Canned, dietetic, (Featherweight) cut stringless, solids & liq.	½ cup (4 oz.)	25	5.0
(Larsen) *Fresh-Lite*, cut, water pack, no salt added	½ cup (4.2 oz.)	18	4.0
Frozen:			
(Frosty Acres)	3 oz.	25	5.0
(Larsen) cut	3 oz.	25	5.0
BEAN & FRANKFURTER, canned:			
(USDA)	1 cup (9 oz.)	367	32.1
(Libby's) *Diner*, micro cup	7¾-oz. serving	330	38.0
BEAN & FRANKFURTER DINNER, frozen:			
(Banquet)	10-oz. dinner	520	57.0
(Morton)	10-oz. dinner	350	45.0
(Swanson) 3-compartment	10½-oz. dinner	440	53.0
BEAN MIX:			
*(Bean Cuisine):			
Florentine, with bow ties	½ cup	199	27.0
French, country, with gemelli	½ cup	214	27.0
Red, Barcelona with radiatore	½ cup	170	27.0
*(Fantastic Foods) black bean, without added ingredients	½ cup	157	28.0
(Knorr) Italian	1 pkg	230	50.0
(Lipton):			
Regular:			
Cajun, with sauce	½ cup	160	28.0
Chicken & sauce	½ cup	150	26.0
Kettle Creations, bean medley with pasta	¼ cup	130	23.0
BEAN SALAD, canned (Green Giant) three bean, solids & liq.	¼ of 17-oz. can	70	18.0
BEAN SOUP (See **SOUP,** Bean)			
BEANS 'N FIXIN'S, canned			

Food	Measure	Cals.	Carbs.
(Hunt's) *Big John's:*			
Beans	3 oz.	100	21.0
Fixin's	1 oz.	50	7.0
BEAN SPROUT:			
Fresh (USDA):			
Mung, raw	½ lb.	80	15.0
Mung, boiled, drained	¼ lb.	32	5.9
Soy, raw	½ lb.	104	12.0
Soy, boiled, drained	¼ lb.	43	4.2
Canned, drained:			
(Chun King)	4 oz.	40	5.9
(La Choy)	⅔ cup (2 oz.)	6	1.4
BEAR CLAWS (Dolly Madison):			
Cherry	2¾-oz. piece	270	36.0
Cinnamon	2¾-oz. piece	290	39.0

BEEF. Values for beef cuts are given below for "lean and fat" and for "lean only." Beef purchased by the consumer at the retail store usually is trimmed to about one-half-inch layer of fat. This is the meat described as "lean and fat." If all the fat that can be cut off with a knife is removed, the remainder is the "lean only." These cuts still contain flecks of fat known as "marbling" distributed through the meat. Cooked meats are medium done.

Food	Measure	Cals.	Carbs.
Choice grade cuts (USDA):			
Brisket:			
Raw	1 lb. (weighed with bone)	1284	0.0
Braised:			
Lean & fat	4 oz.	467	0.0
Lean only	4 oz.	252	0.0
Chuck:			
Raw	1 lb. (weighed with bone)	984	0.0
Braised or pot-roasted:			
Lean & fat	4 oz.	371	0.0
Lean only	4 oz.	243	0.0

Food	Measure	Cals.	Carbs.
Dried (See **BEEF, CHIPPED**)			
Fat, separable, cooked	1 oz.	207	0.0
Filet mignon. There is no data available on its composition. For dietary estimates, the data for sirloin steak, lean only, afford the closest approximation.			
Flank:			
Raw	1 lb.	653	0.0
Braised	4 oz.	222	0.0
Foreshank:			
Raw	1 lb. (weighed with bone)	531	0.0
Simmered:			
Lean & fat	4 oz.	310	0.0
Lean only	4 oz.	209	0.0
Ground:			
Lean:			
Raw	1 lb.	812	0.0
Raw	1 cup (8 oz.)	405	0.0
Broiled	4 oz.	248	0.0
Regular:			
Raw	1 lb.	1216	0.0
Raw	1 cup (8 oz.)	606	0.0
Broiled	4 oz.	324	0.0
Heel of round:			
Raw	1 lb.	966	0.0
Roasted:			
Lean & fat	4 oz.	296	0.0
Lean only	4 oz.	204	0.0
Hindshank:			
Raw	1 lb. (weighed with bone)	604	0.0
Simmered:			
Lean & fat	4 oz.	409	0.0
Lean only	4 oz.	209	0.0
Neck:			
Raw	1 lb. (weighed with bone)	820	0.0
Pot-roasted:			
Lean & fat	4 oz.	332	0.0
Lean only	4 oz.	222	0.0
Plate:			
Raw	1 lb. (weighed with bone)	1615	0.0

Food	Measure	Cals.	Carbs.
Simmered:			
Lean & fat	4 oz.	538	0.0
Lean only	4 oz.	252	0.0
Rib roast:			
Raw	1 lb. (weighed with bone)	1673	0.0
Roasted:			
Lean & fat	4 oz.	499	0.0
Lean only	4 oz.	273	0.0
Round:			
Raw	1 lb. (weighed with bone)	863	0.0
Broiled:			
Lean & fat	4 oz.	296	0.0
Lean only	4 oz.	214	0.0
Rump:			
Raw	1 lb. (weighed with bone)	1167	0.0
Roasted:			
Lean & fat	4 oz.	393	0.0
Lean only	4 oz.	236	0.0
Steak, club:			
Raw	1 lb. (weighed without bone)	1724	0.0
Broiled:			
Lean & fat	4 oz.	515	0.0
Lean only	4 oz.	277	0.0
One 8-oz. steak (weighed without bone before cooking) will give you:			
Lean & fat	5.9 oz.	754	0.0
Lean only	3.4 oz.	234	0.0
Steak, porterhouse:			
Raw	1 lb. (weighed with bone)	1603	0.0
Broiled:			
Lean & fat	4 oz.	527	0.0
Lean only	4 oz.	254	0.0
One 16-oz. steak (weighed with bone before cooking) will give you:			
Lean & fat	10.2 oz.	1339	0.0
Lean only	5.9 oz.	372	0.0

Food	Measure	Cals.	Carbs.
Steak, ribeye, broiled:			
One 10-oz. steak (weighed before cooking without bone) will give you:			
Lean & fat	7.3 oz.	911	0.0
Lean only	3.8 oz.	258	0.0
Steak, sirloin, double-bone:			
Raw	1 lb. (weighed with bone)	1240	0.0
Broiled:			
Lean & fat	4 oz.	463	0.0
Lean only	4 oz.	245	0.0
One 12-oz. steak (weighed before cooking with bone) will give you:			
Lean & fat	6.6 oz.	767	0.0
Lean only	4.4 oz.	268	0.0
One 16-oz. steak (weighed before cooking with bone) will give you:			
Lean & fat	8.9 oz.	1028	0.0
Lean only	5.9 oz.	359	0.0
Steak, sirloin, hipbone:			
Raw	1 lb. (weighed with bone)	1585	0.0
Broiled:			
Lean & fat	4 oz.	552	0.0
Lean only	4 oz.	272	0.0
Steak, sirloin, wedge & round-bone:			
Raw	1 lb. (weighed with bone)	1316	0.0
Broiled:			
Lean & fat	4 oz.	439	0.0
Lean only	4 oz.	235	0.0
Steak, T-bone:			
Raw	1 lb. (weighed with bone)	1596	0.0
Broiled:			
Lean & fat	4 oz.	536	0.0
Lean only	4 oz.	253	0.0
One 16-oz. steak (weighed before cooking with bone) will give you: Broiled:			

Food	Measure	Cals.	Carbs.
Lean & fat	4 oz.	463	0.0
Lean only	4 oz.	245	0.0
***BEEFAMATO* COCKTAIL**,			
canned (Mott's)	6 fl. oz.	80	19.0
BEEF BOUILLON:			
(Borden) *Lite-Line*	1 tsp.	12	2.0
(Herb-Ox):			
Cube	1 cube	6	.7
Packet	1 packet	8	.9
(Knorr)	1 cube	15	.5
(Wyler's)	1 cube	6	1.0
Low sodium (Featherweight)	1 tsp.	18	2.0
BEEF, CHIPPED:			
Cooked, creamed, home recipe			
(USDA)	½ cup (4.3 oz.)	188	8.7
Frozen, creamed:			
(Banquet)	4-oz. pkg.	100	9.0
(Stouffer's)	5½-oz. serving	230	9.0
BEEF DINNER OR ENTREE:			
Canned:			
(Hormel):			
Dinty Moore American Classics, roast, with			
gravy & potatoes	10-oz. serving	260	26.0
Health Selections, &			
mushrooms, micro cup	7-oz. serving	210	25.0
(Libby's) *Diner,* with			
macaroni, microwave cup	7¾-oz. serving	230	34.0
(Top Shelf) microwave bowl:			
Ribs, boneless	1 serving	440	29.0
Roast	1 serving	240	18.0
Freeze dried:			
(AlpineAire)	⅓ cup	106	NA
(Mountain House) with			
rice & onions	1 cup	330	42.0
Frozen:			
(Armour):			
Classic Lite, Steak Diane	10-oz. meal	290	25.0
Dinner Classics:			
Sirloin, roast	10.4-oz. meal	190	21.0
Sirloin tips	10¼-oz. meal	230	20.0
(Banquet):			
Dinner, chopped	11-oz. dinner	420	14.0

Food	Measure	Cals.	Carbs.
Dinner, *Extra Helping*	16-oz. dinner	870	50.0
Entree, patty, with mush-room gravy	8-oz. serving	290	13.0
Platter	10-oz. meal	460	20.0
(Budget Gourmet):			
Sirloin roast	9½-oz. meal	330	36.0
Sirloin tips, with country-style vegetables	10-oz. meal	310	21.0
Tips, in burgundy sauce	11-oz. meal	310	28.0
(Chun King) Szechuan	13-oz. entree	340	57.0
(Freezer Queen):			
Patty, charbroiled:			
Plain	10-oz. meal	300	20.0
With mushroom gravy	7-oz. serving	180	9.0
With mushroom & onion gravy	7-oz. serving	200	10.0
Sliced, with gravy:			
Regular	10-oz. serving	210	18.0
Cook-In-Pouch	4-oz. serving	6	4.0
Deluxe family supper	7-oz. serving	130	10.0
(Goya) ground, with rice	1 pkg.	860	111.0
(Healthy Choice):			
Rib, boneless, with barbecue sauce	11-oz. meal	330	40.0
Sirloin, with barbecue sauce	11-oz. meal	280	44.0
Sirloin tips	11¼-oz. meal	270	29.0
(La Choy) *Fresh & Lite,* & broccoli, with rice	11-oz. meal	260	42.0
(Le Menu):			
Chopped sirloin	12¼-oz. dinner	430	28.0
Sirloin tips	11½-oz. dinner	400	29.0
(Morton) sliced	10-oz. dinner	220	20.0
(Stouffer's):			
Lean Cuisine:			
Oriental, with vegetable & rice	8⅝-oz. meal	290	31.0
Szechuan, with noodles & vegetables	9¼-oz. meal	260	22.0
Right Course:			
Dijon, with pasta & vegetables	9½-oz. meal	290	31.0
Fiesta, with corn & pasta	8⅞-oz. meal	270	23.0
Ragout, with rice pilaf	10-oz. meal	300	38.0
(Swanson):			
4-compartment dinner:			
Regular, & gravy	11¼-oz. dinner	310	38.0

Food	Measure	Cals.	Carbs.
In barbecue sauce	11-oz. dinner	460	51.0
Chopped sirloin	10¾-oz. dinner	340	28.0
Homestyle Recipe, sirloin tips	7-oz. meal	160	16.0
Hungry Man:			
Chopped	16¾-oz. dinner	640	41.0
Sliced	15¼-oz. dinner	450	49.0
(Tyson) premium, champignon	10½-oz. meal	370	30.0
(Weight Watchers):			
Romanoff supreme, with pasta & vegetables	9-oz. meal	230	29.0
Stir-fry:			
Cantonese, with rice	9-oz. meal	200	27.0
Jade garden	9-oz. meal	150	17.0
Ultimate 200:			
London broil	7½-oz. meal	110	4.0
Sirloin tips	7½-oz. meal	200	20.0
BEEF, DRIED, packaged:			
(Carl Buddig) smoked	1 oz.	38	Tr.
(Hormel) sliced	1 oz.	50	Tr.
BEEF, GROUND, SEASONING MIX:			
(Durkee):			
Regular	1 cup	653	9.0
With onion	1 cup	659	6.5
(French's) with onion	1⅛-oz. pkg.	100	24.0
BEEF, PACKAGED:			
(Carl Buddig) smoked	1 oz.	38	Tr.
(Hormel)	1 oz.	50	0.0
(Safeway)	1 oz.	60	1.0
BEEF, PEPPER, ORIENTAL:			
Canned (La Choy)	¾ cup	80	10.0
Frozen:			
(Chun King)	13-oz. entree	310	53.0
(La Choy)	12-oz. dinner	250	45.0
BEEF, POTTED (USDA)	1 oz.	70	0.0
BEEF JERKY:			
(Boar's Head)	.6-oz. serving	100	2.0

Food	Measure	Cals.	Carbs.
(Frito-Lay's):			
Regular	.2-oz. serving	25	1.0
Tender	.7-oz. serving	120	2.0
(Hormel) *Lumberjack*	1-oz. serving	100	0.0
(Pemmican):			
Jalapeño	1.1-oz. serving	90	4.0
Natural	1.3-oz. piece	110	5.0
Peppered	1.3-oz. piece	110	5.0
Steakers:			
Pouch	1.1-oz. pouch	80	4.0
Strip	1 strip	40	2.0
Tabasco	1.3-oz. piece	110	5.0
Tender Tribe	1-oz. serving	80	2.0
(Slim Jim):			
Big Jerk	¼-oz. piece	25	1.0
Giant Jerk	.63-oz. piece	60	2.0
Super Jerk:			
Regular	1 piece	30	1.0
Tabasco	.3-oz. piece	30	1.0
BEEF PIE, frozen:			
(Banquet):			
Regular	7-oz. pie	510	39.0
Supreme Microwave	7-oz. pie	440	30.0
(Empire Kosher)	8-oz. pie	540	51.0
(Morton)	7-oz. pie	400	37.0
(Stouffer's)	10-oz. pie	450	36.0
(Swanson):			
Regular	7-oz. pie	370	36.0
Hungry Man	16-oz. pie	710	71.0
BEEF SOUP (See **SOUP,** Beef)			
BEEF SPREAD, ROAST, canned:			
(Hormel)	1 oz.	62	0.0
(Underwood)	½ of 4¾-oz. can	140	Tr.
BEEF STEW:			
Home recipe, made with lean beef chuck	1 cup (8.6 oz.)	218	15.2
Canned, regular pack:			
(Hormel):			
Regular, micro cup	7½-oz. serving	230	11.0
Dinty Moore:			
Regular	7½-oz. can	190	15.0
Regular	⅕ of 40-oz. can	210	16.0
Microwave bowl	7½-oz. serving	190	15.0

Food	Measure	Cals.	Carbs.
Microwave cup (Libby's):	7½-oz. serving	180	15.0
Regular	½ of 15-oz. can	160	18.0
Diner, microwave cup	7¾-oz. serving	240	22.0
(Pathmark) no frills	8-oz. serving	220	15.0
Canned, dietetic:			
(Estee)	7½-oz. serving	210	15.0
(Featherweight)	7½-oz. can	160	17.0
(Weight Watchers) chunky, microwave cup	7½-oz. serving	120	14.0
Frozen (Banquet) *Family Entree*	8-oz. serving	160	20.6
Mix (Lipton) *Microeasy*, hearty	¼ pkg.	70	14.1

BEEF STEW SEASONING MIX:

Food	Measure	Cals.	Carbs.
*(Durkee)	1 cup	379	16.7
(French's)	1⅛-oz. pkg.	150	30.0

BEEF STOCK BASE (French's)

Food	Measure	Cals.	Carbs.
	1 tsp (.13 oz.)	8	2.0

BEEF STROGANOFF, frozen:

Food	Measure	Cals.	Carbs.
(Armour) *Classics Lite*	11¼-oz. meal	250	30.0
(Budget Gourmet) Light & Healthy	8¾-oz. meal	260	25.0
(Stouffer's) with parsley noodles	9¾-oz. pkg.	390	28.0

BEER & ALE:

Regular:

Food	Measure	Cals.	Carbs.
Anheuser	12 fl. oz.	167	15.4
Black Label	12 fl. oz.	136	11.2
Blatz	12 fl. oz.	142	11.8
Budweiser: Busch Bavarian	12 fl. oz.	142	11.1
C. Schmidt's	12 fl. oz.	136	11.2
Coors:			
Regular	12 fl. oz.	132	11.5
Extra Gold	12 fl. oz.	150	12.5
Michelob, regular	12 fl. oz.	152	13.6
Old Milwaukee	12 fl. oz.	142	13.4
Old Style	12 fl. oz.	147	12.1
Pearl Premium	12 fl. oz.	148	12.3
Rolling Rock, premium	12 fl. oz.	145	10.0
(Schlitz)	12 fl. oz.	150	13.2

Alcohol free:

Food	Measure	Cals.	Carbs.
Cutter	12 fl. oz.	75	19.5
Moussy	12 fl. oz.	54	13.0
Sharp's	12 fl. oz.	86	1.0

Food	Measure	Cals.	Carbs.
Light or low carbohydrate:			
Budweiser Light	12 fl. oz.	108	6.7
Coors	12 fl. oz.	102	4.5
LA	12 fl. oz.	112	15.8
Natural Light	12 fl. oz.	110	6.0
Michelob Light	12 fl. oz.	134	11.5
Old Milwaukee	12 fl. oz.	122	9.2
Pearl Light	12 fl. oz.	68	2.3
Rolling Rock	12 fl. oz.	104	8.0
Schmidt Light	12 fl. oz.	96	3.2
BEER, NEAR:			
Goetz Pale	12 fl. oz.	78	3.9
(Metbrew)	12 fl. oz.	73	13.7
BEER BATTER MIX			
(Golden Dipt)	1 oz.	100	22.0
BEET:			
Raw (USDA):			
Whole	1 lb. (weighed with skins, without tops)	137	31.4
Diced	½ cup (2.4 oz.)	29	6.6
Boiled (USDA) drained:			
Whole	2 beets (2" dia., 3.5 oz.)	32	7.2
Diced	½ cup (3 oz.)	27	6.1
Sliced	½ cup (3.6 oz.)	33	7.3
Canned, regular pack, solids & liq.:			
(Larsen) *Freshlike:*			
Pickled	½ cup (4.3 oz.)	100	25.0
Sliced or whole	½ cup (4.7 oz.)	40	9.0
(Pathmark) sliced	½ cup	45	10.0
(S&W):			
Diced, julienne or small whole	½ cup	40	9.0
Pickled, any style	½ cup	70	16.0
(Town House):			
Regular	½ cup	35	8.0
Pickled	½ cup	80	19.0
Canned, dietetic, solids & liq.:			
(Del Monte) no salt added	½ cup (4 oz.)	35	8.0
(Featherweight) sliced	½ cup	45	10.0
(Larsen) *Fresh-Lite*, sliced, water pack, no salt added	½ cup (4.3 oz.)	40	9.0

Food	Measure	Cals.	Carbs.
(Pathmark) no salt added	½ cup	40	9.0
(S&W) *Nutradiet*, sliced	½ cup	35	9.0
BEET GREENS (USDA):			
Raw, whole	1 lb. (weighed untrimmed)	61	11.7
Boiled, halves & stems, drained	½ cup (2.6 oz.)	13	2.4
BEET PUREE, canned (Larsen) no salt added	½ cup (4.7 oz.)	45	10.0
BÉNÉDICTINE LIQUEUR (Julius Wile) 86 proof	1 fl. oz.	112	10.3
BERRY BEARS, *Fruit Corners* (General Mills)	.9-oz. pouch	100	22.0
BERRY DRINK, MIXED:			
Canned:			
(Hi-C) *Bopin' Berry*	6 fl. oz.	90	23.0
(Johanna Farms) *Scips*	8.45-fl.-oz. container	130	32.0
(Juicy Juice):			
Bottle	6 fl. oz.	90	22.0
Box	8.45-fl.-oz. container	130	30.0
Can	6 fl. oz.	90	22.0
(Minute Maid)	6 fl. oz.	90	23.0
Frozen:			
(Five Alive) citrus	6 fl. oz.	90	22.0
(Minute Maid) punch	6 fl. oz.	90	23.0
*Mix, Crystal Light	8 fl. oz.	4	0.0
BERRY GRAPE JUICE DRINK (Boku) mixed	8 fl. oz.	120	29.0
BERRY NECTAR, MIXED, canned (Santa Cruz Natural) organic	8 fl. oz.	90	22.0
BIG BOY RESTAURANT:			
Beans, green	1 serving	28	6.0
Carrots	1 serving	35	8.0
Chicken dinner:			
Breast, salad without dressing & oat bran bread	1 meal	349	20.0
Breast, with mozzarella, salad without dressing & bread	1 meal	370	24.0
Cajun, salad without dressing & oat bran bread	1 meal	349	20.0

Food	Measure	Cals.	Carbs.
Stir fry, with vegetables	1 meal	562	68.0
Chicken salad dijon	1 serving	391	31.0
Chicken sandwich on pita bread, with mozzarella, *Heart Smart*	1 serving	404	26.0
Corn	1 serving	90	17.0
Fish dinner, cod:			
Baked:			
Regular, salad without dressing & oat bran bread	1 meal	364	20.0
Dijon, salad without dressing & oat bran bread	1 meal	427	21.0
Broiled:			
Regular, salad without dressing & oat bran bread	1 meal	364	20.0
Cajun, salad without dressing & oat bran bread	1 meal	364	20.0
Frozen dessert, *No-no*	1 serving	75	17.0
Peas	1 serving	77	13.0
Potato, baked	1 serving	163	37.0
Rice	1 serving	114	25.0
Roll	1 roll	139	30.0
Salad, dinner, without dressing	1 serving	19	4.0
Salad dressing, buttermilk	1 serving	36	4.0
Spaghetti dinner, salad without dressing & bread	1 meal	450	87.0
Turkey sandwich on pita bread, *Heart Smart*	1 sandwich	224	24.0
Vegetable stir fry	1 serving	408	74.0
Yogurt, frozen:			
Regular	1 serving	72	NA
Shake	1 serving	184	2.0
BIGG MIXX, cereal (Kellogg's):			
Plain	½ cup (1 oz.)	110	24.0
Raisin	½ cup (1.3 oz.)	140	31.0
BIG MAC (See **McDONALD'S**)			
BISCUIT:			
Packaged:			
(Arvey's):			
Country	3" biscuit	160	23.0
Square	1 oz.	80	12.0

Food	Measure	Cals.	Carbs.
(Weight Watchers)			
Buttermilk	1.8-oz. biscuit	100	23.0
(Wonder)	1 biscuit	80	14.0
Refrigerated:			
(Pillsbury)			
Regular:			
Big Premium Heat 'n Eat	1 biscuit	140	16.0
Butter	1 biscuit	50	10.0
Buttermilk	1 biscuit	50	10.0
Ballard, Ovenready	1 biscuit	50	10.0
Big Country	1 biscuit	100	14.0
1869 Brand	1 biscuit	100	12.0
Grands:			
Butter Tastin'	1 biscuit	190	22.0
Cinnamon, raisin	1 biscuit	190	27.0
Flaky	1 biscuit	190	23.0
Hungry Jack,			
Buttermilk:			
Extra rich	1 biscuit	50	9.0
Flaky or fluffy	1 biscuit	90	12.0
(Roman Meal):			
Oat bran, honey nut	1 biscuit	130	19.0
White:			
Regular	1 biscuit	90	16.0
Premium	1 biscuit	125	18.0
BISCUIT MIX:			
(Bisquick)	½ cup	240	37.0
*(Gold Medal), pouch mix,			
prepared with skim milk	⅛ of recipe	90	14.0
BITTERS (Angostura)	1 tsp.	14	2.1
BLACKBERRY:			
Fresh (USDA) includes			
boysenberry, dewberry,			
youngsberry:			
With hulls	1 lb. (weighed		
	untrimmed)	250	55.6
Hulled	½ cup (2.6 oz.)	41	9.4
Canned, regular pack (USDA)			
solids & liq.:			
Juice pack	4-oz. serving	61	13.7
Light syrup	4-oz. serving	82	19.6
Heavy syrup	½ cup (4.6 oz.)	118	28.9
Extra heavy syrup	4-oz. serving	125	30.7
Frozen (USDA):			

Food	Measure	Cals.	Carbs.
Sweetened, unthawed	4-oz. serving	109	27.7
Unsweetened, unthawed	4-oz. serving	55	12.9
BLACKBERRY JELLY:			
Sweetened (Smucker's)	1 T. (.7 oz.)	54	12.0
Dietetic:			
(Diet Delight)	1 T. (.6 oz.)	12	3.0
(Featherweight) imitation	1 T.	16	4.0
BLACKBERRY LIQUEUR			
(Bols)	1 fl. oz.	95	8.9
BLACKBERRY PRESERVE **OR JAM:**			
Sweetened (Smucker's)	1 T. (.7 oz.)	54	12.0
Dietetic:			
(Estee, Louis Sherry)	1 T. (.6 oz.)	6	0.0
(Featherweight)	1 T.	16	4.0
(S&W) *Nutradiet*, red label	1 T.	12	3.0
BLACKBERRY WINE (Mogen David)	3 fl. oz.	135	18.7
BLACK-EYED PEAS:			
Canned, with pork, solids & liq:			
(Allen's) regular	½ cup	100	16.0
(Goya)	½ cup	105	19.5
(Green Giant)	½ cup	90	18.0
(Town House)	½ cup	105	19.5
Frozen:			
(Frosty Acres; McKenzie; Seabrook Farms)	⅓ of pkg. (3.3 oz.)	130	23.0
(Southland)	⅕ of 16-oz. pkg.	120	21.0
BLINTZE, frozen:			
(Empire Kosher):			
Apple	2½ oz.	100	24.0
Blueberry or cherry	2½ oz.	110	25.0
Cheese	2½ oz.	110	20.0
Potato	2½ oz.	130	21.0
(Golden):			
Apple-raisin	1 piece	80	16.0
Cheese	1 piece	80	12.5
Potato	1 piece	105	14.5
(King Kold) cheese:			
Regular	2½-oz. piece	113	18.9
No salt added	1½-oz. piece	95	18.5

Food	Measure	Cals.	Carbs.
BLOODY MARY MIX:			
Dry (Bar-Tender's)	1 serving	26	5.7
Liquid:			
(Holland House) *Smooth N'*			
Spicy	1 fl. oz.	3	<1.0
(Libby's)	6 fl. oz.	40	9.0
(Mr. & Mrs. T):			
Regular	4½ fl. oz.	20	4.0
Rich & spicy	4½ fl. oz.	30	6.0
Tabasco	6 fl. oz.	56	10.0
BLUEBERRY:			
Fresh (USDA):			
Whole	1 lb. (weighed untrimmed)	259	63.8
Trimmed	½ cup (2.6 oz.)	45	11.2
Canned, solids & liq.:			
(USDA):			
Syrup pack, extra heavy	½ cup (4.4 oz.)	126	32.5
Water pack	½ cup (4.3 oz.)	47	11.9
(S&W) in heavy syrup	½ cup	111	30.0
(Thank You Brand):			
Heavy syrup	½ cup (4.3 oz.)	102	25.4
Water pack	½ cup (4.2 oz.)	48	12.0
Frozen (USDA):			
Sweetened, solids & liq.	½ cup (4 oz.)	120	30.2
Unsweetened, solids & liq.	½ cup (2.9 oz.)	45	11.2
BLUEBERRY NECTAR, canned (Knudsen & Sons)	8 fl. oz.	135	34.0
BLUEBERRY PIE (See **PIE,** Blueberry)			
BLUEBERRY PRESERVE OR JAM:			
Sweetened (Smucker's)	1 T.	54	12.0
Dietetic (Estee, Louis Sherry)	1 T.	6	0.0
BLUEBERRY SQUARES, cereal (Kellogg's)	½ cup (1 oz.)	90	23.0
BLUEFISH (USDA):			
Raw:			
Whole	1 lb. (weighed whole)	271	0.0

Food	Measure	Cals.	Carbs.
Meat only	4 oz.	133	0.0
Baked or broiled	4.4-oz. piece (3½" × 3" × ½")	199	0.0
Fried	5.3-oz. piece (3½" × 3" × ½")	308	7.0
BODY BUDDIES, cereal (General Mills) natural fruit flavor	1 cup (1 oz.)	110	24.0
BOJANGLES RESTAURANT:			
Biscuit	1 piece	239	30.0
Chicken, skin free, Southern style:			
Breast	4-oz. serving	270	11.0
Leg	1.8-oz. serving	128	5.0
Thigh	3.2-oz. serving	264	10.0
Chicken sandwich, fillet, grilled, no mayonnaise	1 serving	329	37.0
Coleslaw	1 serving	105	19.0
Pinto beans, Cajun	1 serving	124	25.0
Rice, dirty	1 serving	167	20.0
BOLOGNA:			
(Boar's Head):			
Beef:			
Regular	1 oz.	74	<1.0
Low cholesterol, premium	1 oz.	70	1.0
Beef & pork, regular	1 oz.	80	<1.0
Ham	1 oz.	40	1.0
Lower sodium	1 oz.	75	<1.0
(Eckrich):			
Beef:			
Regular	1 oz.	90	2.0
Smorgas Pak:	¾-oz. slice	70	1.0
Thick slice	1½-oz. slice	140	2.0
Thin slice	1 slice	55	1.0
Garlic	1-oz. slice	90	2.0
German Brand, sliced or chub	1-oz. slice	80	1.0
Lunch chub	1-oz. serving	100	2.0
Meat:			
Regular	1-oz. slice	90	2.0
Thick slice	1.7-oz. slice	160	3.0
Thin slice	1 slice	55	1.0
Ring or sandwich	1-oz. slice	90	2.0
(Healthy Choice) turkey, beef & pork	¾-oz. slice	25	1.0

Food	Measure	Cals.	Carbs.
(Healthy Deli) beef & pork	1 oz.	41	1.1
Hebrew National, beef	1 oz.	90	<1.0
(Hormel):			
Beef:			
Regular	1 slice	85	.5
Coarse grind	1 oz.	80	.5
Meat:			
Regular	1 slice	90	0.0
Light & Lean:			
Regular	1 slice	70	1.0
Thin slice	1 slice	35	.5
(Ohse):			
Beef	1 oz.	85	1.0
Chicken, 15%	1 oz.	90	1.0
Chicken, beef & pork	1 oz.	75	3.0
(Oscar Mayer):			
Beef	.5-oz. slice	48	.5
Beef	1-oz. slice	90	.6
Beef Lebanon	.8-oz. slice	47	.3
Meat	1-oz. slice	90	.7
(Purdue) chicken	1-oz. slice	64	2.0
(Smok-A-Roma):			
Beef	1-oz. slice	90	1.0
Garlic	1-oz. slice	70	1.0
German	1-oz. slice	80	1.0
Meat:			
Regular	1 slice	90	1.0
Thick sliced	1 slice	180	2.0
15% chicken	1-oz. slice	90	1.0
Turkey	1-oz. slice	60	1.0
BOLOGNA & CHEESE:			
(Eckrich)	.7-oz. slice	90	1.0
(Oscar Mayer)	.8-oz. slice	74	.6
BONITO:			
Raw (USDA) meat only	4 oz.	191	0.0
Canned (Star-Kist):			
Chunk	6½-oz. can	605	0.0
Solid	7-oz. can	650	0.0
BOO*BERRY, cereal			
(General Mills)	1 cup (1 oz.)	110	24.0
BORSCHT:			
Regular:			
(Gold's)	8-oz. serving	100	21.0

Food	Measure	Cals.	Carbs.
(Manischewitz) with beets	8-oz. serving	80	20.0
(Rokeach)	1 cup (8 oz.)	96	23.0
Dietetic or low calorie:			
(Gold's)	8-oz. serving	20	5.0
(Manischewitz)	8-oz. serving	20	4.0
(Rokeach):	8-oz. serving	27	6.7
Diet	1 cup (8 oz.)	29	5.8
Unsalted	1 cup (8 oz.)	103	23.0
BOSTON MARKET:			
Apples, hot cinnamon	¾ cup (6.4 oz.)	250	56.0
Beans, BBQ, baked	¾ cup (8.1 oz.)	330	53.0
Bean, casserole, green	¾ cup (6 oz.)	50	10.0
Chicken:			
Dark meat:			
With skin, ¼ chicken	4.6-oz. serving	330	2.0
Without skin, ¼ chicken	3.7-oz. serving	210	1.0
White meat:			
With skin:			
¼ chicken	5.4-oz. serving	330	2.0
½ chicken	10-oz. serving	63	2.0
Without skin, ½ chicken, no wing	3.7-oz. serving	160	0.0
Chicken pot pie	15-oz. serving	750	75.0
Cole slaw	¾ cup (3 oz.)	280	32.0
Cookie:			
Brownie	3.3-oz. piece	450	47.0
Chocolate chip	2.8-oz. piece	340	48.0
Oatmeal raisin	2.8-oz. piece	320	48.0
Corn, whole kernel	¾ cup (5 oz.)	180	30.0
Cornbread	2.4-oz. piece	200	33.0
Gravy, chicken	1 oz.	15	2.0
Ham with cinnamon apples	8-oz. serving	350	36.0
Macaroni & cheese	¾ cup (6.8 oz.)	280	35.0
Meatloaf:			
And brown gravy	7-oz. serving	390	19.0
And chunky tomato sauce	8-oz. serving	370	22.0
Potato:			
Mashed:			
Plain	⅔ cup	180	26.0
With gravy	¾ cup	200	27.0
New potatoes	¾ cup (4.6 oz.)	130	25.0
Rice pilaf	⅔ cup (5.1 oz.)	180	32.0
Roll, honey wheat	1 roll (3.9 oz.)	150	29.0
Salads:			

Food	Measure	Cals.	Carbs.
Caesar:			
Regular, without dressing	7.9-oz. serving	240	14.0
Entree	10-oz. serving	520	16.0
Side salad	4-oz. serving	210	6.0
Chicken:			
Caesar	13-oz. serving	670	16.0
Chunky, entree	5.6-oz. serving	370	3.0
Fruit	¾ cup (5½ oz.)	70	17.0
Pasta, Mediterranean	¾ cup (4.6 oz.)	170	16.0
Tortellini	¾ cup (5.6 oz.)	380	29.0
Sandwich:			
Chicken:			
Without cheese & sauce	11½-oz. serving	430	62.0
With cheese & sauce	12.4-oz. serving	750	72.0
Chicken salad	11½-oz. serving	680	63.0
Ham:			
Without cheese & sauce	9.4-oz. serving	450	66.0
With cheese & sauce	11.9-oz. serving	760	71.0
Ham & turkey club:			
Without cheese & sauce	9.4-oz. serving	430	64.0
With cheese & sauce	13.4-oz. serving	890	76.0
Meatloaf:			
Without cheese & sauce	9.4-oz. serving	450	66.0
With cheese	13.9-oz. serving	860	95.0
Turkey:			
Without cheese & sauce	9.4-oz. serving	400	61.0
With cheese & sauce	11.9-oz. serving	710	68.0
Spinach, creamed	¾ cup (6.4-oz. serving)	293	12.0
Squash, butternut	¾ cup	180	250
Stuffing	¾ cup	310	44.0
Turkey breast, skinless, rotisserie	5-oz. serving	170	1.0
Vegetables, steamed	⅔ cup	35	7.0
Zucchini marinara	¾ cup	80	10.0
BOUILLABAISE SEASONING MIX (Knorr)	1 T.	20	3.0

BOURBON (See **DISTILLED LIQUOR**)

BOSCO (See **SYRUP**)

BOW TIE OR FARFELLE (See **PASTA, DRY OR FRESH, REFRIGERATED**)

Food	Measure	Cals.	Carbs.
BOYSENBERRY:			
Fresh (See **BLACKBERRY**)			
Frozen (USDA) sweetened	10-oz. pkg.	273	69.3
BOYSENBERRY JELLY:			
Sweetened (Smucker's)	1 T. (.7 oz.)	54	12.0
Dietetic (S&W) *Nutradiet*, red label	1 T.	12	3.0
BOYSENBERRY JUICE,			
canned (Smucker's)	8 fl. oz.	120	30.0
BOYSENBERRY NECTAR,			
canned (Knudsen & Sons)	8 fl. oz.	110	33.0
BRAINS, all animals			
(USDA) raw	4 oz.	142	.9
BRAN:			
Crude (USDA)	1 oz.	60	17.5
Miller's (Elam's)	1 T. (.2 oz.)	17	2.8
BRAN BREAKFAST CEREAL:			
(Kellogg's):			
All Bran or *Bran Buds*	⅓ cup (1 oz.)	70	22.0
Cracklin' Oat Bran	½ cup (1 oz.)	110	20.0
40% bran flakes	¾ cup (1 oz.)	90	23.0
Fruitful Bran	¾ cup (1 oz.)	110	27.0
Raisin Bran	¾ cup	110	30.0
(Loma Linda)	1 oz.	90	19.0
(Malt-O-Meal):			
40% bran	⅔ cup (1 oz.)	93	22.5
Raisin	¾ cup (1.4 oz.)	129	29.7
(Post):			
40% bran flakes	⅔ cup (1 oz.)	88	23.0
With raisins	½ cup (1 oz.)	122	32.0
(Ralston Purina):			
Bran Chex	⅔ cup (1 oz.)	90	24.0
Bran News	¾ cup (1 oz.)	100	23.0
Oat	1 cup	130	32.0
(Safeway):			
40% bran flakes	⅔ cup	90	23.0
Raisin	¾ cup	110	29.0

BRANDY (See **DISTILLED LIQUOR**)

Food	Measure	Cals.	Carbs.
BRANDY, FLAVORED (Mr. Boston) 35% alcohol:			
Apricot	1 fl. oz.	94	8.9
Blackberry	1 fl. oz.	92	8.6
Cherry	1 fl. oz.	87	8.4
Coffee	1 fl. oz.	72	10.6
Ginger	1 fl. oz.	72	3.5
Peach	1 fl. oz.	94	8.9
BRAUNSCHWEIGER:			
(Eckrich) chub	1 oz.	70	1.0
(Hormel)	1 oz.	80	0.0
(Jones Dairy Farm):			
Regular:			
Chub	2-oz. serving	150	1.0
Chunk	2-oz. serving	180	1.0
With onion	2-oz. serving	150	2.0
Sliced	1.2-oz. slice	110	1.0
Light, chub or chunk	2-oz. serving	100	1.0
(Oscar Mayer):			
German Brand	1-oz. serving	94	.5
Sliced	1-oz. slice	96	.6
Tube	1-oz. serving	85	1.0
(Swift) 8-oz. chub	1 oz.	109	1.4
BRAZIL NUT:			
Raw (USDA):			
Whole, in shell	1 cup (4.3 oz.)	383	6.4
Shelled	½ cup (2.5 oz.)	458	7.6
Shelled	4 nuts (.6 oz.)	114	1.9
Roasted (Fisher) salted	1 oz. (¼ cup)	193	3.1
BREAD:			
Apple cinnamon (Pritikin)	1-oz. slice	80	14.0
Autumn grain (Interstate Brands) *Merita*	1-oz. slice	75	14.0
Barbecue, *Millbrook*	1.23-oz. slice	100	17.0
Black (Mrs. Wright's)	1 slice	60	11.0
Boston brown:			
(USDA)	3" × ¾" slice (1.7 oz.)	101	21.9
Canned, plain or raisin:			
(B&M)	½" slice (1.6 oz.)	80	18.0
(Friend's)	½" slice	80	18.0
Bran (Roman Meal):			
5 Bran	1-oz. slice	65	13.0
Oat, light	.8-oz. slice	42	9.6

Food	Measure	Cals.	Carbs.
Rice, honey or honey nut	1-oz. slice	71	12.3
Butter & egg (Mrs. Wright's) regular or sesame	1 slice	70	13.0
Buttermilk, *Butternut*	1-oz. slice	80	13.0
Cinnamon (Pepperidge Farm)	1 slice	90	15.0
Cracked wheat:			
(Pepperidge Farm) thin sliced	.9-oz. slice	70	13.0
(Roman Meal)	1-oz. slice	67	12.6
(Wonder)	1 slice	70	13.0
Crispbread, *Wasa*:			
Mora	3.2-oz. slice	333	70.5
Rye:			
Golden	.3-oz. slice	37	7.8
Lite	.3-oz. slice	30	6.2
Sesame	.5-oz. slice	50	10.6
Sport	.4-oz. slice	42	9.1
Date nut roll (Dromedary)	1-oz. slice	80	13.0
Egg, *Millbrook*	1-oz. slice	70	14.0
Flatbread, *Ideal*:			
Bran	.2-oz. slice	19	4.1
Extra thin	.1-oz. slice	12	2.5
Whole grain	.2-oz. slice	19	4.0
French:			
(Arnold) *Francisco*	1/16 of loaf (1 oz.)	70	12.0
(Interstate Brands):			
Eddy's, sour	1.5-oz. slice	110	19.0
Sweetheart, regular	1-oz. slice	70	14.0
(Mrs. Wright's) unsliced	.7-oz. slice	60	10.5
(Pepperidge Farm):			
Fully baked, hearth	1 oz.	75	14.0
Twin	1 oz.	80	15.0
Garlic (Arnold)	1-oz. slice	80	10.0
Hi-fibre (Monks')	1-oz. slice	50	13.0
Hillbilly, Holsum	1-oz. slice	70	13.0
Hollywood:			
Dark	1-oz. slice	72	12.5
Light	1-oz. slice	71	13.1
Honey bran (Pepperidge Farm)	1 slice (1.2 oz.)	90	18.0
Honey & molasses graham (Mrs. Wright's)	1 slice	100	19.0
Hunter's grain (Interstate Brands) *Country Farms*	1.5-oz. slice	120	22.0

Food	Measure	Cals.	Carbs.
Italian:			
(Arnold):			
Regular, Bakery, light	1 slice	45	9.9
Francisco International:			
Regular	1-oz. slice	72	14.1
Thick, sliced	1 slice	66	13.7
(Pepperidge Farm) *Hearth*	1-oz. slice	80	14.0
(Wonder) family	1 slice	70	13.0
Low sodium (Eddy's)	1-oz. slice	80	13.0
Mountain oat (Interstate Brands) *Country Farms*	1.5-oz. slice	130	23.0
Multi-grain:			
(Arnold) *Milk & Honey*	1-oz. slice	70	14.0
(Pritikin)	1-oz. slice	70	12.0
(Weight Watchers)	¾-oz. slice	40	9.4
Natural grains (Arnold)	.8-oz. slice	60	11.0
Oat (Arnold):			
Brannola	1.3-oz. slice	90	14.0
Milk & Honey	1-oz. slice	80	15.0
Oat bran:			
(Awrey's) plain	1 slice	50	10.0
(Roman Meal):			
Honey	1 slice	71	12.7
Honey nut	1 slice	72	12.1
Split-top	1 slice	68	13.2
(Weight Watchers) plain	1 slice	40	10.0
Oatmeal:			
(Mrs. Wright's)	1 slice	80	15.0
(Pepperidge Farm):			
Regular	1 slice	90	17.0
Light	1 slice	49	9.0
Thin sliced	1 slice	40	8.0
Olympian meal (Interstate Brands) *Holsum*	1-oz. slice	70	13.0
Onion dill (Pritikin)	1-oz. slice	70	12.0
Potato (Interstate Brands) *Sweetheart*	1-oz. slice	70	14.0
Pita, Sahara (Thomas'):			
White:			
Regular	2-oz. piece	160	31.0
Mini	1-oz. piece	80	16.0
Large	3-oz. piece	240	48.0
Whole wheat:			
Regular	2-oz. piece	150	28.0
Mini	1-oz. piece	80	14.0
Pumpernickel:			
(Arnold)	1.1-oz. slice	80	14.0

Food	Measure	Cals.	Carbs.
(Levy's)	1.1-oz. slice	80	14.0
(Pepperidge Farm):			
Regular	1.1-oz. slice	80	15.0
Party	.2-oz. slice	15	3.0
Raisin:			
(Arnold) tea	.9-oz. slice	70	13.0
(Interstate Brands) *Butternut*	1-oz. slice	80	15.0
(Monk's) & cinnamon	1-oz. slice	70	10.0
(Pepperidge Farm)	1 slice	90	16.0
(Pritikin)	1-oz. slice	70	13.0
Sun-Maid (Interstate			
Brands)	1-oz. slice	80	15.0
Round top (Roman Meal)	1-oz. slice	69	13.4
Rye:			
(Arnold):			
Jewish	1.1-oz. slice	80	14.0
Melba Thin	.7-oz. slice	40	8.0
(Levy's) real	1.1-oz. slice	80	14.5
(Mrs. Wright's):			
Regular, with or			
without seeds	1 slice	60	11.0
Bavarian	1 slice	60	11.0
Dill, *Grainbelt*	1 slice	100	19.0
Jewish	1 slice	60	9.0
Swedish	1-oz. slice	80	15.0
(Pepperidge Farm):			
Dijon:			
Regular	1 slice	50	9.0
Hearty	1 slice	70	15.0
Family, with or without			
seeds	1 slice	80	16.0
Party	1 slice	15	3.0
(Pritikin)	1-oz. slice	70	12.0
(Weight Watchers)	¾-oz. slice	39	9.5
Salt Rising (USDA)	.9-oz. slice	67	13.0
Sesame seed (Mrs. Wright's)	1 slice	70	14.0
7-Grain, Home Pride	1-oz. slice	72	12.8
Sourdough, *Di Carlo*	1-oz. slice	70	13.6
Split top (Interstate Brands)			
Merita	1-oz. slice	70	12.0
Sunflower & bran (Monk's)	1-oz. slice	70	12.0
Sun grain (Roman Meal)	1-oz. slice	70	12.6
Texas toast (Interstate Brands)			
Holsum	1.4-oz. slice	90	17.0
Wheat (See also Cracked			
Wheat or Whole Wheat):			
America's Own, cottage	1-oz. slice	70	13.0

Food	Measure	Cals.	Carbs.
(Arnold):			
Brannola:			
Dark	1.3-oz. slice	80	13.0
Hearty	1.3-oz. slice	90	13.0
Brick Oven	.8-oz. slice	60	9.0
Brick Oven	1.1-oz. slice	90	14.0
Country	1.3-oz. slice	80	13.0
Less or *Liteway*	.8-oz. slice	40	7.0
Milk & Honey	1-oz. slice	80	15.0
Very thin	.5-oz. slice	40	6.0
Fresh Horizons	1-oz. slice	54	9.6
Fresh & Natural	1-oz. slice	77	13.6
Home Pride	1-oz. slice	73	13.1
(Pepperidge Farm):			
Regular	1 slice	90	18.0
Family	1 slice	70	13.0
Light	1 slice	45	19.0
Very thin slice	1 slice	35	7.0
(Safeway)	1-oz. slice	70	13.0
(Wonder) family	1-oz. slice	75	13.6
(Weight Watchers)	1 slice	40	9.0
Wheatberry, *Home Pride:*			
Honey	1-oz. slice	74	13.3
Regular	1-oz. slice	70	12.5
White:			
America's Own, cottage	1-oz. slice	70	15.0
(Arnold):			
Brick Oven	.8-oz. slice	60	11.0
Brick Oven	1.1-oz. slice	90	14.0
Country	1.3-oz. slice	100	18.0
Less or *Liteway*	.8-oz. slice	40	7.0
Milk & Honey	1-oz. slice	80	15.0
Very thin	.5-oz. slice	40	7.0
Fresh Horizons	1-oz. slice	54	10.0
Home Pride	1-oz. slice	72	13.1
(Interstate Brands):			
Butternut	1-oz. slice	70	14.0
Cookbook	1-oz. slice	75	14.0
Holsum	1-oz. slice	70	14.0
(Monk's)	1-oz. slice	60	10.0
(Pepperidge Farm):			
Family	1 slice	70	13.0
Hearty country	1 slice	95	19.0
Sandwich	1 slice	65	12.0
Thin sliced	1 slice	70	13.0
Toasting	1 slice	90	17.0
Very thin slice	1 slice	40	8.0

Food	Measure	Cals.	Carbs.
(Roman Meal) light	.8-oz. slice	40	10.2
(Weight Watchers) plain	1 slice	40	10.0
Whole wheat:			
(Arnold):			
Brick Oven	.8-oz. slice	60	9.5
Stone ground	.8-oz. slice	50	8.0
Home Pride	1-oz. slice	70	12.2
(Monk's) 100% stone ground	1-oz. slice	70	13.0
(Pepperidge Farm):			
Thin slice	.9-oz. slice	65	12.0
Very thin slice	.6-oz. slice	40	7.5
BREAD CRUMBS:			
(Contadina) seasoned	½ cup (2.1 oz.)	211	40.6
(4C):			
Plain	4 oz.	405	85.2
Seasoned	4 oz.	384	77.3
(Progresso):			
Plain or Italian style	1 T.	30	5.5
Onion	1 T.	27	5.5
*BREAD DOUGH:			
Frozen (Rich's):			
French	¹⁄₂₀ of loaf	59	11.0
Italian	¹⁄₂₀ of loaf	60	11.0
Raisin	¹⁄₂₀ of loaf	66	12.3
Wheat	.5-oz. slice	60	10.5
White	.8-oz. slice	56	9.4
Refrigerated (Pillsbury)			
Poppin' Fresh:			
French	1" slice	60	11.0
Wheat	1" slice	80	12.0
White	1" slice	80	12.0
BREAD MACHINE MIX:			
*(Dromedary):			
Italian herb	½" slice	140	25.0
Wheat, stoneground	½" slice	140	26.0
White, country	½" slice	140	28.0
(Pillsbury) cracked wheat	¹⁄₁₂ of pkg.	130	25.0
*BREAD MIX:			
Home Hearth:			
French	⅜" slice	85	14.5
Rye	⅜" slice	75	14.0
White	⅜" slice	75	14.5

Food	Measure	Cals.	Carbs.
(Pillsbury):			
Banana	¹⁄₁₂ of loaf	170	27.0
Blueberry nut	¹⁄₁₂ of loaf	150	26.0
Cherry nut	¹⁄₁₂ of loaf	180	29.0
Cranberry	¹⁄₁₂ of loaf	160	30.0
Date	¹⁄₁₂ of loaf	160	32.0
Nut	¹⁄₁₂ of loaf	170	28.0
BREAD PUDDING, with	1 cup		
raisins, home recipe (USDA)	(9.3 oz.)	496	75.3
BREADSTICK (Stella D'oro):			
Regular:			
Plain	1 piece	40	7.0
Onion or wheat	1 piece	40	6.0
Pizza	1 piece	45	7.0
Sesame	1 piece	50	6.0
Dietetic:			
Regular	1 piece	45	7.0
Sesame	1 piece	60	7.0
*BREADSTICK DOUGH			
(Pillsbury) soft	1 piece	100	17.0
BREAKFAST DRINK MIX:			
(Lucerne):			
Chocolate	1 envelope	130	26.0
Coffee, strawberry or vanilla	1 envelope	130	28.0
*(Pillsbury):			
Chocolate	8 fl. oz.	290	38.0
Strawberry	8 fl. oz.	290	39.0
Vanilla	8 fl. oz.	300	41.0
BREAKFAST WITH BARBIE,			
cereal (Ralston Purina)	1 cup (1 oz.)	110	25.0
BRIGHT & EARLY	6 fl. oz.	90	20.8
BRITOS, frozen (Patio):			
Beef & bean	½ of 7¼-oz. pkg.	250	33.0
Chicken, spicy	½ of 7¼-oz. pkg.	250	33.0
Chili:			
Green	½ of 7¼-oz. pkg.	250	33.0
Red	½ of 7¼-oz. pkg.	240	31.0
Nacho beef	½ of 7¼-oz. pkg.	270	30.0
Nacho cheese	½ of 7¼-oz. pkg.	250	32.0

Food	Measure	Cals.	Carbs.
BROCCOLI:			
Raw (USDA):			
Whole	1 lb. (weighed untrimmed)	69	16.3
Large leaves removed	1 lb.	113	20.9
Boiled (USDA):			
½" pieces, drained	½ cup (2.8 oz.)	20	3.5
Whole, drained	1 med. stalk (6.3 oz.)	47	8.1
Frozen:			
(Bel Air):			
Chopped	3.3 oz.	25	5.0
Cuts:			
Plain	3.3 oz.	25	5.0
Cheese sauce	3.3 oz.	45	6.0
Spears, cut or whole	3.3 oz.	25	5.0
(Birds Eye):			
With almonds & selected seasonings	⅓ of pkg. (3.3 oz.)	62	5.7
In cheese sauce	⅓ of pkg. (3.3 oz.)	87	8.4
Chopped, cuts or florets	⅓ of pkg. (3.3 oz.)	26	4.9
Spears:			
Regular	⅓ of pkg. (3.3 oz.)	26	5.0
In butter sauce	⅓ of pkg. (3.3 oz.)	58	5.3
Deluxe	⅓ of pkg. (3.3 oz.)	29	5.0
& water chestnuts with selected seasonings	⅓ of pkg. (3.3 oz.)	35	5.8
(Frosty Acres)	3.3-oz. serving	25	5.0
(Green Giant):			
In cream sauce	3.3 oz.	50	7.4
Cuts, *Harvest Fresh*	3 oz.	16	3.0
Cuts, polybag	½ cup	12	3.0
Spears:			
In butter sauce, regular	3⅓ oz.	40	6.0
Harvest Fresh	3 oz.	19	4.0

BROWNIE (See **COOKIE**)

BROWNIE MIX (See **COOKIE MIX**)

Food	Measure	Cals.	Carbs.
BRUSSELS SPROUT:			
Raw (USDA) trimmed	1 lb.	204	37.6
Boiled (USDA) drained	3-4 sprouts	28	4.9
Frozen:			
(USDA) boiled, drained	4 oz.	37	7.4
(Bel-Air)	3.3 oz.	35	7.0
(Birds Eye):			
Regular	⅓ of 10-oz. pkg.	37	7.3
In butter sauce	⅓ of 10-oz. pkg.	59	7.2
Baby, with cheese sauce	⅓ of 10-oz. pkg.	84	8.7
Baby, deluxe	⅓ of 10-oz. pkg.	49	7.3
(Frosty Acres)	3-oz. serving	30	7.0
(Green Giant):			
In butter sauce	3.3 oz.	40	8.0
Polybag	½ cup	25	6.0
(Larsen)	3.3-oz. serving	35	7.0
BUCKWHEAT:			
Flour (See **FLOUR**)			
Groats (Pocono):			
Brown, whole	1 oz.	104	19.4
White, whole	1 oz.	102	20.1
BUC*WHEATS, cereal			
(General Mills)	1 oz. (¾ cup)	110	24.0
BULGUR (form of hard red winter wheat) (USDA):			
Dry	1 lb.	1605	343.4
Canned:			
Unseasoned	4-oz. serving	191	39.7
Seasoned	4-oz. serving	206	37.2
BURGER KING:			
Bagel:			
Bacon, egg & cheese	1 serving	450	46.0
Egg & cheese	1 serving	405	46.0
Ham, egg & cheese	1 serving	435	46.0
Sausage, egg & cheese	1 serving	625	49.0
Biscuit:			
Bacon	1 serving	375	42.0
Bacon & egg	1 serving	465	43.0
Sausage	1 serving	475	44.0
Sausage & egg	1 serving	565	45.0
Breakfast Buddy, with sausage, egg & cheese	3-oz. serving	255	15.0
Cheeseburger:			
Regular	4-oz. serving	318	28.0

Food	Measure	Cals.	Carbs.
Double:			
Regular	5.6-oz. serving	480	29.0
Bacon	5.3-oz. serving	515	26.0
Bacon double, deluxe	5.6-oz serving	590	28.0
Chicken sandwich:			
Regular	8-oz. sandwich	685	57.0
BK Broiler	5.4-oz. sandwich	379	31.0
Chicken Tenders	1 piece	39	2.7
Croissanwich:			
Bacon, egg & cheese	5-oz. serving	353	19.0
Ham, egg & cheese	5-oz. serving	351	20.0
Sausage, egg & cheese	5.6-oz. serving	534	22.0
Danish:			
Apple cinnamon	1 serving	390	62.0
Cheese	1 serving	406	60.0
Cinnamon raisin	1 serving	449	63.0
Egg platter, scrambled:			
Regular	1 serving	549	44.0
Bacon	1 serving	610	44.0
Sausage	1 serving	768	47.0
Fish filet sandwich, *Ocean Catch*	5.8-oz. sandwich	495	49.0
French toast sticks	5-oz. serving	440	60.0
Hamburger, *Burger Buddies*	1 serving	349	31.0
Ice cream bar, *Snickers*	2 fl.-oz serving	220	20.0
Mayonnaise, reduced calorie	1-oz. serving	130	3.0
Muffin, blueberry mini	3.3-oz. serving	292	37.0
Onion rings	3.4-oz. serving	339	38.0
Orange juice	6.5 fl. oz.	82	20.0
Pie:			
Apple	4.5-oz. serving	320	45.0
Cherry	4.5-oz. serving	360	55.0
Lemon	3.2-oz. serving	290	45.0
Potatoes:			
French fries	medium order, salted	372	43.0
Hash browns	2½-oz. serving	213	25.0
Salad, without dressing:			
Chef	9.6-oz serving	178	7.0
Chicken	9-oz. serving	142	8.0
Garden	7.8-oz. serving	90	7.0
Side	4.8-oz. serving	25	5.0
Salad dressing (Newman's Own):			
Regular:			
Blue cheese	2-oz. serving	300	2.0
French	2.2-oz. serving	360	4.0
Ranch	2-oz. serving	350	4.0
Thousand Island	2.2-oz. serving	290	15.0

Food	Measure	Cals.	Carbs.
Dietetic, Italian, light	2-oz. serving	30	6.0
Sauce:			
Barbecue	1-oz. serving	36	9.0
BK Broiler	.5-oz. serving	90	0.0
Bull's Eye barbecue	.5-oz. serving	22	5.0
Honey dipping	1-oz. serving	91	23.0
Ranch dipping	1-oz. serving	171	2.0
Sweet & sour dipping	1-oz. serving	45	11.0
Shake:			
Chocolate	10 fl. oz.	326	49.0
Chocolate, syrup added	11 fl. oz.	409	68.0
Strawberry, syrup added	11 fl. oz.	394	66.0
Vanilla	10 fl. oz.	334	51.0
Whopper:			
Regular	9.5-oz. serving	614	45.0
Regular, with cheese	10.3-oz. serving	706	48.0
Double	12.3-oz. serving	844	45.0
Double, with cheese	13.2-oz. serving	935	48.0
Jr.	4.7-oz. serving	330	29.0
Jr., with cheese	5-oz. serving	380	30.0
BURGUNDY WINE:			
(Carlo Rossi)	3 fl. oz.	69	1.2
(Gallo) regular	3 fl. oz.	66	.6
(Louis M. Martini)			
12½% alcohol	3 fl. oz.	60	.2
(Paul Masson) 12% alcohol	3 fl. oz.	70	2.2
(Taylor) 12½% alcohol	3 fl. oz.	75	3.3
BURGUNDY WINE, SPARKLING:			
(B&G) 12% alcohol	3 fl. oz.	69	2.2
(Great Western) 12% alcohol	3 fl. oz.	82	5.1
(Taylor) 12% alcohol	3 fl. oz.	78	4.2
BURRITO:			
*Canned (Old El Paso)	1 burrito	299	36.0
Frozen:			
(Chi-Chi's Burro):			
Beef	15-oz. meal	570	73.0
Chicken	15-oz. meal	530	73.0
(Fred's Frozen Foods) *Little Juan:*			
Bean & cheese	5-oz. serving	331	46.9
Beef & bean, spicy	10-oz. serving	814	92.2
Beef & potato	5-oz. serving	389	48.9

Food	Measure	Cals.	Carbs.
Chili:			
Green	10-oz. serving	741	87.6
Red	10-oz. serving	799	96.4
Chili dog	5-oz. serving	313	31.4
Red hot	5-oz. serving	433	47.7
(Healthy Choice) quick meal:			
Beef & bean	5.4-oz. meal	270	40.0
Chicken con queso, mild	5.4-oz. meal	280	40.0
(Hormel):			
Cheese	1 burrito	210	32.0
Chicken & rice	1 burrito	200	32.0
Chili, hot	1 burrito	240	33.0
(Old El Paso):			
Regular:			
Bean & cheese	1 piece	340	43.0
Beef & bean:			
Hot	1 piece	340	41.0
Medium	1 piece	330	41.0
Mild	1 piece	330	40.0
Dinner, festive, beef & bean	11-oz. dinner	470	72.0
(Patio):			
Beef & bean:			
Regular	5-oz. serving	370	43.0
Green chili	5-oz. serving	330	43.0
Red chili	5-oz. serving	360	44.0
Red hot	5-oz. serving	360	43.0
(Weight Watchers):			
Beefsteak	7.62-oz. meal	310	36.0
Chicken	7.62-oz. meal	310	34.0
BURRITO, BREAKFAST			
frozen (Swanson) *Great Starts*:			
Original, with cheese & chili			
pepper	3½-oz. serving	200	25.0
Egg, bacon & cheese	1 serving	250	27.0
Egg, ham & cheese	1 serving	210	29.0
Egg, pizza sauce, cheese &			
pepperoni	1 serving	240	28.0
Hot & spicy	1 serving	220	30.0
BURRITO SEASONING MIX			
(Lawry's)	1½-oz. pkg.	132	23.3
BUTTER, salt or unsalted:			
Regular:			
(USDA)	¼ lb.	812	.5
(USDA)	1 T. (.5 oz.)	102	.1

Food	Measure	Cals.	Carbs.
(USDA)	1 pat (5 grams)	36	Tr.
(Breakstone)	1 T.	100	Tr.
(Land O' Lakes)	1 tsp.	35	0.0
(Meadow Gold)	1 tsp.	35	0.0
Whipped (Breakstone)	1 T.	67	Tr.

BUTTERFISH, raw (USDA):
Gulf:

Whole	1 lb. (weighed whole)	220	0.0
Meat only	4 oz.	108	0.0

Northern:

Whole	1 lb. (weighed whole)	391	0.0
Meat only	4 oz.	192	0.0

BUTTERSCOTCH MORSELS

(Nestlé)	1 oz.	150	19.0

BUTTER SUBSTITUTE:
Butter Buds:

Dry	⅛ oz.	12	3.0
Liquid	1 fl. oz.	12	3.0
Sprinkles	1 tsp.	14	2.0
Molly McButter, sprinkles	½ tsp.	4	1.0

C

CABBAGE:
White (USDA):
Raw.

Whole	1 lb. (weighed untrimmed)	86	19.3
Finely shredded or chopped	1 cup (3.2 oz.)	22	4.9
Coarsely shredded or sliced	1 cup (2.5 oz.)	17	3.8
Wedge	3½" × 4½"	24	5.4
Boiled: Shredded, in small amount of water, short time, drained	½ cup (2.6 oz.)	15	3.1

Food	Measure	Cals.	Carbs.
Wedges, in large amount of water, long time, drained	½ cup (3.2 oz.)	17	3.7
Dehydrated	1 oz.	87	20.9
Red:			
Raw (USDA) whole	1 lb. (weighed untrimmed)	111	24.7
Canned, solids & liq:			
(Comstock)	½ cup	60	13.0
(Greenwood)	½ cup	60	13.0
Savory (USDA) raw, whole	1 lb. (weighed untrimmed)	86	16.5
CABBAGE, CHINESE, BOK CHOY:			
Raw:			
Whole	1 lb.	52	8.5
Shredded	½ cup	5	.8
Boiled, drained	½ cup	10	1.5
CABBAGE, STUFFED, frozen (Stouffer's *Lean Cuisine*, with meat & tomato sauce	9½-oz. meal	210	26.0
CABERNET SAUVIGNON:			
(Gallo)	3 fl. oz.	66	0.0
(Louis M. Martini) 12½% alcohol	3 fl. oz.	62	.2
(Paul Masson) 11.9% alcohol	3 fl. oz.	70	.2
CAFE COMFORT, 55 proof	1 fl. oz.	79	8.8
CAKE (See also specific listings such as **DEVIL DOG,** etc.):			
Non-frozen:			
Plain:			
Home recipe, with butter & boiled white icing	⅑ of 9" square	401	70.5
Home recipe, with butter & chocolate icing	⅑ of 9" square	453	73.1
Angel food:			
Home recipe	1/12 of 8" cake	108	24.1
(Dolly Madison)	⅙ of 10½-oz. cake	120	17.0
Apple (Dolly Madison) Dutch, *Buttercrumb*	1½-oz. piece	170	28.0

Food	Measure	Cals.	Carbs.
Apple spice (Entenmann's)			
fat & cholesterol free	1-oz. slice	80	17.0
Apple streusel (Awrey's)	1 piece	160	18.0
Banana crunch (Entenmann's)			
fat & cholesterol free	1-oz. slice	80	18.0
Banana, iced (Awrey's)	1 piece	140	17.0
Banana loaf (Entenmann's)	1.3-oz. serving	90	20.0
Black Forest torte (Awrey's)	1/14 of cake	350	38.0
Blueberry crunch (Entenmann's)			
fat & cholesterol free	1-oz. slice	70	16.0
Butter streusel (Dolly Madison) *Buttercrumb*	1½-oz. piece	150	23.0
Caramel, home recipe:			
Without icing	1/9 of 9" square	322	46.2
With caramel icing	1/9 of 9" square	331	50.2
Carrot (Dolly Madison) *Lunch Cake*	3¼-oz. serving	350	64.0
Carrot supreme (Awrey's) iced	1 piece	210	23.0
Carrot, three-layer (Awrey's) with cream cheese icing	1/12 of cake	390	44.0
Chocolate:			
Home recipe (USDA) 2-layer, with chocolate icing	1/12 of 9" cake	365	55.2
(Awrey's):			
Regular	.8-oz. serving	70	11.0
Devil's food, with white icing	1 piece	150	17.0
Double chocolate:			
Iced	1 piece	130	21.0
Three-layer	1/12 of cake	310	48.0
Torte	1/14 of cake	340	51.0
Two layer	1/12 of cake	250	28.0
German:			
Iced	2" sq.	160	19.0
Three-layer	1/12 of cake	350	46.0
(Dolly Madison) German, *Lunch Cake*	3¼-oz. serving	440	54.0
(Entenmann's) devil's food with fudge icing	1.2-oz. serving	130	19.0
Cinnamon (Dolly Madison) *Buttercrumb*	1½-oz. piece	170	27.0
Coconut (Awrey's) butter cream	1 piece	160	19.0
Coffee:			
(Awrey's) carmel nut	1/12 of cake	140	15.0

Food	Measure	Cals.	Carbs.
(Drake's) small	1 piece	220	33.0
(Entenmann's):			
Regular, cheese	1.6-oz. piece	150	20.0
Fat & cholesterol free, cherry or cinnamon apple	1.3-oz. piece	90	20.0
Creme (Dolly Madison) *Lunch Cake*	7/8-oz. piece	90	17.0
Crumb:			
(Drake's) cinnamon	1.3-oz. serving	150	22.0
(Entenmann's):			
Regular	1.3-oz. serving	160	21.0
Cheese filled	1.4-oz. serving	130	18.0
French, all butter	1.6-oz. serving	180	26.0
(Hostess):			
Regular	1 piece	120	19.0
Light	1 piece	80	19.0
Devil's food, home recipe:			
Without icing	3" × 2" × 1½" piece	201	28.6
With chocolate icing, 2-layer	1/16 of 9" cake	277	41.8
Fruit, home recipe:			
Dark	1/30 of 8" loaf	57	9.0
Light, made with butter	1/30 of 8" loaf	58	8.6
Golden (Entenmann's) with fudge icing	1.2-oz. serving	130	20.0
Hawaiian spice (Dolly Madison) *Lunch Cake*	3¼-oz. piece	350	58.0
Honey (Holland Honey Cake) low sodium:			
Fruit and raisin	½" slice (.9 oz.)	80	19.0
Orange and premium unsalted	½" slice (.9 oz.)	70	17.0
Honey 'n spice (Dolly Madison) *Lunch Cake*	3¼-oz. piece	330	57.0
Lemon (Awrey's) three-layer	1/12 of cake	320	38.0
Louisiana crunch (Entenmann's)	1.7-oz. of cake	180	27.0
Neopolitan torte (Awrey's)	1/14 of cake	380	43.0
Orange (Awrey's) frosty, iced	1 piece	150	19.0
Peanut butter torte (Awrey's)	1/14 of cake	380	44.0
Pineapple crunch (Entenmann's) fat & cholesterol free	1-oz. slice	70	16.0
Pound:			

Food	Measure	Cals.	Carbs.
Home recipe (USDA) equal weights flour, sugar, butter & eggs	3½" × 3½" slice (1.1 oz.)	142	14.1
(Dolly Madison)	⅙ of 14-oz. cake	220	33.0
(Drake's)	⅟₁₀ of cake	16.0	
(Entenmann's) all butter loaf	1-oz. serving	110	15.0
Raisin spice (Awrey's) iced	1 piece	160	21.0
Raspberry nut	⅟₁₆ of cake	310	39.0
Sponge:			
Home recipe (USDA)	⅟₁₂ of 10" cake	196	35.7
(Awrey's)	2" sq.	80	11.0
Strawberry supreme (Awrey's)	⅟₁₄ of cake	270	38.0
Walnut torte (Awrey's)	⅟₁₄ of cake	320	38.0
White, home recipe:			
Made with butter, without icing, 2-layer	⅑ of 9" wide, 3" high cake	353	50.8
Made with butter, with coconut icing, 2-layer	⅟₁₂ of 9" wide, 3" high cake	386	63.1
White & coconut (Dolly Madison), layer	⅟₁₂ of 30-oz. cake	220	37.0
Yellow, home recipe, made with butter, without icing, 2-layer	⅑ of cake	351	56.3
Frozen:			
Banana (Sara Lee) iced	⅛ of cake	170	28.0
Black Forest:			
(Sara Lee) 2-layer	⅛ of cake	190	28.0
(Weight Watchers)	3-oz serving	180	32.0
Boston cream (Pepperidge Farm) supreme	2⅞-oz. serving	290	39.0
Caramel fudge, à la mode (Weight Watchers) *Sweet Celebrations*	3-oz. serving	180	35.0
Carrot:			
(Pepperidge Farm) classic	2½-oz. serving	260	32.0
(Sara Lee):			
Deluxe	1.8-oz. serving	180	26.0
Lights	2½-oz. serving	170	30.0
(Weight Watcher's)	3-oz. serving	170	27.0
Cheesecake:			
(Pepperidge Farm) strawberry, Manhattan	4¼-oz. serving	300	49.0
(Sara Lee):			
Regular, classic	2-oz. serving	200	16.0
Lights, French:			
Plain	3.2-oz. serving	150	24.0

Food	Measure	Cals.	Carbs.
Strawberry	3½-oz. serving	150	29.0
(Weight Watchers) *Sweet Celebrations:*			
Brownie	3½-oz. serving	200	34.0
Strawberry	3.9-oz. serving	180	28.0
Chocolate:			
(Pepperidge Farm):			
Devil's food layer	1⅝-oz. serving	180	24.0
Fudge layer	1⅝-oz. serving	180	23.0
Fudge stripe, layer	1⅝-oz.-serving	170	20.0
German, single layer	1⅝-oz. serving	180	22.0
Supreme	2⅞-oz. serving	300	37.0
(Sara Lee):			
Double, 3-layer	⅛ of cake	220	26.0
Free & Light	⅛ of cake	110	26.0
Mousse, classics	⅛ of cake	260	23.0
Regular	2½-oz. serving	180	31.0
Coconut (Pepperidge Farm):			
Classic	2¼-oz. serving	230	31.0
Layer	1⅝-oz. serving	180	24.0
Coffee (Weight Watchers) cinnamon streusel, *Sweet Celebrations*	1 piece	160	27.0
Devil's food (Pepperidge Farm) layer	⅒ of 17-oz. cake	180	24.0
Golden (Pepperidge Farm) layer	⅒ of 17-oz. cake	180	24.0
Lemon (Pepperidge Farm) *Supreme*	2¾-oz. serving	170	26.0
Lemon cream (Pepperidge Farm)	1⅝-oz. serving	170	21.0
Pineapple cream (Pepperidge Farm)	⅟₁₂ of 24-oz. cake	190	28.0
Pound:			
(Pepperidge Farm) old fashioned, cholesterol free	1 oz.	110	13.0
(Sara Lee) all butter:			
Regular, original	⅒ of cake	130	14.0
Family size	⅕ of cake	130	14.0
Free & Light	⅒ of cake	70	17.0
Strawberry cream (Pepperidge Farm)	⅟₁₂ of 12-oz. cake	190	30.0
Strawberry shortcake:			
(Pepperidge Farm) dessert lights	3-oz. serving	170	30.0

Food	Measure	Cals.	Carbs.
(Sara Lee)	⅛ of cake	190	26.0
(Weight Watchers)			
Sweet Celebrations	1 piece	170	33.0
Vanilla (Pepperidge Farm)			
layer	⅒ of 17-oz. cake	190	25.0
Vanilla fudge swirl			
(Pepperidge Farm)	2¼-oz. serving	250	33.0
CAKE OR COOKIE ICING			
(Pillsbury):			
All flavors			
except chocolate	1 T.	70	12.0
Chocolate	1 T.	60	11.0
CAKE ICING:			
Amaretto almond (Betty			
Crocker) *Creamy Deluxe*	¹⁄₁₂ of can	160	27.0
Butter pecan (Betty Crocker)			
Creamy Deluxe	¹⁄₁₂ of can	170	26.0
Caramel, home recipe (USDA)	4 oz.	408	86.8
Caramel pecan (Pillsbury)			
Frosting Supreme	¹⁄₁₂ of can	160	21.0
Cherry (Betty Crocker) *Creamy*			
Deluxe	¹⁄₁₂ of can	160	27.0
Chocolate:			
(USDA) home recipe	½ cup (4.9 oz.)	519	93.0
(Betty Crocker) *Creamy*			
Deluxe:			
Regular	¹⁄₁₂ of can	160	24.0
With candy-coated			
chocolate chips	¹⁄₁₂ of can	160	24.0
Chip	¹⁄₁₂ of can	170	27.0
With dinosaurs	¹⁄₁₂ of can	160	24.0
Fudge, dark Dutch	¹⁄₁₂ of can	160	22.0
Milk	¹⁄₁₂ of can	160	25.0
Sour cream	¹⁄₁₂ of can	160	23.0
(Duncan Hines):			
Regular	¹⁄₁₂ of can	152	23.3
Fudge, dark Dutch	¹⁄₁₂ of can	149	22.5
Milk	¹⁄₁₂ of can	151	22.9
(Mrs. Wright's) fudge, creamy	¹⁄₁₂ of can	170	25.0
(Pillsbury):			
Regular, fudge	⅛ of can	110	17.0
Frosting Supreme:			
Chip	¹⁄₁₂ of can	150	27.0
Fudge	¹⁄₁₂ of can	150	24.0
Milk	¹⁄₁₂ of can	150	23.0
Mint	¹⁄₁₂ of can	150	24.0

Food	Measure	Cals.	Carbs.
Coconut almond (Pillsbury) *Frosting Supreme*	¹⁄₁₂ of can	150	17.0
Coconut pecan (Pillsbury) *Frosting Supreme*	¹⁄₁₂ of can	160	17.0
Cream cheese:			
(Betty Crocker) *Creamy Deluxe*	¹⁄₁₂ of can	160	27.0
(Duncan Hines)	¹⁄₁₂ of can	152	23.6
(Pillsbury) *Frosting Supreme*	¹⁄₁₂ of can	160	26.0
Double Dutch (Pillsbury) *Frosting Supreme*	¹⁄₁₂ of can	140	22.0
Lemon:			
(Betty Crocker) *Creamy Deluxe*	¹⁄₁₂ of can	170	28.0
(Pillsbury) *Frosting Supreme*	¹⁄₁₂ of can	160	26.0
Polka dot (Duncan Hines):			
Milk chocolate	¹⁄₁₂ of can	168	24.7
Pink vanilla	¹⁄₁₂ of can	154	23.3
Rainbow chip (Betty Crocker) *Creamy Deluxe*	¹⁄₁₂ of can	170	27.0
Rocky road minimorsels (Betty Crocker) *Creamy Deluxe*	¹⁄₁₂ of can	150	20.0
Strawberry (Pillsbury) *Frosting Supreme*	¹⁄₁₂ of can	160	26.0
Vanilla:			
(Betty Crocker) *Creamy Deluxe*	¹⁄₁₂ of can	160	27.0
(Duncan Hines)	¹⁄₁₂ of can	151	23.6
(Pillsbury) *Frosting Supreme*, regular or sour cream	¹⁄₁₂ of can	160	27.0
White:			
Home recipe, boiled (USDA)	4 oz.	358	91.1
Home recipe, uncooked (USDA)	4 oz.	426	92.5
(Betty Crocker) *Creamy Deluxe,* sour cream	¹⁄₁₂ of can	160	27.0
(Mrs. Wright's)	¹⁄₁₂ of can	160	25.0
*CAKE ICING MIX:			
Regular:			
Chocolate:			
(Betty Crocker) creamy:			
Fudge	¹⁄₁₂ of pkg.	180	30.0
Milk	¹⁄₁₂ of pkg.	170	29.0
(Pillsbury)	⅛ of pkg.	50	12.0

Food	Measure	Cals.	Carbs.
Coconut almond (Pillsbury)	¹⁄₁₂ of pkg.	160	16.0
Coconut pecan:			
(Betty Crocker) creamy	¹⁄₁₂ of pkg.	150	19.0
(Pillsbury)	¹⁄₁₂ of pkg.	150	20.0
Lemon (Betty Crocker) creamy	¹⁄₁₂ of pkg.	170	31.0
Vanilla:			
(Betty Crocker) creamy	¹⁄₁₂ of pkg.	170	32.0
(Pillsbury) *Rich 'n Easy*	¹⁄₁₂ of pkg.	150	25.0
White:			
(Betty Crocker) Fluffy	¹⁄₁₂ of pkg.	70	16.0
(Pillsbury) fluffy	¹⁄₁₂ of pkg.	60	15.0
Dietetic (Estee)	1T.	65	13.0
CAKE MEAL (Manischewitz)	½ cup (2.6 oz.)	286	NA
CAKE MIX:			
Regular:			
Angel food:			
(Betty Crocker):			
Confetti, lemon custard or white	¹⁄₁₂ of pkg.	150	34.0
Traditional	¹⁄₁₂ of pkg.	130	30.0
(Duncan Hines)	¹⁄₁₂ of pkg.	124	28.9
*(Mrs. Wright's) deluxe	¹⁄₁₂ of cake	130	31.0
*Apple cinnamon (Betty Crocker) *Supermoist*:			
Regular	¹⁄₁₂ of cake	250	36.0
No cholesterol recipe	¹⁄₁₂ of cake	210	36.0
*Apple streusel (Betty Crocker) *MicroRave*:			
Regular	⅛ of cake	240	33.0
No cholesterol recipe	⅛ of cake	210	33.0
*Banana (Pillsbury) *Pillsbury Plus*	¹⁄₁₂ of cake	250	36.0
*Black Forest cherry (Pillsbury) *Bundt*	¹⁄₁₆ of cake	240	38.0
*Boston cream (Pillsbury) *Bundt*	¹⁄₁₆ of cake	270	43.0
*Butter (Pillsbury) *Pillsbury Plus*	¹⁄₁₂ of cake	260	34.0
Butter Brickle (Betty Crocker) *Supermoist*:			
Regular	¹⁄₁₂ of cake	250	38.0
No cholesterol recipe	¹⁄₁₂ of cake	220	38.0

Food	*Measure*	*Cals.*	*Carbs.*
*Butter pecan (Betty Crocker)			
Supermoist:			
Regular	1/12 of cake	250	35.0
No cholesterol recipe	1/12 of cake	220	35.0
*Carrot (Betty Crocker)			
Supermoist:			
Regular	1/12 of cake	250	35.0
No cholesterol recipe	1/12 of cake	220	35.0
*Carrot'n spice (Pillsbury)			
Pillsbury Plus	1/12 of cake	260	36.0
*Cheesecake:			
(Jello-O)	1/8 of cake	283	36.5
(Royal) No Bake:			
Lite	1/8 of cake	210	23.0
Real	1/8 of cake	280	31.0
*Cherry chip (Betty Crocker)			
Supermoist	1/12 of cake	190	37.0
Chocolate:			
*(Betty Crocker):			
MicroRave:			
Fudge, with vanilla frosting	1/6 of cake	310	40.0
German, with coconut pecan frosting	1/6 of cake	320	37.0
Pudding	1/6 of cake	230	44.0
Supermoist:			
Butter recipe	1/12 of cake	270	35.0
Chip:			
Regular	1/12 of cake	280	36.0
No cholesterol recipe	1/12 of cake	220	36.0
Chocolate chip	1/12 of cake	260	34.0
Fudge	1/12 of cake	260	34.0
German:			
Regular	1/12 of cake	260	35.0
No cholesterol recipe	1/12 of cake	210	35.0
Sour cream:			
Regular	1/12 of cake	260	33.0
No cholesterol recipe	1/12 of cake	220	35.0
(Duncan Hines) fudge	1/12 of pkg.	187	34.8
*(Pillsbury):			
Bundt:			
Macaroon	1/16 of cake	240	36.0
Tunnel of Fudge	1/16 of cake	260	37.0
Microwave:			
Plain	1/8 of cake	210	23.0
Frosted:			

Food	Measure	Cals.	Carbs.
With chocolate frosting	⅛ of cake	300	35.0
With vanilla frosting	⅛ of cake	300	36.0
Supreme, double	⅛ of cake	330	39.0
Tunnel of Fudge	⅛ of cake	290	36.0
Pillsbury Plus:			
Chocolate chip	1/12 of cake	270	33.0
Fudge, dark	1/12 of cake	250	32.0
Fudge, marble	1/12 of cake	270	36.0
German	1/12 of cake	250	36.0
*Cinnamon (Pillsbury) *Streusel Swirl,* microwave	⅛ of cake	240	33.0
*Cinnamon pecan streusel (Betty Crocker) *MicroRave*:			
Regular	⅙ of cake	290	39.0
No cholesterol recipe	⅙ of cake	240	39.0
Coffee cake:			
*(Aunt Jemima)	⅛ of cake	170	29.0
*(Pillsbury) apple cinnamon	⅛ of cake	240	40.0
Devil's food:			
*(Betty Crocker):			
MicroRave, with chocolate frosting:			
Regular	⅙ of cake	310	37.0
No cholesterol recipe	⅙ of cake	240	37.0
Supermoist:			
Regular	1/12 of cake	260	35.0
No cholesterol recipe	1/12 of cake	220	35.0
(Duncan Hines) deluxe	1/12 of pkg.	189	35.6
(Mrs. Wright's) deluxe	1/12 of pkg.	190	32.0
*(Pillsbury) *Pillsbury Plus*	1/12 of cake	270	32.0
Fudge (see Chocolate)			
Gingerbread (See **GINGERBREAD**)			
Golden (Duncan Hines) butter recipe	1/12 of pkg.	188	36.5
*Lemon:			
(Betty Crocker):			
MicroRave, with lemon frosting	⅙ of cake	300	37.0
Pudding	⅙ of cake	230	45.0
Supermoist:			
Regular	1/12 of cake	290	36.0
No cholesterol recipe	1/12 of cake	220	36.0
*(Pillsbury):			
Bundt, Tunnel of Lemon	1/16 of cake	270	45.0

Food	Measure	Cals.	Carbs.
Microwave:			
Plain	⅛ of cake	220	23.0
With lemon frosting	⅛ of cake	300	37.0
Supreme, double	⅛ of cake	300	40.0
Pillsbury Plus	¹⁄₁₂ of cake	250	34.0
Streusel Swirl	¹⁄₁₆ of cake	270	39.0
*Marble (Betty Crocker)			
Supermoist:			
Regular	¹⁄₁₂ of cake	250	35.0
No cholesterol recipe	¹⁄₁₂ of cake	210	35.0
*Pineapple creme (Pillsbury)			
Bundt	¹⁄₁₆ of cake	260	41.0
Pound:			
*(Betty Crocker) golden	¹⁄₁₂ of cake	200	28.0
*(Dromedary)	½" slice		
	(¹⁄₁₂ of pkg.)	150	21.0
*(Mrs. Wright's) deluxe	¹⁄₁₂ of cake	200	32.0
*Spice (Betty Crocker)			
Supermoist:			
Regular	¹⁄₁₂ of cake	260	36.0
No cholesterol recipe	¹⁄₁₂ of cake	220	36.0
*Strawberry (Pillsbury)			
Pillsbury Plus	¹⁄₁₂ of cake	260	37.0
*Upside down			
(Betty Crocker) pineapple:			
Regular	⅑ of cake	250	39.0
No cholesterol recipe	⅑ of cake	240	39.0
*Vanilla (Betty Crocker)			
golden, *Supermoist*	¹⁄₁₂ of cake	280	34.0
White:			
*(Betty Crocker):			
MicroRave, golden,			
with rainbow chip			
frosting	⅙ of cake	320	40.0
Supermoist:			
Regular	¹⁄₁₂ of cake	280	36.0
No cholesterol recipe	¹⁄₁₂ of cake	220	36.0
(Duncan Hines) deluxe	¹⁄₁₂ of pkg.	188	36.1
(Mrs. Wright's)	¹⁄₁₂ of pkg.	180	34.0
*(Pillsbury) *Pillsbury Plus*	¹⁄₁₂ of cake	240	35.0
Yellow:			
*(Betty Crocker):			
MicroRave, with			
chocolate frosting:			
Regular	⅙ of cake	300	36.0
No cholesterol recipe	⅙ of cake	230	36.0
Supermoist:			

Food	Measure	Cals.	Carbs.
Plain:			
Regular	1/12 of cake	260	36.0
No cholesterol recipe	1/12 of cake	220	36.0
Butter recipe	1/12 of cake	260	37.0
(Duncan Hines) deluxe	1/12 of pkg.	188	37.0
(Mrs. Wright's)	1/12 of pkg.	190	33.0
*(Pillsbury):			
Microwave:			
Plain	1/8 of cake	220	23.0
With chocolate frosting	1/8 of cake	300	36.0
Pillsbury Plus	1/12 of cake	260	36.0
*Dietetic (Estee)	1/10 of cake	100	18.0
CALZONE, refrigerated			
(Stefano's):			
Cheese	1 piece (6 oz.)	510	43.0
Pepperoni	1 piece (6 oz.)	520	46.0
Spinach	1 piece (6 oz.)	440	46.0
CAMPARI, 45 proof	1 fl. oz.	66	7.1

CANDY, GENERIC. The following values of candies from the U.S. Department of Agriculture are representative of the types sold commercially. These values may be useful when individual brands or sizes are not known:

Almond:			
Chocolate-coated	1 cup (6.3 oz.)	1024	71.3
Chocolate-coated	1 oz.	161	11.2
Sugar-coated or Jordan	1 oz.	129	19.9
Butterscotch	1 oz.	113	26.9
Candy corn	1 oz.	103	25.4
Caramel:			
Plain	1 oz.	113	21.7
Plain with nuts	1 oz.	121	20.0
Chocolate	1 oz.	113	21.7
Chocolate with nuts	1 oz.	121	20.0
Chocolate-flavored roll	1 oz.	112	23.4
Chocolate:			
Bittersweet	1 oz.	135	13.3
Milk:			
Plain	1 oz.	147	16.1
With almonds	1 oz.	151	14.5
With peanuts	1 oz.	154	12.6
Semisweet	1 oz.	144	16.2

Food	Measure	Cals.	Carbs.
Sweet	1 oz.	150	16.4
Chocolate discs, sugar coated	1 oz.	132	20.6
Coconut center, chocolate-coated	1 oz.	124	20.4
Fondant, plain	1 oz.	103	25.4
Fondant, chocolate-covered	1 oz.	116	23.0
Fudge:			
Chocolate fudge	1 oz.	113	21.3
Chocolate fudge, chocolate-coated	1 oz.	122	20.7
Chocolate fudge with nuts	1 oz.	121	19.6
Chocolate fudge with nuts, chocolate-coated	1 oz.	128	19.1
Vanilla fudge	1 oz.	113	21.2
Vanilla fudge with nuts	1 oz.	120	19.5
With peanuts & caramel, chocolate-coated	1 oz.	130	16.6
Gum drops	1 oz.	98	24.8
Hard	1 oz.	109	27.6
Honeycombed hard candy, with peanut butter, chocolate-covered	1 oz.	131	20.0
Jelly beans	1 oz.	104	26.4
Marshmallow	1 oz.	90	22.8
Mints, uncoated	1 oz.	103	25.4
Nougat & caramel, chocolate-covered	1 oz.	118	20.6
Peanut bar	1 oz.	146	13.4
Peanut brittle	1 oz.	119	23.0
Peanuts, chocolate-covered	1 oz.	159	11.1
Raisins, chocolate-covered	1 oz.	120	20.0
Vanilla creams, chocolate-covered	1 oz.	123	19.9
CANDY, COMMERCIAL:			
Almond, Jordan (Banner)	1¼-oz. box	154	27.9
Almond Joy (Hershey's)	1.76-oz. bar	250	28.0
Apricot Delight (Sahadi)	1 oz.	100	25.0
Baby Ruth	2-oz. piece	260	36.0
Bar None (Hershey's)	1½-oz. serving	240	23.0
Bit-O-Honey (Nestlé)	1.7-oz. serving	200	41.0
Bonkers! (Nabisco)	1 piece	20	5.0
Breath Saver, any flavor	1 piece	8	2.0
Bridge Mix (Nabisco)	1 piece	10	2.0
Butterfinger	2-oz. bar	260	38.0
Butternut (Hollywood Brands)	2¼-oz. bar	310	36.0

Food	Measure	Cals.	Carbs.
Butterscotch (Callard & Bowser)	1-oz. serving	115	25.0
Caramello (Hershey's)	1.6-oz. serving	220	28.0
Caramel Nip (Pearson)	1 piece	30	5.7
Charleston Chew	2-oz. bar	240	44.0
Cherry, chocolate-covered (Welch's):			
Dark	1 piece	90	16.0
Milk	1 piece	85	16.0
Chocolate bar:			
Alpine white (Nestlé)	1 oz.	170	13.0
Brazil Nut (Cadbury's)	2-oz. serving	310	32.0
Caramello (Cadbury's)	2-oz. serving	280	37.0
Crunch (Nestlé)	1⅛-oz. bar	160	19.0
Fruit & nut (Cadbury's)	2-oz. serving	300	33.0
Hazelnut (Cadbury's)	2-oz. serving	310	32.0
Milk:			
(Cadbury's)	2-oz. serving	300	34.0
(Hershey's)	1.55-oz. bar	240	25.0
(Nestlé)	.35-oz. bar	53	6.0
(Nestlé)	1¹⁄₁₆-oz. bar	159	18.1
Special Dark (Hershey's)	1.45-oz. bar	220	25.0
Chocolate bar with almonds:			
(Cadbury's)	2-oz. serving	310	31.0
(Hershey's):			
Milk	1.45-oz. bar	230	20.0
Golden Almond	3.2-oz. bar	520	40.0
(Nestlé)	1-oz.	160	15.0
Chocolate Parfait (Pearson)	1 piece (6.5 grams)	30	5.7
Chocolate, Petite (Andes)	1 piece	26	2.6
Chuckles	1 oz.	100	23.0
Clark Bar	1.5-oz. bar	201	30.4
Coffee Nip (Pearson)	1 piece (6.5 grams)	30	5.7
Coffioca (Pearson)	1 piece (6.5 grams)	30	5.7
Creme De Menthe (Andes)	1 piece	25	2.6
Dutch Treat Bar (Clark)	1¹⁄₁₆-oz. bar	160	20.3
Eggs:			
(Nabisco) *Chuckles*	½ oz.	55	13.5
(Hershey's):			
Creme	1 oz.	136	19.2
Mini	1 oz.	140	20.0
5th Avenue (Hershey's)	2.1-oz. serving	290	39.0
Fruit bears (Flavor Tree) assorted	½ of 2.1-oz. pkg.	117	25.4

Food	Measure	Cals.	Carbs.
Fruit circus (Flavor Tree) assorted	½ of 2.1-oz. pkg.	117	25.4
Fruit roll (Flavor Tree):			
Apple, cherry, grape or raspberry	¾-oz. piece	75	18.5
Apricot	¾-oz. piece	76	17.7
Fruit punch or strawberry	¾-oz. piece	74	18.0
Fudge bar (Nabisco)	1 piece (.7 oz.)	85	14.5
Fun Fruit (Sunkist) any type	.9-oz. piece	100	21.8
Goobers (Nestlé)	1 oz.	160	13.0
Good & Plenty	1 oz.	100	24.8
Good Stuff (Nabisco)	1.8-oz. piece	250	29.0
Halvah (Sahadi) original and marble	1 oz.	150	13.0
Hard (Jolly Rancher):			
All flavors except butterscotch	1 piece	23	5.7
Butterscotch	1 piece	25	5.6
Holidays (M&M/Mars):			
Plain	1 oz.	140	19.0
Peanut	1 oz.	140	16.0
Jelly bar, *Chuckles*	1 oz.	100	25.0
Jelly bean, *Chuckles*	½ oz.	55	13.0
Jelly rings, *Chuckles*	½ oz.	50	11.0
JuJubes, Chuckles	½ oz.	55	12.5
Kisses (Hershey's)	1 piece (.2 oz.)	24	2.5
Kit Kat (Hershey's)	1.65-oz. bar	250	29.0
Krackle Bar	1.55-oz. bar	230	27.0
Licorice:			
Licorice Nips (Pearson)	1 piece (6.5 grams)	30	5.7
(Switzer) bars, bites or stix:			
Black	1 oz.	94	22.1
Cherry or strawberry	1 oz.	98	23.2
Chocolate	1 oz.	97	22.7
Life Savers	1 piece	7	3.0
Lollipops (Life Savers)	.1-oz. pop	45	11.0
Mallo Cup (Boyer)	.6-oz. piece	54	11.2
Mars Bar (M&M/Mars)	1.7-oz. bar	240	30.0
Marshmallow (Campfire)	1 oz.	111	24.9
Marshmallow eggs, *Chuckles*	1 oz.	110	27.0
Mary Jane (Miller):			
Small size	¼-oz. piece	19	3.5
Large size	1½-oz. bar	110	20.3
Milk Duds (Clark)	¾-oz. bar	89	17.8
Milk Shake (Hollywood Brands)	2.4-oz. bar	300	51.0
Milky Way (M&M/Mars)	2.24-oz. bar	290	44.0
Mike & Ikes	1 piece	9	2.1

Food	Measure	Cals.	Carbs.
Mint Parfait:			
(Andes)	.2-oz. piece	27	2.7
(Pearson)	.2-oz. piece	30	5.7
Mint or peppermint:			
Canada Mint (Necco)	.1-oz. piece	12	3.1
Junior Mint pattie (Nabisco)	1 piece (.1 oz.)	10	2.0
Peppermint pattie:			
(Nabisco)	1 piece (.5 oz.)	55	12.5
York (Hershey's)	1¼-oz. serving	160	28.0
M&M's:			
Peanut	1.83-oz. pkg.	270	30.0
Plain	1.69-oz. pkg.	240	33.0
Mounds (Hershey's)	1.9-oz. bar	260	31.0
Mr. Goodbar (Hershey's)	1.85-oz. bar	300	24.0
Munch bar (M&M/Mars)	1.42-oz. bar	220	19.0
My Buddy (Tom's)	1.8-oz. piece	250	30.0
Naturally Nut & Fruit Bar (Planters):			
Almond/apricot; almond/ pineapple; peanut/raisin	1 oz.	140	17.0
Walnut/apple	1 oz.	150	16.0
Necco Wafers:			
Assorted	2.02-oz. roll	227	56.5
Chocolate	2.02-oz. roll	228	56.3
Nougat centers, *Chuckles*	1 oz.	110	26.0
Oh Henry! (Nestlé)	1 oz.	140	16.0
$100,000 Bar (Nestlé)	1¼-oz. bar	175	23.8
Orange slices, *Chuckles*	1 oz.	110	24.0
Park Avenue (Tom's)	1.8-oz. piece	230	34.0
Payday (Hollywood Brands):			
Regular	1.9-oz. piece	250	28.0
Chocolate coated	2-oz. piece	290	30.0
Peanut bar (Planters)	1.6-oz. piece	240	21.0
Peanut, chocolate-covered:			
(Curtiss)	1 piece	5	1.0
(Nabisco)	1 piece (4.1 grams)	11	1.0
Peanut butter cup:			
(Boyer)	1.5-oz. pkg.	148	17.4
(Reese's)	.9-oz. cup	140	13.0
Peanut Butter Pals (Tom's)	1.3-oz. serving	200	19.0
Peanut crunch (Sahadi)	¾-oz. bar	110	9.0
Peanut Parfait:			
(Andes)	1 piece	28	2.5
(Pearson)	1 piece	30	5.7
Peanut Plank (Tom's)	1.7-oz. piece	230	28.0
Peanut Roll (Tom's)	1.7-oz. piece	230	29.0

Food	Measure	Cals.	Carbs.
Pom Poms (Nabisco)	1 oz.	100	15.0
Powerhouse (Hershey's)	2-oz. serving	260	38.0
Raisin, chocolate-covered (Nabisco)	1 piece	5	.7
Raisinets (Nestlé)	1 oz.	120	20.0
Reese's Pieces (Hershey's)	1.95-oz. pkg.	270	31.0
Reggie Bar	2-oz. bar	290	29.0
Rolo (Hershey's)	1 piece (6 grams)	34	4.6
Royals, mint chocolate (M&M/Mars)	1.52-oz. pkg.	212	29.5
Sesame Crunch (Sahadi)	¾-oz. bar	110	7.0
Sesame Tahini (Sahadi)	1 oz.	190	4.0
Skittles (M&M/Mars)	1 oz.	113	26.3
Skor (Hershey's)	1.4-oz. bar	220	22.0
Sky Bar (Necco)	1.5-oz. bar	198	31.5
Snickers (M&M/Mars)	2.16-oz. bar	290	36.0
Solitaires (Hershey's)	½ of 3.2-oz. pkg.	260	20.0
Spearmint leaves, *Chuckles*	1 oz.	110	15.0
Starburst (M&M/Mars)	1-oz. serving	120	24.0
Sugar Babies (Nabisco):	1⅝-oz. pkg.	180	40.0
Sugar Daddy (Nabisco) caramel sucker	1⅜-oz.	150	33.0
Sugar Mama (Nabisco)	1 piece (.8 oz.)	90	17.0
Symphony (Hershey's):			
Almond	1.4-oz. serving	220	20.0
Milk	1.4-oz. serving	220	22.0
3 Musketeers	2.13-oz. bar	260	46.0
Ting-A-Ling (Andes)	1 piece	24	2.8
Tootsie Roll:			
Chocolate	.23-oz. midgee	26	5.3
Chocolate	¹⁄₁₆-oz. bar	72	14.3
Chocolate	1-oz. bar	115	22.9
Flavored	.6-oz. square	19	3.8
Pop, all flavors	.49-oz. pop	60	12.5
Pop drop, all flavors	4.7-gram piece	19	4.2
Twizzler (Y & S) strawberry	1-oz. serving	100	23.0
Whatchamacallit (Hershey's)	1.8-oz. bar	260	30.0
Wispa (Hershey's)	1 oz.	150	17.0
Y & S Bites	1 oz.	100	23.0
Zagnut Bar (Clark)	.7-oz. bar	85	12.5
Zero (Hollywood Brands)	2-oz. bar	210	34.0
CANDY, DIETETIC:			
Caramel (Estee)	1 piece	30	5.0
Chocolate or chocolate-flavored:			

Food	Measure	Cals.	Carbs.
(Estee):			
Coconut	.2-oz. square	30	2.0
Crunch	.2-oz. square	22	2.0
Fruit & nut	.2-oz. square	30	2.5
Milk	.2-oz. square	30	2.5
(Louis Sherry):			
Bittersweet	.2-oz. piece	30	3.0
Coffee-flavored	.2-oz. piece	22	2.0
Estee-ets, with peanuts (Estee)	1 piece		
	(1.4 grams)	7	.8
Gum drops (Estee) any flavor	1 piece		
	(1.8 grams)	6	1.5
Gummy Bears (Estee)	1 piece	7	1.3
Hard candy:			
(Estee) assorted fruit	1 piece (.1 oz.)	12	3.0
(Louis Sherry)	1 piece (.1 oz.)	12	3.0
Lollipop (Estee)	1 piece (.2 oz.)	25	6.0
Peanut brittle (Estee)	¼ oz.	35	5.0
Peanut butter cup (Estee)	1 cup (.3 oz.)	40	3.0
Raisins, chocolate-covered	1 piece		
(Estee)	(1.2 grams)	3	.5
CANDY APPLE COOLER			
DRINK, canned (Hi-C)	6 fl. oz.	94	23.1
CANNELONI			
Canned (Chef Boyardee)	7 ½ oz. serving	230	33.0
Frozen:			
(Armour) *Dining Lite,*			
cheese	9-oz. meal	310	38.0
(Celentano) florentine	12-oz. pkg.	350	48.0
(Stouffer's) *Lean Cuisine:*			
Beef with tomato sauce	9⅝-oz. pkg.	200	28.0
Cheese with tomato sauce	9⅛-oz. pkg.	270	27.0
CANTALOUPE, fresh (USDA):			
Whole, medium	1 lb. (weighed		
	with skin &		
	cavity contents)	68	17.0
Cubed or diced	½ cup (2.9 oz.)	24	6.1
CAPERS (Crosse & Blackwell)	1 T.	5	1.0
CAP'N CRUNCH, cereal			
(Quaker):			
Regular	¾ cup (1 oz.)	121	22.9
Crunchberry	¾ cup (1 oz.)	120	22.9

Food	Measure	Cals.	Carbs.
Peanut butter	¾ cup (1 oz.)	127	20.9
CARAWAY SEED (French's)	1 tsp (1.8 grams)	8	.8
CARL'S JR. **RESTAURANT:**			
Bacon	2 strips (10 grams)	40	0.0
Brownie, fudge	4½-oz. serving	597	88.0
Burrito, breakfast	1 serving	430	29.0
Cake, chocolate	3-oz. serving	300	49.0
California Roast Beef'n Swiss			
Sandwich	7.3-oz. serving	360	43.0
Cheese:			
American	.6-oz. serving	63	1.0
Swiss	.6-oz. serving	57	1.0
Chicken sandwich:			
Charbroiler BBQ, lite	6.3-oz. serving	310	34.0
Charbroiler Club	8.2-oz. serving	570	42.0
Santa Fe	7.9-oz. serving	530	36.0
Teriyaki, light	1 serving	330	42.0
Chicken stars	1 piece	38	1.8
Cookie, chocolate chip	2¼-oz. serving	370	48.0
Danish	1 serving	520	75.0
Eggs, scrambled	2.4-oz. serving	160	1.0
Fish sandwich, filet	7.9-oz. serving	550	58.0
French toast dips, excluding syrup	4.7-oz. serving	410	40.0
Hamburger:			
Plain:			
Regular	4.3-oz. serving	320	33.0
Famous Star	8.6-oz. serving	610	42.0
Happy Star	3.0-oz. serving	220	26.0
Old Time Star	6.9-oz. serving	400	38.0
Super Star	11¼-oz. serving	820	41.0
Cheeseburger, *Western Bacon*:			
Regular	8-oz. serving	730	59.0
Double	11.6-oz. serving	970	58.0
Hot cakes, with margarine, excluding syrup	5½-oz. serving	360	59.0
Milk, 1% lowfat	10 fl. oz.	150	20.0
Muffins:			
Blueberry	4.2-oz. muffin	340	49.0
Bran	4.7-oz. muffin	370	61.0
English, with margarine	1 muffin	230	28.0
Onion rings	3.2-oz. serving	310	38.0
Orange juice, small	8 fl. oz.	94	21.0
Potato:			
Baked:			

Food	Measure	Cals.	Carbs.
Bacon & cheese	14.1-oz. serving	630	76.0
Broccoli & cheese	14-oz. serving	530	75.0
Cheese	14.2-oz. serving	550	72.0
Lite, plain	9.8-oz. serving	290	65.0
Sour cream & chive	10.4-oz. serving	430	70.0
French fries, regular	6-oz. serving	360	43.0
Hash brown nuggets	3-oz. serving	270	27.0
Quesadilla, breakfast	1 serving	300	25.0
Salad-to-go:			
Chef's	10.7-oz. serving	180	11.0
Chicken:			
Regular	12-oz. serving	260	11.0
Lite menu	1 serving	200	8.0
Garden:			
Regular	1 serving	50	4.0
Lite menu	1 serving	50	4.0
Taco	14.3-oz. serving	356	18.0
Salad dressing:			
Regular:			
Blue cheese	1-oz. serving	150	0.0
House	1-oz. serving	110	2.0
1000 Island	1-oz. serving	110	4.0
Dietetic, Italian	1-oz. serving	40	.5
Sauce:			
Barbecue or sweet & sour	1 serving	50	11.0
Honey	1 serving	90	23.0
Mustard	1 serving	45	10.0
Salsa	1 serving	10	2.0
Sausage	1½-oz. patty	190	1.0
Shakes	1 regular size shake	353	61.0
Soft drink:			
Regular	1 regular size soft drink	243	62.0
Dietetic	1 regular size soft drink	2	0.0
Soup:			
Broccoli, cream of	6 fl. oz.	140	14.0
Chicken & noodle	6 fl. oz.	80	11.0
Chowder, clam, Boston	6 fl. oz.	140	12.0
Vegetable, Lumber Jack mix	6 fl. oz.	70	10.0
Steak sandwich, *Country Fried*	7.2-oz. serving	610	54.0
Sunrise Sandwich:			
Bacon	4½-oz. serving	370	32.0
Sausage	6.1-oz. serving	500	31.0
Tea, iced	1 regular size drink	2	0.0

Food	Measure	Cals.	Carbs.
Turkey club sandwich	9.3-oz. serving	530	50.0
Zucchini	4.3-oz. serving	300	33.0
CARNATION DO-IT-YOURSELF DIET PLAN:			
Chocolate	2 scoops (1.1 oz.)	110	21.0
Vanilla	2 scoops (1.1 oz.)	110	22.0
CARNATION INSTANT BREAKFAST:			
Bar:			
Chocolate chip	1 bar (1.44 oz.)	200	20.0
Chocolate crunch	1 bar (1.34 oz.)	190	20.0
Honey nut	1 bar (1.35 oz.)	190	18.0
Peanut butter with chocolate chips	1 bar (1.4 oz.)	200	20.0
Peanut butter crunch	1 bar (1.35 oz.)	200	20.0
Drink packets:			
Chocolate or egg nog	1 packet	130	24.0
Chocolate malt	1 packet	130	22.0
Coffee, strawberry or vanilla	1 packet	130	25.0
CARROT:			
Raw (USDA):			
Whole	1 lb. (weighed with full tops)	112	26.0
Partially trimmed	1 lb. (weighed without tops, with skins)	156	36.1
Trimmed	5½" × 1" carrot (1.8 oz.)	21	4.8
Trimmed	25 thin strips (1.8 oz.)	21	4.8
Chunks	½ cup (2.4 oz.)	29	6.7
Diced	½ cup (1½ oz.)	30	7.0
Grated or shredded	½ cup (1.9 oz.)	23	5.3
Slices	½ cup (2.2 oz.)	27	6.2
Strips	½ cup (2 oz.)	24	5.6
Boiled, drained (USDA):			
Chunks	½ cup (2.9 oz.)	25	5.8
Diced	½ cup (2½ oz.)	24	5.2
Slices	½ cup (2.7 oz.)	24	5.4
Canned, regular pack, solids & liq.:			
(Comstock)	½ cup (4.2 oz.)	35	6.0
(Larsen) *Freshlike*	½ cup	30	6.0

Food	Measure	Cals.	Carbs.
(S&W) any style	½ cup	30	7.0
Canned, dietetic pack, solids & liq.:			
(Featherweight) sliced	½ cup	30	6.0
(Larsen) *Fresh-Lite,* sliced, low sodium	½ cup (4.4 oz.)	25	6.0
(S&W) *Nutradiet,* green label	½ cup	30	7.0
Frozen:			
(Bel-Air) whole, baby	3.3 oz.	40	9.0
(Birds Eye) whole, baby deluxe	⅓ of pkg. (3.3 oz.)	32	7.0
(Frosty Acres) cut or whole	3.3-oz. serving	40	9.0
(Green Giant) cuts, in butter sauce	½ cup	80	16.0
CARROT JUICE, canned (Hollywood)	6 fl. oz.	80	16.0
CASABA MELON (USDA):			
Whole	1 lb. (weighed whole)	61	14.7
Flesh only, cubed or diced	4 oz.	31	7.4
CASHEW BUTTER			
(Hain) raw or toasted	1 T.	95	4.0
CASHEW NUT:			
(USDA)	1 oz.	159	8.3
(USDA)	½ cup (2.5 oz.)	393	20.5
(USDA)	5 large or 8 med.	60	3.1
(Beer Nuts)	1 oz.	170	8.0
(Eagle Snacks):			
Honey Roast:			
Regular	1 oz.	170	9.0
With peanuts	1 oz.	170	8.0
Lightly salted	1 oz.	170	7.0
(Fisher):			
Dry roasted	¼ cup (1.2 oz.)	160	8.0
Honey roasted	1 oz.	150	7.0
Oil roasted	¼ cup (1.2 oz.)	170	8.0
(Party Pride) dry roasted	1 oz.	170	9.0
(Planters):			
Dry roasted, salted or unsalted	1 oz.	160	9.0
Honey roasted:			
Plain	1 oz.	170	11.0
With peanuts	1 oz.	170	9.0

Food	Measure	Cals.	Carbs.
Oil roasted	1 oz.	170	8.0
(Tom's)	1 oz.	178	7.8
CATFISH, freshwater (USDA)			
raw fillet	4 oz.	117	0.0
CATSUP:			
Regular:			
(Heinz)	1 T.	18	4.0
(Hunt's)	1 T. (.5 oz.)	15	4.0
(Smucker's)	1 T.	24	6.0
(Town House)	1 T.	15	4.0
Dietetic or low calorie:			
(Estee)	1 T. (.5 oz.)	6	1.0
(Heinz) lite	1 T.	8	2.0
(Hunt's) no salt added	1 T.	20	5.0
(Weight Watchers)	1 T.	12	3.0
CAULIFLOWER:			
Raw (USDA):			
Whole	1 lb. (weighed untrimmed)	49	9.2
Flowerbuds	½ cup (1.8 oz.)	14	2.6
Slices	½ cup (1.5 oz.)	11	2.2
Boiled (USDA) flowerbuds, drained	½ cup (2.2 oz.)	14	2.5
Frozen:			
(Birds Eye):			
Regular or florets, deluxe	⅓ of 10-oz. pkg.	23	5.0
With cheese sauce	½ of 10-oz. pkg.	130	12.0
(Budget Gourmet) *Side Dish,* in cheese sauce	5-oz. serving	110	6.0
(Frosty Acres)	3.3-oz. serving	25	5.0
(Green Giant):			
In cheese sauce, regular	3.3 oz.	50	7.5
Cuts, polybag	½ cup	12	3.0
(Larsen)	3.3 oz. serving	25	5.0
CAULIFLOWER, PICKLED			
(Vlasic) hot & spicy	1 oz.	4	1.0
CAVATELLI, frozen			
(Celentano)	⅕ of 16-oz. pkg.	250	52.0
CAVIAR, STURGEON			
(USDA):			
Pressed	1 oz.	90	1.4

Food	Measure	Cals.	Carbs.
Whole eggs	1 T. (.6 oz.)	42	.5
CELERIAC ROOT, raw (USDA):			
Whole	1 lb. (weighed unpaired)	156	39.2
Pared	4 oz.	45	9.6
CELERY, all varieties (USDA):			
Fresh:			
Whole	1 lb. (weighed untrimmed)	58	13.3
1 large outer stalk	8" × 1½" at root end (1.4 oz.)	7	1.6
Diced, chopped or cut in chunks	½ cup (2.1 oz.)	10	2.3
Slices	½ cup (1.9 oz.)	9	2.1
Boiled, drained solids:			
Diced or cut in chunks	½ cup (2.7 oz.)	10	2.4
Slices	½ cup (3 oz.)	12	2.6
Frozen (Larsen)	3½ oz. serving	14	3.0
CELERY SALT (French's)	1 tsp.	2	Tr.
CELERY SEED (French's)	1 tsp.	11	1.1
CEREAL (See individual listings such as **BRAN BREAKFAST CEREAL;** *COCOA PUFFS;* **CORN FLAKES; NATURAL CEREAL;** *NUTRI-GRAIN;* **OATMEAL;** etc.)			
CEREAL BAR			
(Kellogg's) *Smart Start:*			
Common Sense, oat bran, with raspberry filling	1.5-oz. bar	170	28.0
Cornflakes with mixed berry filling	1.5-oz. bar	170	27.0
Nutri-Grain, blueberry or strawberry	1.5-oz. bar	180	26.0
Raisin bran	1.5-oz. bar	160	28.0
Rice Krispies, with almonds	1-oz. bar	130	18.0
CERTS	1 piece	6	1.5

Food	Measure	Cals.	Carbs.
CERVELAT:			
(USDA):			
Dry	1 oz.	128	.5
Soft	1 oz.	87	.5
(Hormel) Viking	1-oz. serving	90	0.0
CHABLIS WINE:			
(Almaden) light	3 fl. oz.	42	DNA
(Carlo Rossi)	3 fl. oz.	66	1.5
(Gallo):			
White	3 fl. oz.	60	.5
Pink	3 fl. oz.	60	3.0
(Louis M. Martini) 12½%			
alcohol	3 fl. oz.	59	.2
(Paul Masson):			
Regular, 11.8% alcohol	3 fl. oz.	71	2.7
Light, 7.1% alcohol	3 fl. oz.	45	2.7
CHAMPAGNE:			
(Great Western):			
Regular, 12% alcohol	3 fl. oz.	71	2.5
Brut, 12% alcohol	3 fl. oz.	74	3.4
Pink, 12% alcohol	3 fl. oz.	81	4.9
(Taylor) dry, 12½% alcohol	3 fl. oz.	78	3.9
CHARD, Swiss (USDA):			
Raw, whole	1 lb. (weighed untrimmed)	104	19.2
Raw, trimmed	4 oz.	29	5.2
Boiled, drained solids	½ cup (3.4 oz.)	17	3.2
CHARDONNAY WINE (Louis M. Martini) 12½% alcohol	3 fl. oz.	60	.2
CHARLOTTE RUSSE, homemade recipe (USDA)	4 oz.	324	38.0
CHEERIOS, cereal (General Mills):			
Regular	1¼ cups (1 oz.)	110	20.0
Apple cinnamon	¾ cup (1 oz.)	110	22.0
Honey & nut	¾ cup (1 oz.)	110	23.0
CHEERIOS-TO-GO (General Mills):			
Plain	¾-oz. pkg.	80	15.0
Apple cinnamon	1-oz. pkg.	110	22.0

Food	Measure	Cals.	Carbs.
Honeynut	1-oz. pkg.	110	23.0

CHEESE:
American or cheddar:
(USDA):

Food	Measure	Cals.	Carbs.
Regular	1 oz.	105	.5
Cube, natural	1" cube (.6 oz.)	68	.3
(Alpine Lace):			
Regular	1 oz.	80	2.0
Ched-R-Lo	1 oz.	80	1.0
Free 'N Lean	1 oz.	40	1.0
(Borden) Lite-Line	1 oz.	70	1.0
(Churny) cheddar, lite,			
mild or sharp	1 oz.	80	1.0
(Dorman's):			
American:			
Lo-chol	1 oz.	90	1.0
Low sodium	1 oz.	110	1.0
Cheddar:			
Light, regular or			
Cheddar-Jack	1 oz.	80	1.0
Lo-chol	1 oz.	100	1.0
(Healthy Choice) cheddar,			
shredded, fat free	1 oz.	40	1.0
(Kraft):			
American singles	1 oz.	90	2.0
Cheddar, regular or Old			
English	1 oz.	110	1.0
Laughing Cow, natural	1 oz.	100	Tr.
(Land O' Lakes):			
American, process:			
Regular	1 oz.	110	1.0
Sharp	1 oz.	100	1.0
Cheddar, natural:			
Regular	1 oz.	110	<1.0
& bacon	1 oz.	110	1.0
Extra sharp	1 oz.	100	1.0
(Lucerne):			
American slices	1 oz.	110	1.0
Cheddar	1 oz.	110	0.0
(Polly-O) cheddar, shredded	1 oz.	110	1.0
(Safeway) American	1 oz.	110	1.0
(Weight Watchers) cheddar,			
mild, natural, regular,			
low sodium or shredded	1 oz.	80	1.0
Wispride	1 oz.	115	1.0

Food	Measure	Cals.	Carbs.
Blue:			
(USDA) natural	1 oz.	104	.6
(Dorman's):			
Castello 70%	1 oz.	134	0.1
Danabler 50%	1 oz.	100	0.3
(Kraft)	1 oz.	100	1.0
Laughing Cow	¾-oz. wedge	55	.5
(Safeway)	1 oz.	100	1.0
(Sargento) cold pack or crumbled	1 oz.	100	1.0
Bonbino, *Laughing Cow*, natural	1 oz.	103	Tr.
Brick:			
(USDA) natural	1 oz.	105	.5
(Land O' Lakes)	1 oz.	110	1.0
(Safeway) mild	1 oz.	100	1.0
Brie (Sargento) *Danish Danko*	1 oz.	80	.1
Burgercheese (Sargento) *Danish Danko*	1 oz.	106	1.0
Camembert (USDA) domestic	1 oz.	85	.5
Colby:			
(Alpine Lace) *Colby-Lo*	1 oz.	80	1.0
(Churny) lite	1 oz.	80	1.0
(Dorman's) *Lo-chol*	1 oz.	100	1.0
(Kraft)	1 oz.	110	1.0
(Land O' Lakes)	1 oz.	110	1.0
(Lucerne) loaf or shredded	1 oz.	110	0.0
(Safeway)	1 oz.	110	0.0
(Weight Watchers) natural	1 oz.	80	1.0
Cottage:			
Unflavored:			
Creamed:			
(USDA)	½ cup (4.3 oz.)	130	3.5
(Breakstone):			
Regular	4 oz.	110	4.0
Low fat	4 oz.	100	4.0
(Friendship):			
California style	½ cup	120	4.0
Low fat, lactose reduced or no salt added	½ cup	90	4.0
(Land O'Lakes)	4 oz.	120	4.0
(Lucerne) low fat, regular or unsalted	½ cup	100	4.0
Uncreamed:			
(Breakstone) dry curd, unsalted, non fat	4 oz.	90	6.0
(Johanna Farms):			

Food	Measure	Cals.	Carbs.
Large or small curd	½ cup	120	4.0
Low fat or no salt added	½ cup	90	4.0
Flavored:			
(Friendship) pineapple:			
4% fat	½ cup	140	15.0
low fat, 1%	½ cup	110	15.0
(Knudsen):			
4% fat, with pineapple	4 oz.	140	14.0
Low fat, 2%:			
Fruit cocktail	4 oz.	130	16.0
Peach	4 oz.	113	12.7
Pineapple	4 oz.	113	12.0
Strawberry	4 oz.	113	12.7
Non fat	4 oz.	70	3.0
Cream:			
(USDA)	1 oz.	106	.6
(Friendship) soft	1 oz.	103	.8
(Healthy Choice) fat free:			
Plain	1 oz.	30	2.0
Herb & garlic	1 oz.	30	2.0
(Kraft) *Philadelphia Brand:*			
Regular	1 oz.	100	1.0
With chive & onion	1 oz.	100	2.0
Light	1 oz.	60	2.0
Olive & pimento	1 oz.	90	2.0
(Lucerne) plain, regular or soft	1 oz.	100	1.0
Edam:			
(Churny) *May-Bud*	1 oz.	100	0.0
(Kaukauna)	1 oz.	100	<1.0
(Land O' Lakes)	1 oz.	100	<1.0
Laughing Cow	1 oz.	100	Tr.
Farmer:			
(Churny) *May-Bud*	1 oz.	90	1.0
(Friendship) regular or no salt added	1 oz.	40	1.0
(Kaukauna)	1 oz.	100	<1.0
Wispride	1 oz.	100	1.0
Feta:			
(Churny)	1 oz.	75	1.2
(Safeway)	1 oz.	75	1.0
Gjetost (Sargento) Norwegian	1 oz.	118	13.0
Gouda:			
(Churny) *May-Bud:*			
Regular	1 oz.	100	1.0
Lite	1 oz.	81	1.0
(Kaukauna)	1 oz.	100	<1.0

Food	Measure	Cals.	Carbs.
(Land O' Lakes)	1 oz.	100	1.0
Laughing Cow:			
Regular	1 oz.	110	Tr.
Mini, waxed	¾ oz.	80	Tr.
(Lucerne)	1 oz.	100	1.0
Gruyère, *Swiss Knight*	1 oz.	100	Tr.
Havarti (Sargento):			
Creamy	1 oz.	90	.2
Creamy, 60% milk	1 oz.	177	.2
Hoop (Friendship) natural	1 oz.	21	.5
Hot pepper (Sargento) sliced	1 oz.	112	1.0
Jalapeño Jack (Land O' Lakes)	1 oz.	90	1.0
Jarlsberg (Safeway) Norwegian	1 oz.	100	0.0
Kettle Moraine (Sargento)	1 oz.	100	1.0
Limburger (Sargento) natural	1 oz.	93	14.0
Longhorn:			
(Lucerne)	1 oz.	110	0.0
(Safeway)	1 oz.	110	0.0
Monterey Jack:			
(Alpine Lace) *Monti Jack Lo*	1 oz.	80	1.0
(Churny) lite	1 oz.	80	0.0
(Kaukauna)	1 oz.	110	<1.0
(Kraft)	1 oz.	110	0.0
(Land O' Lakes)	1 oz.	110	<1.0
(Lucerne)	1 oz.	105	0.0
(Safeway)	1 oz.	105	0.0
(Weight Watchers) natural	1 oz.	80	1.0
Mozzarella:			
(Alpine Lace) *Free 'N Lean*	1 oz.	40	0.0
(Dorman's) light	1 oz.	80	1.0
(Healthy Choice) chunk, fat			
free	1 oz.	40	1.0
(Kraft)	1 oz.	80	0.0
(Land O' Lakes) part skim milk	1 oz.	80	1.0
(Lucerne) shredded, sliced or			
whole	1 oz.	80	0.0
(Polly-O):			
Fior di Latte	1 oz.	80	1.0
Lite	1 oz.	70	1.0
Part skim milk, regular or			
shredded	1 oz.	80	1.0
Smoked	1 oz.	85	1.0
Whole milk:			
Regular	1 oz.	90	1.0
Old fashioned, regular	1 oz.	70	1.0
(Sargento):			
Bar, rounds, shredded			

Food	Measure	Cals.	Carbs.
regular or with spices, sliced for pizza or square	1 oz.	79	1.0
Whole milk	1 oz.	100	1.0
Munester:			
(Alpine Lacc)	1 oz.	100	1.0
(Dorman's):			
Light	1 oz.	80	0.0
Lo-chol	1 oz.	100	1.0
Low sodium	1 oz.	110	0.0
(Kaukauna)	1 oz.	110	<1.0
(Land O' Lakes)	1 oz.	100	<1.0
(Safeway)	1 oz.	105	0.0
Wispride	1 oz.	100	Tr.
Parmesan:			
(USDA):			
Regular	1 oz.	111	.8
Grated	½ cup (not packed)	169	1.2
(Lucerne) grated	1 oz.	110	1.0
(Polly-O) grated	1 oz.	130	1.0
(Progresso) grated	1 T.	23	*1.0
Pot (Sargento) regular, French onion or garlic	1 oz.	30	1.0
Provolone:			
(Alpine Lace) *Provo-Lo*	1 oz.	70	1.0
(Frigo)	1 oz.	90	1.0
Laughing Cow:			
Cube	⅙ oz.	12	.1
Wedge	¾ oz.	55	.5
Ricotto:			
(Frigo) part skim milk	1 oz.	43	.9
(Poly-O):			
Lite	1 oz.	40	1.5
Old-fashioned	1 oz.	50	1.0
Part skim milk	1 oz.	45	1.0
Whole milk	1 oz.	50	1.0
(Sargento):			
Part skim milk	1 oz.	39	1.0
Whole milk	1 oz.	49	1.0
Romano (Polly-O) wedge	1 oz.	130	1.0
Roquefort, natural (USDA)	1 oz.	104	.6
Samsoe (Sargento) Danish	1 oz.	101	.2
Scamorze (Frigo)	1 oz.	79	.3
Semisoft:			
Bel Paese	1 oz.	90	.3

Food	Measure	Cals.	Carbs.
Laughing Cow:			
Babybel:			
Regular	1 oz.	91	Tr.
Mini	¾ oz.	74	Tr.
Bonbel:			
Regular	1 oz.	100	Tr.
Mini	¾ oz.	74	Tr.
Reduced calorie	1 oz.	45	Tr.
Slim Jack (Dorman's)	1 oz.	80	1.0
Swiss:			
(USDA) domestic, natural			
or process	1 oz.	105	.5
(Alpine Lace) *Swiss-Lo*	1 oz.	90	1.0
(Churny) lite	1 oz.	90	1.0
(Dorman's) light	1 oz.	90	0.0
(Lucerne)	1 oz.	100	0.0
(Safeway)	1 oz.	100	0.0
(Weight Watchers) natural	1 oz.	90	1.0
Taco (Sargento) shredded	1 oz.	105	1.0

CHEESE ENTREE (See
**MACARONI & CHEESE;
SOUFFLE,** Cheese; **WELSH
RAREBIT**)

CHEESE FONDUE,

Food	Measure	Cals.	Carbs.
Swiss Knight	1 oz.	60	1.0

CHEESE FOOD:

Food	Measure	Cals.	Carbs.
American or cheddar:			
(USDA) process	1 oz.	92	2.0
(Borden) *Lite-Line*	1 oz.	50	1.0
(Fisher) *Ched-O-Mate* or			
Sandwich-Mate	1 oz.	90	1.0
(Land O' Lakes)	¾-oz. slice	70	2.0
(Lucerne)	1 oz.	90	2.0
(Shedd's) *Country Crock*	1 oz.	70	3.0
Cheez-ola (Fisher)	1 oz.	90	1.0
Chef's Delight (Fisher)	1 oz.	70	4.0
Garlic & Herb, *Wispride*	1 oz.	90	4.0
Hot pepper (Lucerne)	1 oz.	90	2.0
Italian herb (Land O' Lakes)	1 oz.	90	2.0
Jalapeño (Borden) *Lite-Line*	1 oz.	50	1.0
Low sodium (Borden) *Lite-Line*	1 oz.	70	2.0
Muenster (Borden) *Lite-Line*	1 oz.	50	1.0
Mun-chee (Pauly)	1 oz.	100	2.0
Neufchatel (Shedd's) *Country*			
Crock	1 oz.	70	1.0

Food	Measure	Cals.	Carbs.
Onion (Land O' Lakes)	1 oz.	90	2.0
Pepperoni (Land O' Lakes)	1 oz.	90	1.0
Pimiento (Lucerne)	1 oz.	80	2.0
Salami (Land O' Lakes)	1 oz.	90	2.0
Swiss:			
(Borden) *Lite-Line*	1 oz.	50	1.0
(Kraft) reduced fat	1 oz.	90	1.0
(Pauly)	.8-oz. slice	74	1.6
CHEESE SPREAD:			
American or cheddar:			
(USDA)	1 T. (.5 oz.)	40	1.1
(Fisher)	1 oz.	80	2.0
Laughing Cow	1 oz.	72	.7
(Nabisco) *Easy Cheese*	1 tsp.	16	.4
Blue, *Laughing Cow*	1 oz.	72	.7
Brick (Sargento) cracker snacks	1 oz.	100	1.0
Cheese 'n Bacon (Nabisco)			
Easy Cheese	1 tsp.	16	.4
Golden velvet (Land O' Lakes)	1 oz.	80	2.0
Gruyère, *Laughing Cow,*			
La Vache Que Rit:			
Regular	1 oz.	72	.7
Reduced calorie	1 oz.	46	1.3
Nacho (Nabisco) *Easy Cheese*	1 tsp.	16	.4
Pimiento:			
(Nabisco) *Snack Mate*	1 tsp.	15	.3
(Price)	1 oz.	80	2.0
Provolone, *Laughing Cow*	1 oz.	72	.7
Velveeta (Kraft)	1 oz.	80	2.0
CHENIN BLANC WINE (Louis M. Martini) 12½% alcohol	3 fl. oz.	56	.9
CHERRY:			
Sour:			
Fresh (USDA):			
Whole	1 lb. (weighed with stems)	213	52.5
Whole	1 lb. (weighed without stems)	242	59.7
Pitted	½ cup (2.7 oz.)	45	11.1
Canned, syrup pack, pitted: (USDA):			
Light syrup	4 oz. (with liq.)	84	21.2
Heavy syrup	½ cup (with liq.)	116	29.5
Extra heavy syrup	4 oz. (with liq.)	127	32.4

Food	Measure	Cals.	Carbs.
(Thank You Brand)	½ cup (4.5 oz.)	123	29.4
Canned, water pack, pitted, solid & liq.	½ cup (4.3 oz.)	52	13.1
Frozen, pitted:			
Sweetened	½ cup (4.6 oz.)	146	36.1
Unsweetened	4 oz.	62	15.2
Sweet:			
Fresh (USDA):			
Whole	1 lb. (weighed with stems)	286	71.0
Whole, with stems	½ cup (2.3 oz.)	41	10.2
Pitted	½ cup (2.9 oz.)	57	14.3
Canned, syrup pack:			
(USDA):			
Light syrup, pitted	4 oz. (with liq.)	74	18.7
Heavy syrup, pitted	½ cup (with liq., 4.2 oz.)	96	24.2
Extra heavy syrup, pitted	4 oz. (with liq.)	113	29.0
(Del Monte) solids & liq.:			
Dark	½ cup (4.3 oz.)	90	23.0
Light	½ cup (4.3 oz.)	100	26.0
Stokely-Van Camp) pitted, solids & liq.	½ cup (4.2 oz.)	50	11.0
(Thank You Brand) heavy syrup	½ cup (4.5 oz.)	98	23.0
Canned, dietetic or water pack, solids & liq.:			
(Diet Delight)	½ cup (4.4 oz.)	70	17.0
(Featherweight):			
Dark	½ cup	60	13.0
Light	½ cup	50	11.0
(Thank You Brand) water pack	½ cup (4.5 oz.)	61	14.1
CHERRY, CANDIED (USDA)	1 oz.	96	24.6
CHERRY, MARASCHINO (USDA)	1 oz. (with liq.)	33	8.3
CHERRY DRINK:			
Canned:			
(Hi-C) chilled	6 fl. oz.	100	24.7
(Johanna Farms) *Ssips*	8.45-fl.-oz. container	130	32.0
(Lincoln) cherry berry	6 fl. oz.	100	25.0
(Smucker's)	8 fl. oz.	130	31.0

Food	Measure	Cals.	Carbs.
Squeezit (General Mills)	6¾-fl.-oz. container	110	27.0
*Mix (Funny Face)	8 fl. oz.	88	22.0
CHERRY-GRAPE JUICE DRINK, canned (Boku)	8 fl. oz.	120	29.0
CHERRY HEERING (Hiram Walker)	1 fl. oz.	80	10.0
CHERRY JELLY:			
Sweetened (Smucker's)	1 T. (.5 oz.)	54	12.0
Dietetic (Featherweight)	1 T.	16	4.0
CHERRY JUICE, canned:			
(Juicy Juice)	8.45-fl.-oz. container	130	32.0
(Knudsen & Sons):			
Black	8 fl. oz	150	38.0
Tart	8 fl. oz	125	30.0
(Santa Cruz Natural) organic	8 fl. oz.	125	29.0
(Welch's) *Orchard*	6 fl. oz.	180	45.0
CHERRY JUICE DRINK, canned (Hi-C)	8.45-fl.-oz. container	141	34.8
CHERRY LIQUEUR (DeKuyper) 50 proof	1 fl. oz.	75	8.5
CHERRY PRESERVES OR JAM:			
Sweetened (Smucker's)	1 T. (.7 oz.)	54	12.0
Dietetic:			
(Estee)	1 T. (.6 oz.)	6	0.0
(Louis Sherry)	1 T. (.6 oz.)	6	0.0
(S&W) *Nutradiet,* red label	1 T. (.6 oz.)	12	3.0
CHESTNUT (USDA):			
Fresh:			
In shell	1 lb. (weighed in shell)	713	154.7
Shelled	4 oz.	220	47.7
Dried:			
In shell	1 lb. (weighed in shell)	1402	292.4
Shelled	4 oz.	428	89.1

Food	Measure	Cals.	Carbs.
CHEWING GUM:			
Sweetened:			
Bazooka, bubble	1 slice	18	4.5
Beechies	1 piece	6	2.0
Beech Nut; Beeman's,			
Big Red; Black Jack;			
Clove; Doublemint;			
Freedent; Fruit Punch;			
Juicy Fruit, Spearmint			
(Wrigley's); *Teaberry*	1 stick	10	2.3
Bubble Yum	1 piece	25	7.0
Dentyne	1 piece	4	1.2
Extra (Wrigley's)	1 piece	8	Tr.
Hubba Bubba (Wrigley's)	1 piece		
	(8 grams)	23	5.8
Dietetic:			
Bubble Yum	1 piece	20	5.0
(*Care*Free*)	1 piece	8	2.0
(Estee) bubble or regular	1 piece	5	1.4
Orbit (Wrigley's)	1 piece	8	Tr.
CHEX, cereal (Ralston Purina):			
Bran (See **BRAN**			
BREAKFAST CEREAL)			
Corn	1 cup (1 oz.)	110	25.0
Double	⅔ cup (1 oz.)	100	24.0
Honey graham	⅔ cup (1 oz.)	110	25.0
Oat, honey nut	½ cup (1 oz.)	100	22.0
Rice	1⅛ cups (1 oz.)	110	25.0
Wheat	⅔ cup (1 oz.)	110	23.0
CHIANTI WINE (Italian Swiss			
Colony) 13% alcohol	3 fl. oz.	64	1.5
CHICKEN (USDA):			
Broiler, cooked, meat only	4 oz.	154	0.0
Capon, raw, with bone	1 lb. (weighed		
	ready-to-cook)	937	0.0
Fryer:			
Raw:			
Ready-to-cook	1 lb. (weighed		
	ready-to-cook)	382	0.0
Breast	1 lb. (weighed		
	with bone)	394	0.0
Leg or drumstick	1 lb. (weighed		
	with bone)	313	0.0

Food	Measure	Cals.	Carbs.
Thigh	1 lb. (weighed with bone)	-435	.0.0
Fried. A 2½-lb. chicken (weighed before cooking with bone) will give you:			
Back	1 back (2.2 oz.)	139	2.7
Breast	⅓ breast (3⅓ oz.)	154	1.1
Leg or drumstick	1 leg (2 oz.)	87	.4
Neck	1 neck (2.1 oz.)	121	1.9
Rib	1 rib (.7 oz.)	42	.8
Thigh	1 thigh (2¼ oz.)	118	1.2
Wing	1 wing (1¾ oz.)	78	.8
Fried, frozen (See **CHICKEN, FRIED,** frozen)			
Fried skin	1 oz.	199	2.6
Hen and cock:			
Raw	1 lb. (weighed ready-to-cook)	987	0.0
Stewed:			
Meat only	4 oz.	236	0.0
Chopped	½ cup (2.5 oz.)	150	0.0
Diced	½ cup (2.4 oz.)	139	0.0
Ground	½ cup (2 oz.)	116	0.0
Roaster:			
Raw	1 lb. (weighed ready-to-cook)	791	0.0
Roasted:			
Dark meat without skin	4 oz.	209	0.0
Light meat without skin	4 oz.	206	0.0
CHICKEN, BONED, canned:			
Regular:			
(USDA)	1 cup (7.2 oz.)	406	0.0
(Hormel) chunk:			
Breast	6¾-oz. serving	350	0.0
Dark	6¾-oz. serving	327	0.0
White & dark:			
Regular	6¾-oz. serving	340	0.0
Low salt	6¾-oz. serving	330	0.0
(Swanson) chunk:			
Mixin' chicken	2½ oz.	130	1.0
White	2½ oz.	90	0.0
Low sodium (Featherweight)	2½ oz.	154	0.0
CHICKEN, CREAMED, frozen (Stouffer's)	6½ oz. pkg.	300	5.9

Food	Measure	Cals.	Carbs.
CHICKEN, FRIED, frozen:			
(Banquet):			
Assorted	2-lb. pkg.	1650	145.0
Breast portion	11½-oz. pkg.	440	26.0
Hot & spicy	32-oz. pkg.	1650	145.0
Thigh & drumstick	25-oz. pkg.	1000	56.0
(Country Pride) southern fried:			
Chunks	3 oz.	276	14.0
(Swanson):			
Assorted	3¼-oz. serving	270	16.0
Breast portion	4½-oz. serving	360	21.0
Nibbles	3¼-oz. serving	300	19.0
Thighs & drumsticks	3¼-oz. serving	290	17.0
CHICKEN, PACKAGED:			
(Boar's Head) low fat	1 oz.	25	Tr.
(Carl Buddig) smoked, sliced	1 oz.	60	1.0
(Eckrich) breast	1 slice	20	.5
(Louis Rich) breast, oven			
roasted	1-oz. slice	40	Tr.
(Oscar Mayer) breast:			
Oven roasted	1-oz. slice	30	.6
Smoked	1-oz. slice	26	.5
(Weaver):			
Bologna	1 slice	44	.5
Breast	1 slice	25	.5
Roll	1 slice	46	.5
CHICKEN, POTTED (USDA)	1 oz.	70	0.0
CHICKEN À LA KING:			
Home recipe (USDA)	1 cup (8.6 oz.)	468	12.3
Canned (Swanson)	½ of 10½-oz. can	190	9.0
Frozen:			
(Armour) *Classics Lite*	11¼-oz. meal	290	38.0
(Banquet) Cookin' Bag	4-oz. pkg.	110	9.0
(Freezer Queen):			
Cook-in-Pouch	4-oz. serving	70	6.0
Single serve	9-oz. serving	270	37.0
(Le Menu):			
Regular	10¼-oz. dinner	320	29.0
Healthy entree	10¼-oz. dinner	330	29.0
(Stouffer's) with rice	8¼-oz. entree	240	29.0
(Weight Watchers)	9½-oz. pkg.	290	34.0
	9-oz. pkg.	220	15.0
CHICKEN BOUILLON:			
Regular:			

Food	Measure	Cals.	Carbs.
(Herb-Ox):			
Cube	1 cube	6	.6
Packet	1 packet	12	1.9
(Knorr)	1 packet	16	.6
(Maggi) cube	1 cube	7	1.0
(Wyler's)	1 cube	8	1.0
Low sodium:			
(Borden) *Lite-Line,*	1 tsp.	12	2.0
(Featherweight)	1 tsp.	18	2.0
CHICKEN CHUNKS, frozen			
(Country Pride):			
Regular	3 oz.	240	15.0
Southern fried	3 oz.	280	14.0
CHICKEN DINNER OR ENTREE:			
Canned:			
(Hormel) *Dinty Moore,* &			
dumplings, microwave cup	7½-oz. can	190	20.0
(Swanson) & dumplings	7½-oz. serving	220	19.0
(Top Shelf):			
Acapulco	1 serving	390	41.0
Breast:			
Glazed	10-oz. meal	170	19.0
With Spanish rice	10-oz. meal	400	38.0
Cacciatore	10-oz. meal	210	25.0
Sweet & sour	1 serving	270	41.0
(Ultra Slim Fast)			
Mesquite	12-oz. meal	350	61.0
Roasted, in mushroom sauce	12-oz. meal	280	30.0
Sweet & sour	12-oz. meal	330	57.0
& vegetables	12-oz. meal	290	45.0
Frozen:			
(Armour):			
Classics Lite:			
Breast medallion			
marsala	10½-oz. meal	250	27.0
Burgundy	10½-oz. meal	210	25.0
Oriental	10-oz. meal	180	24.0
Sweet & sour	11-oz. meal	240	39.0
Dining Lite, glazed	9-oz. meal	220	30.0
Dinner Classics:			
Glazed	10¾-oz. dinner	300	24.0
Mesquite	9½-oz. dinner	370	42.0
Parmigiana	11½-oz. dinner	370	27.0
With wine and mush-			
room sauce	10¾-oz. dinner	280	24.0

Food	Measure	Cals.	Carbs.
(Banquet):			
Cookin' Bag & vegetable primavera	4-oz. serving	100	14.0
Dinner:			
Regular:			
& dumplings	10-oz. dinner	430	34.0
Fried	10-oz. dinner	400	45.0
Extra Helping:			
Fried	16-oz. dinner	570	70.0
Fried, all white meat	16-oz. dinner	570	70.0
Nuggets:			
BBQ sauce	10-oz. dinner	640	56.0
Sweet & Sour Sauce	10-oz. dinner	650	54.0
Family Entree:			
& dumplings	¼ of 28-oz. pkg.	280	28.0
& vegetable primavera	¼ of 28-oz. pkg.	140	18.0
Microwave, nuggets, with sweet & sour sauce	4½-oz. serving	360	22.0
Platter:			
Boneless:			
Drumsnacker	7-oz. meal	430	49.0
Nuggets	6.4-oz. meal	430	46.0
Patty	7½-oz. meal	380	34.0
Fried, all white meat, any type	9-oz. meal	430	21.0
(Budget Gourmet):			
Regular:			
Marsala	9-oz. meal	260	31.0
Sweet & sour	10-oz. meal	340	55.0
Light & Healthy:			
Au gratin	9.1-oz. meal	230	23.0
Breast:			
Herbed, with fettucini	11-oz. meal	240	30.0
Mesquite	11-oz. meal	250	33.0
Parmigiana	11-oz. meal	270	30.0
Mandarin	10-oz. meal	240	38.0
Orange glazed	9-oz. meal	270	45.0
Roast, with home-style gravy	11-oz. meal	280	36.0
Teriyaki	11-oz. meal	300	40.0
(Celentano):			
Parmigiana, cutlets	9-oz. pkg.	400	21.0
Primavera	11½-oz. pkg.	260	26.0
(Chun King):			
Imperial	13-oz. entree	300	54.0
Walnut, crunchy	13-oz. entree	310	49.0

Food	Measure	Cals.	Carbs.
(Freezer Queen):			
Cacciatore, single serve	9-oz. serving	270	37.0
Croquettes, breaded with gravy, Family Supper	7-oz. serving	240	20.0
Primavera, sliced, with gravy, cook-in-pouch	5-oz. serving	80	6.0
Sweet & sour, with rice, single serve	9-oz. serving	300	48.0
(Healthy Choice):			
À l'orange	9½-oz. meal	260	39.0
Glazed	8½-oz. meal	230	28.0
Herb roasted	11-oz. meal	260	38.0
Mesquite	10½-oz. meal	310	52.0
Oriental	11¼-oz. meal	220	31.0
Parmigiana	11½-oz. meal	280	38.0
& pasta divan	11½ oz. meal	310	45.0
Sweet & sour	11½-oz. meal	280	44.0
(Kid Cuisine):			
Fried	7¼-oz. meal	420	41.0
Nuggets	6¼-oz. meal	400	46.0
(La Choy) *Fresh & Lite:*			
Almond, with rice & vegetables	9¾-oz. meal	270	40.1
Imperial	11-oz. meal	260	45.0
Oriental, spicy	9¾-oz. meal	270	52.0
Sweet & sour	10-oz. meal	260	50.1
(Le Menu):			
Regular, dinner:			
Cordon bleu	11-oz. dinner	460	47.0
Parmigiana	11¾-oz. dinner	410	31.0
Sweet & sour	11¼-oz. dinner	400	41.0
In wine sauce	10-oz. dinner	280	27.0
Healthy style dinner:			
Glazed breast	10-oz. dinner	230	25.0
Herb roasted	10-oz. dinner	240	18.0
Sweet & sour	10-oz. dinner	250	29.0
Healthy style entree:			
Dijon	8-oz. entree	240	21.0
(Morton):			
Regular:			
Boneless	11-oz. dinner	329	44.7
Boneless	17-oz. dinner	627	84.0
Fried	11-oz. dinner	431	64.1
Light, boneless	11-oz. dinner	250	30.0
(Stouffer's):			
Regular:			
Cashew, in sauce with rice	9½-oz. meal	380	29.0

Food	Measure	Cals.	Carbs.
Creamed	6½-oz. meal	300	8.0
Divan	8½-oz. meal	320	11.0
Escalloped, & noodles	10-oz. meal	420	27.0
Lean Cuisine:			
À l'orange, with almond rice	8-oz. meal	260	30.0
Breast, in herbed cream sauce	9½-oz. meal	260	11.0
Breast, marsala, with vegetables	8⅛-oz. meal	190	11.0
Breast, Parmesan	10-oz. meal	260	19.0
Cacciatore, with vermicelli	10⅞-oz. meal	250	26.0
Fiesta	8½-oz. meal	250	29.0
Glazed, with vegetable rice	8½-oz. meal	270	23.0
Oriental	9⅜-oz. meal	230	23.0
& vegetables with vermicelli	11¾-oz. meal	270	29.0
Right Course:			
Italiano, with fettucini & vegetables	9⅝-oz. meal	280	29.0
Sesame	10-oz. meal	320	34.0
Tenderloins in barbecue sauce with rice pilaf	8¾-oz. meal	270	38.0
Tenderloins in peanut sauce with linguini & vegetables	9¼-oz. meal	330	32.0
(Swanson):			
Regular, 4-compartment dinner:			
Fried:			
BBQ flavor	10-oz. dinner	540	61.0
Dark meat	9¾-oz. dinner	560	55.0
White meat	10¼-oz. dinner	550	60.0
Nuggets	8¾-oz. dinner	470	47.0
Homestyle Recipe, entrees:			
Cacciatore	10.95 oz. meal	260	33.0
Fried	7-oz. meal	390	33.0
Nibbles	4¼-oz. meal	340	29.0
Hungry Man, dinner:			
Boneless	17¾-oz. dinner	700	65.0
Fried:			
Dark meat	14½-oz. dinner	860	77.0
White meat	14½-oz. dinner	870	80.0
(Tyson):			
Regular:			
Breast, boneless, Marinated:			

Food	Measure	Cals.	Carbs.
Barbecue	3¾ oz. serving	120	5.0
Butter garlic	3¾ oz. serving	160	3.0
Italian or teriyaki	3¾ oz. serving	130	6.0
Breast strips, boneless, Oriental	2¾ oz. serving	110	6.0
Chick 'n Cheddar	2.6 oz. serving	220	11.0
Mesquite breast tenders, boneless	2¾ oz. serving	110	4.0
Chicken Meal:			
Herb	13¾-oz. meal	340	43.0
Honey mustard	13¾oz. meal	390	52.0
Italian style	13¾-oz. meal	310	38.0
Mesquite	13¼-oz. meal	330	38.0
Salsa	13¾-oz. meal	370	52.0
Gourmet Selection:			
A l'orange	9½-oz. meal	300	36.0
& beef luau	10½-oz. meal	330	42.0
Dijon	8½-oz. meal	310	22.0
Francais	9½-oz. meal	280	20.0
Glazed, with sauce	9¼-oz. meal	240	29.0
Honey roasted	9-oz. meal	220	23.0
Mesquite	9-oz. meal	320	39.0
Oriental	10¼-oz. meal	270	32.0
Parmigiana	9-oz. meal	270	32.0
Sweet & sour	11-oz. meal	420	50.0
Healthy Portion, sesame	13½-oz. meal	390	58.0
Looney Tunes:			
Bugs Bunny, chunks	7.7-oz. meal	290	31.0
Road Runner	6.7-oz. meal	300	42.0
Tazmanian Devil, drumettes	8-oz. meal	310	31.0
Yosemite, Sam, barbecue	7.38-oz. meal	230	28.0
Microwave, tenders (Weight Watchers).	3½ oz. serving	230	19.0
Smart Ones:			
A l'orange	8-oz. meal	190	34.0
Fiesta, with Spanish rice	8-oz. meal	210	37.0
Francais, with garlic vegetables	8½-oz. meal	150	18.0
Grilled & glazed	8-oz. meal	130	17.0
Honey mustard, with sauce	7½-oz. meal	140	20.0
Piccata, lemon herb	7½-oz. meal	160	25.0
Stir fry:			
Ginger with vegetables	9-oz. meal	160	21.0

Food	Measure	Cals.	Carbs.
Orange glazed, with rice	9-oz. meal	170	25.0
Polynesian	9-oz. meal	190	34.0
Sesame with lo mein noodles	9-oz. meal	200	23.0
Teriyaki, with spring vegetables	9-oz. meal	140	16.0
Ultimate 200:			
Barbecue, glazed	6½-oz. meal	180	16.0
Cordon bleu	7.7-oz. meal	170	15.0
Grilled, glazed	7½-oz. meal	150	17.0
Imperial	8½-oz. meal	200	25.0
Kiev	7-oz. meal	190	22.0
Southern baked	6.3-oz. meal	170	10.0
Teriyaki	7.6-oz. meal	150	7.0
Refrigerated (Perdue):			
Raw, breast, boneless, seasoned:			
Barbecue	4 oz.	130	8.0
Lemon pepper	4 oz.	110	2.0
Italian	4 oz.	110	4.0
Oriental	4 oz.	120	4.0
Cooked, breast, boneless, seasoned:			
Barbecue	3 oz.	110	5.0
Lemon pepper	3 oz.	90	2.0

CHICKEN DINNER MIX
(Chicken Helper) Skillet Dinner:

Cheesy broccoli	7-oz. serving	310	34.0
Creamy chicken	8¼-oz. serving	330	29.0
Creamy mushroom	8-oz. serving	320	31.0
Stir fry	7-oz. serving	370	36.0
(Lipton) Microeasy:			
Barbecue style	¼ of pkg.	220	24.0
Country style	¼ of pkg.	190	15.0

CHICKEN FRICASEE (USDA)

home recipe	1 cup (8.5 oz.)	386	7.7

CHICKEN GIZZARD (USDA):

Raw	4 oz.	128	.8
Simmered	4 oz.	168	.8

CHICKEN & NOODLES,
frozen:

Food	Measure	Cals.	Carbs.
(Armour):			
Dining Lite	9-oz. meal	240	28.0
Dinner Classics	11-oz. meal	230	23.0
(Budget Gourmet)	10-oz. meal	440	28.0
(Stouffer's) homestyle	10-oz. meal	310	21.0
(Weight Watchers)	9-oz. meal	240	25.0
CHICKEN NUGGETS, frozen:			
(Country Pride)	3-oz. serving	250	14.0
(Empire Kosher)	12-oz. pkg.	708	56.0
(Freezer Queen):			
Deluxe Family Supper	3-oz. serving	270	15.0
Platter	6-oz. serving	410	36.0
(Swanson)	3-oz. serving	230	14.0
(Weight Watchers)	5.9-oz. meal	220	23.0
CHICKEN PATTY, frozen:			
(County Pride) regular	12-oz. pkg.	1000	56.0
(Empire Kosher)	12-oz. pkg.	792	52.0
(Freezer Queen) platter	7½-oz. serving	360	30.0
CHICKEN PIE, frozen:			
(Banquet)	7-oz pie	550	39.0
(Empire Kosher)	8-oz. pie	463	49.0
(Morton)	7-oz. pie	420	27.0
(Stouffer's)	10-oz. pie	530	35.0
(Swanson):			
Regular	7-oz. pie	380	35.0
Hungry Man	16-oz. pie	630	57.0
CHICKEN SALAD (Carnation)	¼ of 7½-oz. can	120	3.8
CHICKEN SANDWICH, frozen:			
(Croissant Pockets) with broc-coli & cheddar cheese	1 piece	300	37.0
(Hormel) *Quick Meal*:			
Regular	1 piece	340	42.0
Grilled	1 piece	300	35.0
(Hot Pockets) & cheddar cheese with broccoli	1 piece	300	37.0
(Lean Pockets):			
Glazed, supreme	1 piece	240	34.0
Parmesan	1 piece	260	34.0

CHICKEN SOUP (See **SOUP,**
Chicken)

Food	Measure	Cals.	Carbs.
CHICKEN STEW:			
Canned:			
(Hormel) *Dinty Moore*:			
Regular	7½ oz. can	260	15.0
Microwave cup	7½ oz. can	260	15.0
(Swanson)	7⅝-oz. can	160	15.0
*Freeze-dried (Mountain			
House)	1 cup	230	30.0
CHICKEN STICKS, frozen			
(Country Pride)	12-oz. pkg.	960	64.0
CHICK-FIL-A:			
Brownie, fudge, with nuts	2.8 oz.	350	40.0
Cheesecake:			
Plain	1 serving	270	7.0
With topping:			
Blueberry	1 serving	290	9.0
Strawberry	1 serving	290	8.0
Chicken nuggets	8-pack serving	287	12.5
Icedream	1 small cup	134	18.9
Lemonade	10 oz.	124	32.0
Pie, lemon	4.1-oz. slice	329	63.8
Potato, *Waffle Fries*	3-oz. serving	270	33.0
Salad:			
Carrot and raisin	1 cup	116	17.9
Chicken:			
Garden salad,			
chargrilled	1 serving	128	8.3
Salad plate	1 serving	291	9.8
Tossed without dressing	1 serving	21	4.2
Salad dressing, regular:			
Blue cheese	1 serving	222	1.8
Honey french	1 serving	256	16.8
Salad dressing, dietetic:			
Italian, lite	1 serving	22	2.8
Ranch, lite	1 serving	93	9.0
Sandwich; chicken:			
Regular	1 serving	360	28.1
Chargrilled:			
Regular	1 serving	258	23.7
Deluxe	1 serving	266	25.5
Chick-Fil-A:			
With bun	1 serving	426	40.0
Without bun	1 serving	219	2.0
Chick-N-Q	1 serving	409	40.9
Deluxe	1 serving	368	29.8

Food	Measure	Cals.	Carbs.
Salad, on wheat bread	1 serving (5.7 oz.)	449	35.0
Soup, chicken, hearty breast:			
Small	1 serving	152	11.0
Medium	1 serving (14 fl. oz.)	230	19.0
Large	1 serving (17½ oz.)	432	36.0
CHICK-PEAS OR GARBANZOS:			
Dry (USDA)	1 cup (7.1 oz.)	720	122.0
Canned, regular pack, solids & liq.:			
(Allen's)	½ cup	110	18.0
(Furman's)	⅓ cup (2.6 oz.)	237	13.5
(Goya)	½ cup (4 oz.)	110	17.0
(Old El Paso)	½ cup	190	16.0
(Progresso)	½ cup	120	22.0
Canned, dietetic pack, solids & liq. (S&W) *Nutradiet*	½ cup	105	19.0
CHILI, OR CHILI CON CARNE:			
Canned, regular pack:			
Beans only:			
(Comstock)	½ cup (4.4 oz.)	140	23.0
(Hormel) in sauce	5 oz.	130	19.0
(Hunt's)	½ cup (3.5 oz.)	100	18.0
(S&W)	½ cup	130	23.0
(Town House)	½ cup	110	20.0
With beans:			
(Gebhardt) hot	½ of 15-oz. can	470	46.0
(Hormel):			
Regular, hot or mild	½ of 7½-oz. can	150	13.5
Micro Cup:			
Regular, hot	½ of 7.4-oz.	125	12.0
With macaroni, *Chili Mac*	½ of 7½-oz. can	86	9.0
(Hunt's) *Just Rite:*			
Regular	4 oz.	200	16.0
Hot	4 oz.	195	16.0
(Old El Paso)	1 cup	349	12.3
Without beans:			
(Gebhardt)	½ of 15-oz. can	410	13.0
(Hunt's) *Just Rite*	4 oz.	180	9.0
Canned, dietetic pack:			
(Estee) with beans	7½-oz. serving	370	27.0

Food	Measure	Cals.	Carbs.
(Featherweight) with beans	7½-oz.	270	25.0
(Healthy Choice) turkey, with beans	½ of 7½-oz. can	100	10.0
Frozen:			
(Stouffer's):			
Regular, with beans	8⅓-oz. meal	260	24.0
Right Choice, vegetarian	9¾-oz. meal	280	45.0
(Swanson) *Homestyle Recipe*	8¼-oz. meal	270	26.0
Mix, *Manwich, Chili Fixins:*			
Sauce only	5.3 oz.	110	20.0
*Prepared	8-oz. serving	290	20.0
CHILI SAUCE:			
(USDA)	½ cup (4.8 oz.)	142	33.8
(El Molino) green, mild	1 T.	5	1.0
(Heinz)	1 T.	17	3.0
(LaVictoria) green	1 T.	3	1.0
(Ortega) green:			
Hot	1 oz.	9	1.9
Medium or mild	1 oz.	7	1.7
CHILI SEASONING MIX:			
(French's) *Chili-O:*			
Plain	⅙ of pkg.	25	5.0
Onion	⅙ of pkg.	35	7.0
(Gebhardt) Chili Quick	1 tsp.	10	2.0
(Lawry's)	1.6-oz. pkg.	143	26.6
(Old El Paso)	⅕ of pkg.	20	4.0
CHIMICHANGA, frozen:			
(Fred's) *Marquez:*			
Beef, shredded	5-oz. serving	351	35.0
Chicken	5-oz. serving	350	42.0
(Old El Paso):			
Regular:			
Beef	1 piece	370	37.0
Chicken	1 piece	360	33.0
Dinner, festive:			
Beef	11-oz. dinner	540	65.0
Beef & cheese	11-oz. dinner	510	53.0
Entree:			
Bean & cheese	1 piece	350	36.0
Beef	1 piece	380	35.0
Beef & pork	1 piece	340	35.0
Chicken	1 piece	370	35.0

Food	Measure	Cals.	Carbs.
CHIPS (See **CRACKERS, PUFFS & CHIPS**)			
CHIVES (USDA) raw	1 T. (3 grams)	1	.2
CHOCO-DILES (Hostess)	1 piece	240	32.0
CHOCOLATE, BAKING:			
(Baker's):			
Bitter or unsweetened	1-oz. square	180	8.6
Semi-sweet:			
Regular	1-oz. square	156	16.8
Chips	¼ cup (1½ oz.)	207	31.7
Sweetened, *German's*	1 oz. square	158	17.3
(Hershey's):			
Bitter or unsweetened	1 oz.	190	7.0
Sweetened:			
Dark chips, regular or mini	1 oz.	151	17.8
Milk, chips	1 oz.	150	18.0
Semi-sweet, chips	1 oz.	147	17.3
(Nestlé):			
Bitter or unsweetened, *Choco-bake*	1-oz. packet	180	8.0
Sweet or semi-sweet, morsels	1 oz.	150	17.0
CHOCOLATE DRINK:			
Canned (Yoo-hoo)	8 fl. oz	130	28.0
*Mix (Lucerne)	8 fl. oz	240	32.0
CHOCOLATE ICE CREAM (See **ICE CREAM,** Chocolate)			
CHOCOLATE SYRUP (See **SYRUP,** Chocolate)			
CHOP SUEY:			
Home recipe (USDA) with meat	1 cup (8.8 oz.)	300	12.8
Frozen:			
(Stouffer's) beef, with rice	12-oz. pkg.	340	43.0
CHOWDER (See **SOUP,** Chowder)			
CHOW CHOW (USDA):			
Sour	1 cup (8.5 oz.)	70	9.8
Sweet	1 cup (8.6 oz.)	284	66.2

Food	Measure	Cals.	Carbs.
CHOW MEIN:			
Canned:			
(Chun King) Divider-pak:			
Beef	¼ of pkg.	91	11.6
Chicken	½ of 24-oz. pkg.	110	12.7
Pork	¼ of pkg.	116	11.2
Shrimp	¼ of pkg.	91	13.0
(La Choy):			
Regular:			
Beef	7 oz.	60	6.0
Chicken	7 oz.	70	6.0
Meatless	¾ cup	35	6.0
Shrimp	¾ cup	45	4.0
*Bi-pack:			
Beef	¾ cup	70	8.0
Beef pepper oriental or			
shrimp	¾ cup	80	10.0
Chicken	¾ cup	80	8.0
Pork	¾ cup	80	7.0
Vegetable	¾ cup	50	8.0
Frozen:			
(Armour) *Dining Lite*,			
chicken, & rice	9-oz. meal	180	31.0
*(Chun King) chicken	13-oz. entree	370	53.0
(Empire Kosher)	7½-oz. serving	97	12.0
(Healthy Choice) chicken	8½-oz. meal	220	31.0
(La Choy):			
Chicken:			
Dinner	12-oz. dinner	260	44.0
Entree	⅔ cup	90	11.0
Shrimp:			
Dinner	12-oz. dinner	220	47.0
Entree	¾ cup	70	11.0
(Morton) chicken, light:			
Dinner	11-oz. meal	260	43.0
Entree	8-oz. meal	210	35.0
(Stouffer's):			
Regular, chicken	8-oz. pkg.	130	11.0
Lean Cuisine, chicken,			
with rice	11¼-oz. serving	250	36.0
*Mix (Betty Crocker)	¼ pkg.	260	43.0
CHOW MEIN SEASONING			
MIX (Kikkoman)	1⅛-oz. pkg.	98	13.8
CHURCH'S FRIED CHICKEN:			
Biscuit	2.1-oz. serving	250	25.6

Food	Measure	Cals.	Carbs.
Chicken:			
Breast:			
Boneless	2.8-oz. serving	200	4.3
Fried	4.3-oz. serving	278	9.0
Breast & wing, fried	4.8-oz. serving	303	9.0
Leg:			
Regular	2.9-oz. serving	147	5.0
Boneless	2-oz. serving	140	2.4
Thigh:			
Regular	4.2-oz. serving	306	9.0
Boneless	2.8-oz. serving	230	5.3
Wing, boneless	3.1-oz. serving	250	7.7
Chicken fillet, breast:			
Plain	1 serving	608	46.0
Cheese	1 serving	661	47.0
Coleslaw	3-oz. serving	92	8.4
Corn on the cob:			
Plain	5.7-oz. serving	190	32.4
With butter oil	1 serving	237	33.0
Fish fillet:			
Plain	1 serving	430	45.0
Cheese	1 serving	483	46.0
Frozen dessert	1 serving	180	27.0
Hot dog:			
Regular:			
Cheese	1 serving	330	21.0
Chili	1 scrving	320	23.0
Super:			
Regular	1 serving	520	44.0
Cheese	1 serving	580	45.0
Chili	1 serving	570	47.0
Hushpuppy	1 piece	78	11.5
Okra	2.8-oz. serving	210	19.1
Onion rings	1 serving	280	30.0
Pie, apple	3.1-oz. serving	280	40.5
Potatoes:			
French fries	regular order (2.7 oz.)	210	28.5
Mashed, with gravy	3.7-oz. serving	90	14.0
Rice, cajun	3.1-oz. serving	130	15.6

CINNAMON, GROUND

(French's)	1 tsp. (1.7 grams)	6	1.4

CINNAMON SUGAR

(French's)	1 tsp. (4.3 grams)	16	4.0

Food	Measure	Cals.	Carbs.
CINNAMON TOAST CRUNCH, cereal (General Mills)	¾ cup (1 oz.)	120	22.0
CITRON, candied (S&W)	1 piece	2	.6
CITRUS COOLER DRINK, canned (Hi-C)	6 fl. oz.	95	23.3
CITRUS DRINK, chilled or *frozen (Five Alive)	6 fl. oz.	87	21.8
CITRUS JUICE, canned (Santa Cruz), natural, organic	8 fl. oz.	125	29.0
CITRUS PUNCH, canned or chilled (Minute Maid)	6 fl. oz.	90	23.0
CLAM:			
Raw (USDA):			
Hard or round:			
Meat & liq.	1 lb. (weighed in shell)	71	6.1
Meat only	1 cup (8 oz.)	182	13.4
Soft:			
Meat & liq.	1 lb. (weighed in shell)	142	5.3
Meat only	1 cup (8 oz.)	186	3.0
Canned:			
(Doxsee):			
Chopped or minced:			
Drained solids	½ cup	97	1.9
Solids & liq.	½ cup	59	3.2
Whole:			
Drained solids	½ cup	97	1.9
Solids & liq.	½ cup	58	3.1
(Gorton's) minced, drained solids	1 can	140	8.0
(Progresso) minced	½ cup	70	2.0
Frozen:			
(Gorton's) fried strips, crunchy	3½ oz.	330	24.0
(Matlaw's) stuffed	1 clam	90	10.0
(Mrs. Paul's) fried, light	2½-oz. serving	200	21.0
CLAMATO COCKTAIL (Mott's)	6 fl. oz.	96	23.0

Food	Measure	Cals.	Carbs.
CLAM JUICE (USDA)	½ cup	23	2.5
CLARET WINE:			
(Gold Seal) 12% alcohol	3 fl. oz.	82	.4
(Taylor) 12.5% alcohol	3 fl. oz.	72	2.4
CLUSTERS, cereal			
(General Mills)	½ cup (1 oz.)	110	20.0
COBBLER:			
Non-frozen (Awrey's) deep dish:			
Apple	⅛ of pkg.	320	48.0
Blueberry	⅛ of pkg.	310	45.0
Frozen (Pet-Ritz):			
Apple	4.3-oz. serving	290	50.0
Blackberry crumb	4.3-oz. serving	260	45.0
Blueberry	4.3-oz. serving	370	50.0
Peach	4.3-oz. serving	300	48.0
Strawberry	4.3-oz. serving	290	50.0
COCKTAIL (See individual listings)			
COCKTAIL MIX (See individual listings such as **PIÑA COLADA COCKTAIL** or **WHISKEY SOUR COCKTAIL**)			
COCOA:			
Dry, unsweetened:			
(USDA):			
Low fat	1 T. (5 grams)	10	3.1
High fat	1 T. (5 grams)	14	2.8
(Hershey's) American process	1 T. (5 grams)	22	2.3
Mix, regular:			
(Carnation) all flavors	1-oz. pkg.	110	23.0
(Hershey's)	1 T.	27	5.7
(Nestlé)	1¼ oz.	150	26.0
(Ovaltine) hot'n rich	1 oz.	120	22.0
Swiss Miss:			
Regular:			
Double rich	1 envelope	110	19.1
Milk chocolate or with mini marshmallows	1 envelope or 3-4 heaping tsps.	110	20.0

Food	Measure	Cals.	Carbs.
European creme:			
Amaretto or chocolate	1 envelope	150	29.0
Creme de menthe	1¼-oz. envelope	145	25.0
Mocha	1¼-oz. envelope	140	24.0
Mix, dietetic:			
(Carnation):			
70 Calorie	¾-oz. packet	70	15.0
Sugar free	.5-oz. envelope	50	8.0
*(Estee)	6 fl. oz.	50	9.0
(Lucerne)	1 envelope	50	8.0
(Ovaltine) reduced calorie	.45-oz. envelope	50	8.0
Swiss Miss:			
Lite	1 envelope	70	17.0
Milk chocolate	.5-oz. envelope	50	10.0
With sugar-free mini			
marshmallows	.5-oz. envelope	50	9.0
(Weight Watchers)	1 envelope	60	10.0
COCOA KRISPIES, cereal			
(Kellogg's)	¾ cup (1 oz.)	110	25.0
COCOA PUFFS, cereal			
(General Mills)	1 cup (1 oz.)	110	25.0
COCONUT:			
Fresh (USDA):			
Whole	1 lb. (weighed in shell)	816	22.2
Meat only	4 oz.	392	10.7
Grated or shredded, loosely packed	½ cup (1.4 oz.)	225	6.1
Dried, canned or packaged:			
(Baker's):			
Angel Flake:			
Packaged in bag	⅓ cup (.9 oz.)	118	10.6
Canned	⅓ cup (.9 oz.)	120	10.4
Cookie cut	⅓ cup (1.3 oz.)	186	17.1
Premium shred	⅓ cup (1 oz.)	138	12.4
Southern style	⅓ cup (.9 oz.)	118	10.3
(Town House) flakes or shredded	1 oz.	150	12.0
COCONUT, CREAM OF, canned:			
(Coco Lopez)	1 T.	60	10.0
(Holland House)	1 oz.	81	18.0

Food	Measure	Cals.	Carbs.
COCONUT NECTAR, canned			
(Knudsen & Sons)	8 fl. oz.	150	29.0
COCO WHEATS, cereal (Little			
Crow):			
Regular	1 T. (.42 oz.)	43	9.3
Instant	1¼-oz. serving	130	29.0
COD:			
(USDA):			
Raw, meat only	4 oz.	88	0.0
Broiled	4 oz.	193	0.0
Dehydrated, lightly salted	4 oz.	425	0.0
Frozen:			
(Captain's Choice) fillet	3-oz. fillet	89	0.0
(Frionor) *Norway Gourmet*	4-oz. fillet	70	0.0
(Gorton's) *Fishmarket Fresh*	5 oz.	110	0.0
(National Sea Products):			
Plain	5 oz. raw	110	0.0
Butter crumb, center cut or			
loin	5 oz. raw	160	4.0
Lemon pepper crumb, cen-			
ter cut or loin	5 oz. raw	170	6.0
Marinara crumb, center cut			
or loin	5 oz. raw	160	5.0
(Van de Kamp's) *Today's*			
Catch	4 oz.	80	0.0
COD DINNER OR ENTREE,			
Frozen:			
(Armour) *Dinner Classics,*			
almondine	12-oz. meal	360	33.0
(Mrs. Paul's) fillet, light	1 piece	240	22.0
(Frionor) *Norway Gourmet:*			
With dill sauce	4½-oz. fillet	80	1.0
With toasted bread crumbs	4½-oz. fillet	160	3.0
COD LIVER OIL			
(Hain) regular, cherry or mint	1 T.	120	0.0
COFFEE:			
Regular:			
*Max-Pax; Maxwell House			
Electra Perk; Yuban,*			
Yuban Electra Matic	6 fl. oz.	2	0.0
Mellow Roast	6 fl. oz.	8	2.0

Food	Measure	Cals.	Carbs.
Decaffeinated:			
*Brim, regular or electric perk	6 fl. oz.	2	0.0
*Brim, freeze-dried; Decaf; Nescafe	6 fl. oz.	4	1.0
*Sanka, regular or electric perk	6 fl. oz.	2	0.0
Instant:			
(Maxwell House)	6 fl. oz.	4	1.0
*Mellow Roast	6 fl. oz.	8	2.0
*Sunrise	6 fl. oz.	6	1.0
*Mix (General Foods)			
International Coffee:			
Café Amaretto	6 fl. oz.	59	7.0
Café Français	6 fl. oz.	59	6.6
Café Vienna, Orange Cappuccino	6 fl. oz.	65	10.3
Irish Mocha Mint	6 fl. oz.	55	7.4
Suisse Mocha	6 fl. oz.	58	7.6
COFFEE CAKE (See **CAKE**, Coffee)			
COFFEE LIQUEUR			
(DeKuyper)	1 fl. oz.	93	12.4
COFFEE SOUTHERN	1 fl. oz.	79	8.8
COGNAC (See **DISTILLED LIQUOR**)			
COLA SOFT DRINK (See **SOFT DRINK**, Cola)			
COLD DUCK WINE (Great Western) pink, 12% alcohol	3 fl. oz.	92	7.7
COLESLAW, solids & liq. (USDA):			
Prepared with commercial French dressing	4-oz. serving	108	8.6
Prepared with homemade French dressing	4-oz. serving	146	5.8
Prepared with mayonnaise	4-oz. serving	163	5.4
Prepared with mayonnaise type salad dressing	1 cup (4.2 oz.)	119	8.5

Food	Measure	Cals.	Carbs.
*COLESLAW MIX (Libby's)			
Super Slaw	½ cup	240	11.0
COLLARDS:			
Raw (USDA):			
Leaves, including stems	1 lb.	181	32.7
Leaves only	½ lb.	70	11.6
Boiled (USDA) drained:			
Leaves, cooked in large amount of water	½ cup (3.4 oz.)	29	4.6
Leaves & stems, cooked in small amount of water	½ cup (3.4 oz.)	31	4.8
Canned (Allen's) chopped, solids & liq.	½ cup (4.1 oz.)	25	2.0
Frozen, chopped:			
(Bel-Air)	3.3 oz.	25	4.0
(Birds Eye)	⅓ pkg. (3.3 oz.)	31	4.4
(Frosty Acres)	3.3-oz. serving	25	4.0
(McKenzie)	⅓ pkg. (3.3 oz.)	25	4.0
CONCORD WINE (Gold Seal)			
13–14% alcohol	3 fl. oz.	125	9.8
COOKIE:			
Home recipe (USDA):			
Brownie with nuts	1¾" × 1¾" × ⅞"	97	10.2
Chocolate chip	1 oz.	146	17.0
Sugar, soft, thick	1 oz.	126	19.3
Frozen:			
(Pepperidge Farm) classic, hot fudge	1 piece	370	46
(Weight Watchers) *Sweet Celebrations*:			
À la mode	1 piece	180	35.0
Chocolate	1 piece	100	16.0
Swiss mocha fudge	1 piece	90	18.0
Packaged:			
Almond toast (Stella D'oro)	1 piece	60	10.0
Angel bar (Stella D'oro)	1 piece	80	7.0
Angelic Goodies (Stella D'oro)	1 piece	110	16.0
Angel wings (Stella D'oro)	1 piece	70	7.0
Anginetti (Stella D'oro)	1 piece	30	5.0
Animal:			
(USDA)	1 piece (3 grams)	11	2.1
(FFV)	1 piece (.1 oz.)	14	3.0

Food	Measure	Cals.	Carbs.
(Gerber)	.2-oz. piece	30	5.0
(Nabisco) *Barnum's Animals*	1 piece	12	1.9
(Ralston)	1 piece (2 grams)	8	1.5
(Sunshine)	1 piece	8	1.4
(Tom's)	1.7 oz.	210	37.0
Anisette sponge (Stella D'oro)	1 piece	50	10.0
Anisette toast (Stella D'oro):			
Regular	1 piece	50	9.0
Jumbo	1 piece	110	23.0
Apple cinnamon bar (Tastykake)	1 piece	180	29.0
Apple cinnamon oat bran (Frookie)	1 piece	45	6.5
Apple Newtons (Nabisco)	1 piece	73	14.0
Apple N' Raisin (Archway)	1 cookie	120	20.0
Apple-raisin (Health Valley) Fruit Chunks	1 cookie	80	16.0
Apricot, filled (Archway)	1 piece	110	19.0
Apricot Raspberry (Pepperidge Farm)	1 piece (.4 oz.)	50	7.5
Assortment:			
(Nabisco) Famous:			
Baronet	1 piece	47	6.7
Butter flavor	1 piece	22	3.3
Biscos sugar wafer	1 piece	19	2.5
Cameo creme sandwich	1 piece	47	7.0
Kettle cookie	1 piece	32	5.0
Lorna Doone	1 piece	35	4.5
Oreo, chocolate	1 piece	47	6.7
(Stella D'oro) Hostess or *Lady Stella*	1 piece	40	6.0
Blueberry Newtons (Nabisco)	1 piece	73	14.0
Bordeaux (Pepperidge Farm)	1 piece (7.1 grams)	35	5.5
Breakfast Treats (Stella D'oro)	1 piece	100	15.0
Brown edge wafer (Nabisco)	1 piece (.2 oz.)	28	4.0
Brownie:			
(Little Debbie) fudge	1 piece	310	46.0
(Nabisco) *Almost Home*, fudge & nut	1 piece	160	23.0
(Pepperidge Farm):			
Chocolate nut	.4-oz. piece	55	5.5
Nut, large	.9-oz. piece	140	15.0
(Tastykake) fudge walnut	1 piece	370	52.0

Food	Measure	Cals.	Carbs.
Brussels (Pepperidge Farm):			
Regular	1 piece	55	6.5
Mint	1 piece	65	8.5
Butter flavored:			
(Nabisco)	1 piece (.2 oz.)	22	3.3
(Sunshine)	1 piece (.2 oz.)	30	4.5
Cappuccino (Pepperidge Farm)	9 grams	50	6.0
Capri (Pepperidge Farm)	1 piece (.5 oz.)	80	10.0
Caramel Patties (FFV)	1 piece	75	10.0
Carob chip (Health Valley)			
Healthy Chip	1 piece	26	6.0
Cherry Newtons (Nabisco)	1 piece	73	13.3
Chessman (Pepperidge Farm)	1 piece (.3 oz.)	45	6.0
Chinese dessert (Stella D'oro)	1 piece	170	20.0
Chocolate & chocolate-covered:			
(Keebler)			
Fudge strips	1 piece (.4 oz.)	50	7.0
(Nabisco):			
Famous wafer	1 piece (.2 oz.)	22	5.2
Pinwheel, cake	1 piece (1.1 oz.)	130	20.0
Snap	1 piece (.14 oz.)	19	3.0
(Sunshine) nuggets	1 piece	23	3.3
Chocolate chip or chunk:			
(Archway) & toffee	.1-oz. piece	150	21.0
(Frookie) regular,			
Mandarin or mint	1 piece	45	6.5
(Keeblcr):			
Chips deluxe	1 piece (.5 oz.)	90	10.0
Rich 'n chips	1 piece (.5 oz.)	80	10.0
(Nabisco):			
Almost Home, fudge or real	1 piece (.5 oz.)	65	10.0
Chips Ahoy!:			
Regular	1 piece (.3 oz.)	47	6.0
Chewy	1 piece (.5 oz.)	65	9.0
Chips 'n More:			
Coconut	1 piece (.5 oz.)	75	9.0
Fudge	1 piece (.3 oz.)	47	6.3
Original	1 piece (.5 oz.)	75	9.0
Snaps	1 piece (.2 oz.)	22	3.5
(Pepperidge Farm):			
Regular	1 piece (.3 oz.)	50	6.0
Chesapeake, with pecans	1 piece	120	14.0
Family Request	1 piece	45	7.5
Nantucket	1 piece	120	15.0

Food	Measure	Cals.	Carbs.
Pecan	1 piece	70	8.0
Mocha	1 piece	40	5.3
(Sunshine):			
Chip-A-Roos:			
Regular	1 piece (.5 oz.)	60	8.0
Chocolate	1 piece (.5 oz.)	60	7.0
Chippy Chews	1 piece	50	8.0
(Tom's)	1.7-oz. serving	230	34.0
Chocolate peanut bar (Nabisco) Ideal	1 piece (.6 oz.)	75	8.5
Cinnamon raisin (Nabisco) *Almost Home*	1 piece (.5 oz.)	70	8.0
Coconut fudge (FFV)	1 piece	80	10.0
Como Delights (Stella D'oro)	1 piece	150	18.0
Danish (Nabisco) imported	1 piece (.2 oz.)	30	3.6
Date pecan (Pepperidge Farm)	1 piece (.4 oz.)	55	7.5
Devil's food cake (Nabisco)	1 piece	140	30.0
Dinosaurs (FFV)	1 oz.	130	20.0
Dutch apple bar (Stella D'oro)	1 piece	110	19.0
Dutch cocoa (Archway)	1 piece	110	19.0
Egg biscuit (Stella D'oro):			
Regular	1 piece	80	14.0
Roman	1 piece	140	20.0
Fig bar:			
(FFV)	1 piece	70	12.0
(Nabisco) *Fig Newtons*	1 piece (.5 oz.)	50	10.0
(Sunshine) Chewies	1 piece (.5 oz.)	50	11.0
(Tom's) bar	1 oz.	100	21.0
Frookwich (Frookie):			
Chips & creme & vanilla sandwich	1 piece	50	7.0
Chocolate sandwich	1 piece	50	7.0
Lemon sandwich	1 piece	50	7.0
PB	1 piece	50	7.0
Fruitins (Frookie) Apple	1 piece	50	11.0
Fruit stick (Nabisco) *Almost Home*	1 piece (.7 oz.)	70	14.0
Fudge (Stella D'oro):			
Deep night	1 piece	65	8.0
Swiss	1 piece	70	9.0
Fudge bar (Tastykake)	1 piece	190	29.0
Funky Monkeys (Frookie):			
Chocolate	1 piece	7	1.2
Vanilla	1 piece	7	1.2

Food	Measure	Cals.	Carbs.
Geneva (Pepperidge Farm)	1 piece (.4 oz.)	65	7.0
Gingerboys (FFV)	1 oz.	120	20.0
Gingerman (Pepperidge Farm)	1 piece	35	5.0
Gingersnap:			
(Archway)	1 piece (.5oz.)	25	4.0
(FFV)	1 oz.	130	22.0
(Nabisco)	1 piece	30	5.5
(Sunshine)	1 piece (.2 oz.)	20	3.0
Golden bars (Stella D'oro)	1 piece	110	16.0
Golden fruit raisin (Sunshine)	1 piece (smallest portion after breaking on scoreline) (.6 oz.)	70	14.0
Hazelnut (Pepperidge Farm)	1 piece (.4 oz.)	55	7.5
Heyday (Nabisco)	1 piece	140	15.0
Jelly tart (FFV)	1 piece	60	11.0
Ladyfinger (USDA)	3¼" × 1⅜" × 1⅛" (.4 oz.)	40	7.1
Lemon (Archway)	1 piece	155	23.0
Lemon Cooler (Sunshine)	1 piece (.2 oz.)	30	4.3
Lemon nut crunch (Pepperidge Farm)	1 piece (.4 oz.)	55	6.5
Lido (Pepperidge Farm)	1 piece (.6 oz.)	90	10.0
Linzer (Pepperidge Farm)	1 piece	120	20.0
Macaroon (Nabisco) soft	1 piece	190	23.0
Mallo Puffs (Sunshine)	1 piece (.6 oz.)	70	12.0
Margherite (Stella D'oro)	1 piece	70	10.0
Marshmallow:			
(Nabisco):			
Mallomars	1 piece (.5 oz.)	65	9.0
Puffs, cocoa covered	1 piece (.1 oz.)	120	20.0
Sandwich	1 piece (.3 oz.)	30	5.5
Twirls cakes	1 piece (1 oz.)	130	19.0
(Planters) banana pie	1 oz.	127	22.0
Milano (Pepperidge Farm)	1 piece (.4 oz.)	75	8.5
Mint fudge (FFV)	1 piece	80	11.0
Molasses (Nabisco) *Pantry*	1 piece (.5 oz.)	65	10.5
Molasses crisp (Pepperidge Farm)	1 piece (.2 oz.)	35	4.0
Nassau (Pepperidge Farm)	1 piece (.5 oz.)	80	9.0
Nilla wafer (Nabisco)	1 piece (.1 oz.)	19	3.0
Oatmeal:			
(Archway):			
Regular	1 piece	110	19.0
Apple bran	1 piece	107	18.0

Food	Measure	Cals.	Carbs.
Apple filled	1 piece	90	18.0
Date filled, raisin or raisin bran	1 piece	100	18.0
Golden, *Ruth's*	1 piece	120	20.0
Iced	1 piece	140	22.0
(FFV):			
Regular	1 piece	26	4.0
Bar	1 piece	70	11.0
(Frookie) raisin or 7-grain	1 piece	45	6.5
(Keebler) old fashioned	1 piece (18 grams)	80	12.0
(Nabisco) *Bakers Bonus*	1 piece (.5 oz.)	65	10.0
Cookie Little	1 piece (.1 oz.)	6	1.0
(Pepperidge Farm):			
Irish	1 piece	45	6.5
Milk chocolate, Dakota	1 piece	110	15.0
Raisin:			
Regular	1 piece	55	7.5
Santa Fe	1 piece	100	16.0
(Sunshine):			
Country style	1 piece	60	8.0
Peanut sandwich	1 piece	70	9.0
Orbits (Sunshine):			
Butter flavored	1 piece	15	2.5
Chocolate	1 piece	15	2.3
Orleans (Pepperidge Farm) regular	1 piece (.2 oz.)	30	3.6
Peanut & peanut butter: (Nabisco):			
Almost Home	1 piece	70	8.0
Nutter Butter:			
Creme pattie	1 piece (.3 oz.)	37	4.3
Sandwich	1 piece (.5 oz.)	70	9.0
(Sunshine) wafer	1 piece	40	5.0
Pecan Sandies (Keebler)	1 piece (16 grams)	80	9.0
Pfeffernusse (Stella D'oro)	1 piece	40	7.0
Pirouettes (Pepperidge Farm)	1 piece	35	4.5
Praline Pecan (FFV)	1 piece	40	10.0
Raisin (USDA)	1 oz.	107	22.9
Raisin bran (Pepperidge Farm)	1 piece (.4 oz.)	53	6.5
Rocky road (Archway)	1 piece	130	20.0
Royal Dainty (FFV)	1 piece	60	7.0
Royal Nuggets (Stella D'oro)	1 piece	2	.1
Sandwich:			

Food	Measure	Cals.	Carbs.
(Keebler):			
Fudge creme	1 piece (12 grams)	60	8.0
Oatmeal cream	(.5 oz.)	80	11.0
Pitter Patter	1 piece (17 grams)	90	11.0
(Nabisco):			
Almost Home	1 piece	140	20.0
Baronet	1 piece (.3 oz.)	47	6.7
Cameo	1 piece (.3 oz.)	47	7.0
Gaity, fudge chocolate	1 piece (.3 oz.)	50	6.3
Giggles	1 piece (.3 oz.)	70	8.5
I Screams	1 piece (.5 oz.)	75	10.0
Mystic Mint	1 piece (.5 oz.)	75	9.5
Oreo:			
Regular	1 piece (.3 oz.)	47	6.7
Double Stuf	1 piece (.5 oz.)	70	9.5
Mini	1 piece	14	2.0
Mint	1 piece (.5 oz.)	70	10.0
Vanilla, *Cookie Break*	1 piece (.3 oz.)	47	6.7
(Sunshine):			
Regular:			
Chocolate fudge or cup custard	1 piece (.5 oz.)	70	9.0
Hydrox	1 piece (.4 oz.)	50	7.0
Vienna Fingers	1 piece	70	11.0
Chips 'n Middles:			
Fudge	1 piece (.5 oz.)	70	10.0
Peanut butter	1 piece (.5 oz.)	70	9.0
Tru Blue, any flavor	1 piece (.6 oz.)	80	11.0
Sesame (Stella D'oro)			
Regina	1 piece	50	6.0
Shortbread or shortcake:			
(FFV) country	1 piece	70	9.0
(Nabisco):			
Fudge striped	1 piece	50	6.3
Lorna Doone	1 piece (.3 oz.)	35	4.5
Pecan	1 piece (.5 oz.)	75	8.0
(Pepperidge Farm):			
Regular	1 piece	75	8.5
Pecan	1 piece	70	7.0
Social Tea, biscuit (Nabisco)	1 piece	22	3.5
Sprinkles (Sunshine)	1 piece (.6 oz.)	70	12.0
Strawberry (Pepperidge Farm)	1 piece (.4 oz.)	50	7.5
Sugar:			
(Nabisco) rings, *Bakers Bonus*	1 piece (.5 oz.)	65	10.0

Food	Measure	Cals.	Carbs.
(Pepperidge Farm)	1 piece (.4 oz.)	50	6.5
Sugar wafer:			
(Dutch Twin) any flavor	1 piece (.3 oz.)	36	4.7
(Nabisco) *Biscos*	1 piece (.1 oz.)	19	2.5
(Sunshine)	1 piece (.3 oz.)	45	6.0
Super Heroes (Nabisco)	1 piece (.1 oz.)	12	1.8
Tahiti (Pepperidge Farm)	1 piece (.5 oz.)	90	9.0
Tango (FFV)	1 piece	80	13.0
Toy (Sunshine)	1 piece (.1 oz.)	12	2.0
Trolley Cakes (FFV)	1 piece	60	12.5
Vanilla wafer (Keebler)	1 piece (4 grams)	20	2.7
Waffle creme:			
(Dutch Twin)	1 piece (.3 oz.)	45	5.7
(Nabisco)	1 piece (.3 oz.)	50	6.7
Zanzibar (Pepperidge Farm)	1 piece (.3 oz.)	40	4.3

COOKIE, DIETETIC:

Food	Measure	Cals.	Carbs.
Apple pastry (Stella D'oro)	1 piece	90	14.0
Apple raisin bar (Weight Watchers)	1 piece	100	18.0
Apple spice (Frookie) fat free	1 piece	50	11.0
Banana (Frookie) fat free	1 piece	45	10.0
Brownie:			
(Entenmann's) fat free	1/10 strip	110	27.0
(Little Debbie) low fat	1 piece	190	39.0
Chocolate chip:			
(Estee)	1 piece	30	4.0
(Nabisco) *SnackWells*, bite size, reduced fat	1 piece	10	1.6
Coconut:			
(Estee)	1 piece	30	4.0
(Stella D'oro)	1 piece	50	6.0
Devil's food cookie cake (Nabisco) *SnackWells*	1 piece	50	13.0
Egg biscuit (Stella D'oro)	1 piece	40	7.0
Fruit filled (Health Valley) mini fruit center, fat free	1 piece	14	2.0
Fruit & honey (Entenmann's) fat & cholesterol free	1 piece	40	9.0
Fruitins (Frookie) fat free	1 piece	45	10.5
Fudge (Estee)	1 piece	30	4.0
Kichel (Stella D'oro)	1 piece	8	.7
Lemon (Estee) thin	1 piece (.2 oz.)	30	4.0
Oatmeal raisin:			

Food	Measure	Cals.	Carbs.
(Entenmann's) fat & choles-			
terol free	1 piece (.4 oz.)	40	8.5
(Estee)	1 piece (.2 oz.)	30	4.0
(Frookie) raisin, fat free	1 piece	50	11.0
(Nabisco) *SnackWells*	1 piece	55	10.0
Peach apricot pastry (Stella D'oro)	1 piece	90	13.0
Prune pastry (Stella D'oro)	1 piece	90	13.0
Sandwich:			
(Estee)	1 piece	45	6.0
(Nabisco) *SnackWells*:			
Chocolate with chocolate creme, reduced fat	1 piece	50	10.0
Creme, reduced fat	1 piece	55	10.5
Sesame (Stella D'oro)			
Regina	1 piece	40	6.0
Wafer, chocolate-covered (Estee)	1 piece (.85 oz.)	130	14.0
Wafer, creme filled (Estee):			
Assorted	1 piece	20	3.0
Chocolate or vanilla	1 piece	20	3.0
COOKIE CRISP, cereal (Ralston Purina) any flavor	1 cup (1 oz.)	110	25.0
*COOKIE DOUGH:			
Refrigerated (Pillsbury):			
Brownie, fudge microwave	⅑ of pkg.	70	9.0
Chocolate chip or sugar	1 cookie	70	9.0
Peanut butter	1 cookie	70	8.0
Frozen (Rich's):			
Chocolate chip	1 cookie	138	20.3
Oatmeal	1 cookie	125	18.3
Oatmeal & raisins	1 cookie	122	19.1
Peanut butter	1 cookie	128	14.6
Sugar	1 cookie	118	17.4
COOKIE MIX:			
Regular:			
Brownie:			
*(Betty Crocker):			
Regular:			
Chocolate chip	¹⁄₂₄ of pan	140	20.0
Frosted	¹⁄₂₄ of pan	160	26.0
Fudge:			
Regular size	¹⁄₁₆ of pan	150	23.0

Food	*Measure*	*Cals.*	*Carbs.*
Family size	1/24 of pan	140	22.0
Supreme	1/24 of pan	120	21.0
German chocolate	1/24 of pan	160	24.0
Walnut	1/16 of pan	140	18.0
MicroRave:			
Frosted	1 piece	180	27.0
Fudge	1 piece	150	22.0
Walnut	1 piece	160	21.0
(Duncan Hines):	1/24 of pkg.	119	22.0
Chewey recipe	1/24 of pkg.	98	17.9
Fudge, original	1/24 of pkg.	122	22.4
Milk chocolate	1/24 of pkg.	128	22.1
Peanut butter	1/24 of pkg.	120	16.6
Truffle	1/16 of pkg.	200	32.4
Turtle	1/16 of pkg.	166	32.4
*(Pillsbury) fudge:			
Deluxe:			
Plain	1/16 of pkg.	150	21.0
Family size	1/24 of pkg.	150	20.0
With walnuts	1/16 of pkg.	150	19.0
Microwave	1/9 of pkg.	190	25.0
Ultimate:			
Caramel chunk or chunky triple	1/16 of pkg.	170	25.0
Double	1/16 of pkg.	160	24.0
Rocky road	1/16 of pkg.	170	24.0
**Robin Hood* (General Mills) fudge	1/16 of pkg.	100	16.0
Chocolate (Duncan Hines) double	1/36 of pkg.	67	9.2
Chocolate chip:			
*(Betty Crocker) *Big Batch*	1 cookie	60	8.0
(Duncan Hines)	1/36 of pkg.	73	9.2
Date bar (Betty Crocker)	1/24 of pkg.	60	9.0
Oatmeal (Duncan Hines) raisin	1/36 of pkg.	68	9.1
Peanut butter (Duncan Hines)	1/36 pkg.	68	7.5
Sugar (Duncan Hines) golden	1/36 of pkg.	59	8.4
*Dietetic (Estee) brownie	2" × 2"-sq. cookie	50	8.0
COOKING SPRAY:			
Mazola No Stick	2½-second spray	6	0.0
Pam	1-second spray	2	0.0

Food	Measure	Cals.	Carbs.
(Weight Watchers) any type	1-second spray	2	0.0
Wesson Lite	2-second spray	<1	0.0
CORIANDER SEED (French's)	1 tsp. (1.4 grams)	6	.8
CORN:			
Fresh, white or yellow (USDA):			
Raw:			
Untrimmed, on the cob	1 lb. (weighed in husk)	167	36.1
Trimmed, on cob	1 lb. (husk removed)	240	55.1
Boiled:			
Kernels, cut from cob, drained	1 cup (5.8 oz.)	137	31.0
Whole	4.9-oz. ear (5" × 1¾")	70	16.2
Trimmed, on the cob	5" × 1¾" ear	70	16.2
Canned, regular pack: (USDA):			
Golden or yellow, whole kernel, solids & liq., vacuum pack	½ cup (3.7 oz.)	87	21.6
Golden or yellow, whole kernel, wet pack	½ cup (4.5 oz.)	84	20.1
Golden or yellow, whole kernel, drained solids, wet pack	½ cup (3 oz.)	72	16.4
White kernel, drained solids	½ cup (2.8 oz.)	70	16.4
White, whole kernel, drained liq., wet pack	4 oz.	29	7.8
Cream style	½ cup (4.4 oz.)	105	25.6
(Allen's) whole kernel, golden	½ cup (4.2 oz.)	80	3.0
(Green Giant) solids & liq.:			
Cream style	½ cup	100	24.0
Whole kernel or shoe peg, golden	4¼ oz.	90	18.0
Whole kernel, vacuum pack	½ cup	80	16.0
Whole kernel, *Mexicorn*	3½ oz.	80	19.0
Whole kernel, white, vacuum pack	½ cup	80	20.0
(Larsen) *Freshlike:*			
Whole kernel, vacuum pack	½ cup (3.9 oz.)	100	22.0

Food	Measure	Cals.	Carbs.
Whole kernel, vacuum pack, with pepper	½ cup (4 oz.)	90	23.0
(Pathmark):			
Cream style, No Frills	½ cup	105	25.5
Golden	½ cup	50	12.5
Vacuum pack	½ cup	60	12.5
Whole kernel, No Frills	½ cup	80	19.0
(Stokely-Van Camp) solids & liq.:			
Cream style, golden	½ cup (4.5 oz.)	105	23.5
Cream style, white	½ cup (4.6 oz.)	110	24.5
Whole kernel, golden	½ cup	90	19.5
(S&W):			
Cream style, *Premium Homestyle*:			
No added starch	½ cup	120	24.0
Starch added	½ cup	105	25.0
White, premium	½ cup	90	20.0
(Town House):			
Cream style	½ cup	80	18.0
Whole kernel	½ cup	70	17.0
Canned, dietetic pack, solids & liq.:			
(Diet Delight) whole kernel	½ cup	60	15.0
(Green Giant)	½ cup	80	18.0
(Larsen) *Fresh-Lite*, whole kernel, no salt added	½ cup (4.5 oz.)	80	19.0
(Pathmark) No Frills, no salt added	½ cup	70	8.0
Frozen:			
(Bel-Air):			
On the cob:			
Regular	1 ear	120	29.0
Short ears	1 ear	65	15.0
Whole kernel	3.3 oz.	80	20.0
(Birds Eye):			
On the cob:			
Regular	4.4-oz. ear	120	28.7
Big Ears	5.7-oz. ear	156	37.0
Little Ears	4.6-oz. ear	126	30.0
Whole kernel:			
Cob corn, deluxe baby	⅓ of 8-oz. pkg.	23	4.0
Deluxe, petite	⅓ of 8-oz. pkg.	66	1.6
Sweet:			
Regular	¼ of 12-oz. pkg.	74	18.0
Butter sauce	⅓ of 10-oz. pkg.	85	17.0
Deluxe, tender	⅓ of 10-oz. pkg.	82	20.0

Food	Measure	Cals.	Carbs.
(Frosty Acres):			
On the cob	1 ear	120	29.0
Whole kernel	3.3-oz. serving	80	20.0
(Green Giant):			
On the cob:			
Nibbler, regular	1 car	60	13.0
Niblet Ear, regular	1 ear	120	26.0
Cream style	½ cup	110	25.0
Whole kernel, *Niblets:*			
In butter sauce, golden	½ cup	100	19.0
Harvest Fresh, golden	3 oz.	80	17.0
Polybag, white	½ cup	70	15.0
(Larsen):			
On the cob:			
3-inch piece	2.2-oz. piece	60	15.0
5-inch piece	4.4-oz. piece	120	29.0
Cut	3.3 oz.	80	20.0
CORNBREAD:			
Home recipe (USDA):			
Corn pone, prepared with white, whole-ground cornmeal	4 oz.	231	41.1
Johnnycake, prepared with yellow, degermed cornmeal	4 oz.	303	51.6
Southern style, prepared with degermed cornmeal	2½" × 2½" × 1⅝" piece	186	28.8
Southern style, prepared with whole-ground cornmeal	4 oz.	235	33.0
Spoon bread, prepared with white, whole-ground cornmeal	4 oz.	221	19.2
*Mix:			
(Aunt Jemima)	⅙ of pkg.	220	34.0
(Dromedary)	2" × 2" piece (¹⁄₁₆ of pkg.)	130	20.0
Gold Medal	⅙ of pkg.	150	22.0
(Pillsbury) *Ballard*	⅛ of recipe	140	25.0
*CORN DOG, frozen:			
(Fred's) *Little Juan*	2¾-oz. serving	231	24.6
(Hormel)	1 piece	220	21.0
CORN DOG BATTER MIX			
(Golden Dipt)	1 oz.	100	22.0

Food	Measure	Cals.	Carbs.
CORNED BEEF:			
Cooked (USDA), boneless, medium fat	4-oz. serving	422	0.0
Canned, regular pack:			
Dinty Moore (Hormel)	2-oz. serving	130	0.0
(Libby's)	⅕ of 12-oz. can	160	2.0
Packaged:			
(Eckrich) sliced	1-oz. slice	40	1.0
(Carl Buddig) smoked, sliced	1 oz.	40	Tr.
(Oscar Mayer)	.6-oz. slice	16	.1
CORNED BEEF HASH, canned:			
(Libby's)	⅓ of 24-oz. can	420	21.0
Mary Kitchen (Hormel)	½ of 15-oz. can	360	19.0
CORNED BEEF SPREAD, canned:			
(Hormel)	1 oz.	70	0.0
(Underwood)	½ of 4½-oz. can	120	Tr.
CORN FLAKE CRUMBS			
(Kellogg's)	¼ cup (1 oz.)	100	24.0
CORN FLAKES, cereal:			
(General Mills) *Country*	1 cup (1 oz.)	110	25.0
(Kellogg's):			
Regular	1 cup (1 oz.)	100	24.0
Sugar Frosted Flakes	¾ cup (1 oz.)	110	26.0
(Malt-O-Meal):			
Plain	1 cup (1 oz.)	106	24.8
Sugar coated	¾ cup (1 oz.)	109	26.0
(Post) *Post Toasties*	1¼ cups (1 oz.)	111	24.0
(Safeway) plain	1 cup (1 oz.)	110	25.0
CORNMEAL, WHITE OR YELLOW:			
Dry:			
Bolted:			
(USDA)	1 cup (4.3 oz.)	442	90.9
(Aunt Jemima/Quaker)	1 cup (4 oz.)	408	84.8
Degermed:			
(USDA)	1 cup (4.9 oz.)	502	108.2
(Aunt Jemima/Quaker)	1 cup (4 oz.)	404	88.8
Self-rising degermed:			
(USDA)	1 cup (5 oz.)	491	105.9
(Aunt Jemima)	1 cup (6 oz.)	582	126.0
Self-rising, whole ground			
(USDA)	1 cup (5 oz.)	489	101.4

Food	Measure	Cals.	Carbs.
Whole ground, unbolted (USDA)	1 cup (4.3 oz.)	433	90.0
Cooked:			
(USDA)	1 cup (8.5 oz.)	120	25.7
(Albers) degermed	1 cup	119	25.5
Mix (Aunt Jemima/Quaker) bolted	1 cup (4 oz.)	392	80.4
CORN POPS, cereal (Kellogg's)	1 cup (1 oz.)	110	26.0
CORN PUDDING, home recipe (USDA)	1 cup (8.6 oz.)	255	31.9
CORN PUREE, canned (Larsen) no salt added	½ cup	100	22.5
CORNSTARCH (Argo; Kingsford's)	1 tsp. (8 grams)	10	8.3
CORN SYRUP (See **SYRUP,** Corn)			
COTTAGE PUDDING, home recipe (USDA):			
Without sauce	2 oz.	180	30.8
With chocolate sauce	2 oz.	195	32.1
With strawberry sauce	2 oz.	166	27.4
COUGH DROP:			
(Beech-Nut)	1 drop	10	2.5
(Pine Bros.)	1 drop	10	2.4
COUNT CHOCULA, cereal (General Mills)	1 oz. (1 cup)	110	24.0
COUSCOUS:			
Dry (Fantastic Foods):			
Regular	¼ cup	210	43.0
Whole wheat	¼ cup	180	42.0
Mix:			
(Casbah):			
Almond chicken	1 pkg.	160	29.0
Asparagus au gratin	1 pkg.	150	28.0
Pilaf	1 oz.	100	20.0
Tomato parmesan	1 pkg.	170	34.0
(Fantastic Foods):			
Black bean salsa	1 pkg.	240	46.0
Cheddar, nacho, cup	1 pkg.	200	36.0
Pilaf, savory	1 pkg.	240	50.0

Food	Measure	Cals.	Carbs.
Vegetable, creole	1 pkg.	220	41.0
*(Near East) Moroccan	½ cup	52	9.2
COWPEA (USDA):			
Immature seeds:			
Raw, whole	1 lb. (weighed in pods)	317	54.4
Raw, shelled	½ cup (2.5 oz.)	92	15.8
Boiled, drained solids	½ cup (2.9 oz.)	89	15.0
Canned, solids & liq.	4 oz.	79	14.1
Frozen (See **BLACK-EYED PEAS,** frozen)			
Young pods with seeds:			
Raw, whole	1 lb. (weighed untrimmed)	182	39.2
Boiled, drained solids	4 oz.	39	7.9
Mature seeds, dry:			
Raw	1 lb.	1556	279.9
Raw	½ cup (3 oz.)	292	52.4
Boiled	½ cup (4.4 oz.)	95	17.2
CRAB:			
Fresh, steamed (USDA):			
Whole	½ lb. (weighed in shell)	202	1.1
Meat only	4 oz.	105	.6
Canned:			
(USDA) drained	4 oz.	115	1.2
(S&W) dungeness	3¼ oz.	81	1.0
Frozen (Wakefield's)	4 oz.	86	.7
CRAB, DEVILED:			
Home recipe (USDA)	4 oz.	213	15.1
Frozen (Mrs. Paul's):			
Regular	1 cake	180	18.0
Miniature	3½ oz.	240	25.0
CRAB, IMITATION			
(Louis Kemp) *Crab Delights,* chunks, flakes or legs	2-oz. serving	60	7.0
CRAB APPLE, flesh only (USDA)	¼ lb.	71	20.2
CRAB APPLE JELLY (Smucker's)	1 T. (.7 oz.)	53	13.5

Food	Measure	Cals.	Carbs.
CRAB CAKE SEASONING			
MIX (Old Bay)	1 pkg.	133	18.0
CRAB IMPERIAL:			
Home recipe (USDA)	1 cup (7.8 oz.)	323	8.6
Frozen (Gorton's) Light			
Recipe, stuffed	1 pkg.	340	36.0
CRACKER CRUMBS, graham:			
(Nabisco)	⅛ of 9" pie shell		
	(2 T.)	60	11.0
(Sunshine)	½ cup	275	47.5
CRACKER MEAL (Nabisco)	2 T.	50	12.0
CRACKERS, PUFFS & CHIPS:			
Animal (FFV)	1 oz.	130	21.0
Arrowroot biscuit (Nabisco)	1 piece (.2 oz.)	22	3.5
Bacon-flavored thins (Nabisco)	1 piece (.1 oz.)	10	1.3
Bravos (Wise)	1 oz.	150	18.0
Bugles (Tom's)	1 oz.	150	18.0
Butter (Pepperidge Farm) thin	1 piece	17	2.5
Cafe Cracker (Sunshine)	1 piece (smallest portion after breaking on scoreline)	20	2.3
Cheese flavored:			
American Heritage (Sunshine):			
Cheddar	1 piece	16	1.6
Parmesan	1 piece	18	1.8
Better Blue Cheese (Nabisco)	1 piece	7	.8
Better Cheddar (Nabisco)	1 piece	6	.7
Better Nacho (Nabisco)	1 piece	8	.9
Better Swiss (Nabisco)	1 piece	7	.8
Cheddar Sticks (Flavor Tree)	1 oz.	160	12.0
Cheese Bites (Tom's)	1½ oz.	200	26.0
Cheese 'n Crunch (Nabisco)	1 piece	4	.4
Cheese Doodles (Wise):			
Crunchy	1 oz.	160	16.0
Fried	1 oz.	150	16.0
Chee-Tos, crunchy or puffy	1 oz.	160	15.0
Cheez Balls (Planters)	1 oz.	160	14.0
Cheez Curls (Planters)	1 oz.	160	14.0
Cheez-It (Sunshine)	1 piece	6	.6
Corn cheese (Tom's):			
Crunchy	⅝ oz.	280	25.0

Food	Measure	Cals.	Carbs.
Puffed, baked	1⅛ oz.	180	18.0
Curls (Old Dutch)	1 oz.	160	14.0
Dip In A Chip (Nabisco)	1 piece (.1 oz.)	9	1.0
(Dixie Belle)	1 piece	6	.7
(Eagle)	1 oz.	130	18.0
Nacho cheese cracker (Old El Paso)	1 oz.	76	15.3
Nips (Nabisco)	1 piece (.04 oz.)	5	.7
(Planters) squares	1 oz.	140	15.0
(Ralston Purina)	1 piece (1.1 grams)	6	.7
Sandwich (Nabisco)	1 piece	35	4.0
Tid-Bit (Nabisco)	1 piece	4	.5
Chicken in a Biskit (Nabisco)	1 piece (.1 oz.)	11	1.1
Chipsters (Nabisco)	1 piece	2	.3
Cinnamon Treats (Nabisco)	1 piece	30	5.5
Classic golden (Nabisco) *SnackWells,* reduced fat	1 piece	10	1.9
Club cracker (Keebler)	1 piece (3.2 grams)	15	2.0
Corn chips:			
Dippy Doodle (Wise)	1 oz.	160	12.0
(Flavor Tree)	1 oz.	150	17.0
Fritos:			
Regular	1 oz.	160	16.0
Barbecue flavor	1 oz.	150	15.5
Happy Heart (TKI Foods)	⅜-oz. pkg.	40	8.0
Heart Lovers (TKI Foods)	⅜-oz. pkg.	40	8.0
(Laura Scudder's)	1 oz.	160	15.0
(Old Dutch)	1 oz.	160	15.0
(Tom's) regular	1 oz.	105	17.0
Corn Smackers (Weight Watchers)	.5-oz. pkg.	60	10.0
Corn Pops (Energy Food Factory) original, fat free or nacho	1 oz.	100	22.0
Corn Stick (Flavor Tree)	1 oz.	160	15.0
Country Cracker (Nabisco)	1 piece	16	1.8
Crown Pilot (Nabisco)	1 piece (.6 oz.)	70	11.0
Diggers (Nabisco)	1 piece	4	.5
Dip In A Chip (Nabisco)	1 piece	9	1.0
Doo Dads (Nabisco)	1 oz.	140	18.0
English Water Biscuit (Pepperidge Farm)	1 piece (.1 oz.)	27	3.2
Escort (Nabisco)	1 piece (.1 oz.)	23	3.0
Flutters (Pepperidge Farm):			
Garden herb	¾ oz.	100	14.0

Food	Measure	Cals.	Carbs.
Golden sesame or toasted wheat	¾ oz.	110	13.0
Original butter	¾ oz.	100	15.0
Goldfish (Pepperidge Farm):			
Thins, cheese	1 piece	12	2.0
Tiny:			
Cheddar cheese or parmesan	1 oz.	120	19.0
Original	1 oz.	130	18.0
Pizza flavored	1 oz.	130	19.0
Pretzel	1 oz.	110	20.0
Graham:			
(Dixie Belle) sugar-honey coated	1 piece	15	2.6
FlavorKist (Schulze and Burch) sugar-honey coated	1 double cracker	57	10.0
Honey Maid (Nabisco)	1 piece (.25 oz.)	30	5.5
(Keebler):			
Cinnamon Crisp	1 piece	17	2.7
Honey coated	1 piece	17	3.0
(Nabisco):			
Party Graham	1 piece	47	6.0
SnackWells, cinnamon snack, reduced fat	1 piece	5	1.3
(Ralston Purina) sugar-honey coated	1 piece	15	2.6
(Rokeach)	8 pieces	120	21.0
(Sunshine):			
Cinnamon	1 piece (.1 oz.)	17	2.8
Honey	1 piece	15	2.5
Graham, chocolate or cocoa-covered (Keebler) deluxe	1 piece (.3 oz.)	40	5.5
Great Crisps (Nabisco):			
Cheese & chive, real bacon, sesame or tomato & celery	1 piece	8	.9
French onion	1 piece	10	1.1
Nacho	1 piece	9	1.0
Savory garlic	1 piece	9	1.1
Great Snackers (Weight Watchers)	.5-oz. pkg.	60	8.0
Hi Ho Crackers (Sunshine)	1 piece	20	2.0
Meal Mates (Nabisco)	1 piece	23	3.0
Melba Toast (See **MELBA TOAST**)			

Food	Measure	Cals.	Carbs.
Nachips (Old El Paso)	1 piece	17	1.7
Nacho Rings (Tom's)	1 oz.	160	15.0
Oat thins (Nabisco)	1 piece (.1 oz.)	9	1.2
Ocean Crisp (FFV)	1 piece	60	10.0
Onion rings (Wise)	1 oz.	130	21.0
Oyster:			
(Dixie Belle)	1 piece (.03 oz.)	4	.6
(Keebler) *Zesta*	1 piece	2	.3
(Nabisco) *Dandy* or			
Oysterettes	1 piece (.03 oz.)	3	.5
(Ralston Purina)	1 piece	4	.6
(Sunshine)	1 piece	4	.6
Party Mix (Flavor Tree)	1 oz.	160	11.0
Peanut butter & cheese (Eagle)	1.8-oz. serving	280	26.0
Pepper (Nabisco) *SnackWells*,			
fat free	1 piece	8	1.8
Pizza Crunchies (Planters)	1 oz.	160	15.0
Potato chips (see **POTATO**			
CHIPS)			
Ritz (Nabisco)	1 piece (.1 oz.)	17	2.3
Ritz Bits (Nabisco):			
Regular, low salt			
or cheese	1 piece	3	.4
Cheese or peanut butter			
sandwich	1 piece	13	1.2
Rich & Crisp (Dixie Bell;			
Ralston Purina)	1 piece	14	1.9
Roman Meal Wafer, boxed	1 piece	11	1.3
Royal Lunch (Nabisco)	1 piece	60	10.0
Rye toast (Keebler)	1 piece	16	2.0
RyKrisp (Ralston Purina):			
Natural	1 triple cracker	20	5.5
Seasoned	1 triple cracker	22	5.5
Saltine:			
(Dixie Belle) regular or			
unsalted	1 piece (.1 oz.)	12	2.0
Flavor Kist (Schulze			
and Burch)	1 piece	12	2.0
Krispy (Sunshine)	1 piece	12	2.2
Premium (Nabisco):			
Regular, low salt,			
unsalted top or whole			
wheat	1 piece	12	2.0
Bits	1 piece	4	.6

Food	Measure	Cals.	Carbs.
(Ralston Purina) regular or			
unsalted	1 piece	12	2.0
(Rokeach)	1 piece	12	2.0
Zesta (Keebler)	1 piece	13	2.1
Schooners (FFV):			
Regular	½ oz.	60	10.0
Whole wheat	½ oz.	70	8.0
Sea Rounds (Nabisco)	1 piece (.5 oz.)	50	10.0
Sesame:			
(Estee)	½ oz.	70	9.0
(Flavor Tree):			
Chip	1 oz.	150	13.0
Crunch	1 oz.	150	10.0
Sticks:			
Plain	1 oz.	150	13.0
With bran	1 oz.	160	11.0
No salt added	1 oz.	160	12.0
(Keebler) toasted	1 piece	16	2.0
(Sunshine) *American Heritage*	1 piece	17	2.0
Sesame wheat (Natures			
Cupboard)	1 piece	11	1.4
Snack Cracker (Rokeach)	1 piece (.1 oz.)	14	2.1
Snackers (Dixie Bell; Ralston			
Purina)	1 piece	17	2.2
Snacks Sticks			
(Pepperidge Farm):			
Cheese, three	1 piece	16	2.4
Pretzel	1 piece	15	2.9
Pumpernickel or			
sesame	1 piece	17	2.5
Sociables (Nabisco)	1 piece	12	1.5
Sour cream & onion stick			
(Flavor Tree)	1 oz.	150	13.0
Spirals (Wise)	1 oz.	160	15.0
Taco chips (Laura Scudder)			
mini	1 oz.	150	17.0
Tortilla chips:			
Doritos, nacho or taco:	1 oz.	140	18.0
Regular or *Salsa Rio*	1 oz.	140	19.0
Cool Ranch:			
Regular	1 oz.	140	18.0
Light	1 oz.	120	21.0
Nacho cheese:			
Regular	1 oz.	140	18.0
Light	1 oz.	120	21.0

Food	Measure	Cals.	Carbs.
Taco	1 oz.	140	18.0
(Eagle)	1 oz.	150	17.0
(Guiltless Gourmet) original, salted or unsalted, nacho or white corn	1 oz.	110	24.0
(Nabisco):			
Nacho	1 piece	12	1.3
Toasted corn	1 piece	11	1.4
(Old Dutch):			
Nacho	1 oz.	156	15.0
Taco	1 oz.	152	15.0
(Old El Paso)	1 oz.	150	17.0
(Planters)	1 oz.	150	18.0
(Tom's) nacho	1 oz.	140	18.0
Tostitos:			
Jalapeño & cheese or sharp nacho	1 oz.	150	17.0
Traditional	1 oz.	140	18.0
Town House Cracker (Keebler)	1 piece (3.1 grams)	16	1.8
Triscuit (Nabisco):			
Regular, low salt or wheat & bran	1 piece	20	3.3
Bits	1 piece	7	1.2
Tuc (Keebler)	1 piece (.2 oz.)	23	2.7
Twiddle Sticks (Nabisco)	1 piece	53	7.0
Twigs (Nabisco)	1 piece (.1 oz.)	14	1.6
Uneeda Biscuit (Nabisco)	1 piece	30	5.0
Unsalted (Estee)	1 piece (.1 oz.)	15	2.5
Vegetable thins (Nabisco)	1 piece	10	1.1
Waverly (Nabisco)	1 piece	17	2.5
Wheat:			
(Dixie Belle) snack	1 piece	9	1.2
(Estee) *6 calorie*	1 piece	6	2.0
(Featherweight) wafer, unsalted	1 piece	13	2.3
(Flavor Tree) nuts	1 oz.	200	5.0
(Nabisco):			
SnackWells, fat free	1 piece	12	2.5
Wheat Thins:			
Regular or low salt	1 piece (.1 oz.)	9	1.1
Cheese	1 piece (.1 oz.)	8	1.0
Nutty	1 piece (.1 oz.)	11	1.1
Wheatsworth	1 piece	14	1.9
(Pepperidge Farm):			

Food	Measure	Cals.	Carbs.
Cracked	1 piece	33	4.7
Hearty	1 piece	25	3.2
Toasted, with onion	1 piece	20	3.0
(Sunshine):			
American Heritage	1 piece	15	2.0
Wafer	1 piece	10	1.2
CRANAPPLE JUICE DRINK			
(Ocean Spray) canned:			
Regular	6 fl. oz.	127	31.1
Dietetic	6 fl. oz.	41	10.0
CRANBERRY, fresh			
(Ocean Spray)	½ cup (2 oz.)	25	6.0
CRANBERRY-APPLE COCKTAIL:			
Canned (Minute Maid) *Juices To Go*	6 fl. oz.	120	30.0
*Frozen (Welch's)	6 fl. oz.	120	30.0
CRANBERRY-APPLE DRINK, canned (Town House)	6 fl. oz.	130	32.0
CRANBERRY JUICE COCKTAIL:			
Canned:			
Regular pack:			
(Ardmore Farms)	6 fl. oz.	77	19.1
(Ocean Spray)	6 fl. oz.	103	25.4
(Town House)	6 fl. oz.	110	26.0
Dietetic (Ocean Spray)	6 fl. oz.	41	9.8
*Frozen (Sunkist)	6 fl. oz.	110	28.2
CRANBERRY NECTAR, canned (Knudsen & Sons)	8 fl. oz.	110	28.0
CRANBERRY-RASPBERRY JUICE DRINK, canned:			
Regular:			
(Ocean Spray)	6 fl. oz.	110	27.0
(Tropicana) *Twister*	6 fl. oz.	110	27.0
Dietetic:			
(Ocean Spray)	6 fl. oz.	40	10.0

Food	Measure	Cals.	Carbs.
(Tropicana) *Twister*, with strawberry	6 fl. oz.	30	7.0
CRANBERRY SAUCE:			
Home recipe (USDA) sweetened, unstrained	4 oz.	202	51.6
Canned:			
(Ocean Spray):			
Regular:			
Jellied	2 oz.	87	21.7
Whole berry	2 oz.	93	23.1
Cran-Fruit:			
& apple	2 oz.	100	24.0
& orange, raspberry or strawberry	2 oz.	100	23.0
(Town House) jellied	2 oz.	100	25.0
CRANICOT (Ocean Spray)	6 fl. oz.	110	26.0
***CRAN-BLUEBERRY* JUICE DRINK,** canned (Ocean Spray)	6 fl. oz.	120	30.0
***CRANTASTIC* JUICE DRINK,** canned (Ocean Spray)	6 fl. oz.	110	27.0
CREAM:			
Half & half (Dairylea)	1 fl. oz.	40	1.0
Light, table or coffee (Sealtest) 16% fat	1 T.	26	.6
Light, whipping, 30% fat (Sealtest)	1 T. (.5 oz.)	45	1.0
Heavy, whipping:			
(Johanna Farms) 36% butterfat	1 T. (.5 oz.)	52	1.0
(Land O' Lakes)	1 T. (.5 oz.)	50	1.0
Sour:			
(Friendship):			
Regular	1 T. (.5 oz.)	27	.5
Light	1 T. (.5 oz.)	17	.1
(Johanna Farms)	¼ cup	123	1.4
(Land O' Lakes):			
Regular	1 T. (.5 oz.)	30	1.0
Light, plain or with chives	1 T.	20	2.0
(Lucerne) light	1 T.	22	1.0
(Weight Watchers)	1 T. (.5 oz.)	17	1.0
Substitute (See **CREAM SUBSTITUTE**)			

Food	Measure	Cals.	Carbs.
CREAM PUFF, home recipe			
(USDA) custard filling	3½" × 2" piece	303	26.7
CREAM SUBSTITUTE:			
Coffee Mate (Carnation)	1 tsp.	11	1.1
Coffee Rich (Rich's)	½ oz.	22	2.2
Coffee Tone (Lucerne):			
Regular	1 tsp.	10	1.0
Frozen	1T.	24	2.0
Non-dairy	½ fl. oz.	16	1.0
Cremora (Borden)	1 tsp.	12	1.0
Dairy Light (Alba)	2.8-oz. envelope	10	1.0
Mocha Mix (Presto Food			
Products)	1 T. (.5 oz.)	19	1.2
N-Rich	1 tsp.	10	2.0
CREAM OF TARTAR			
(Tone's)	1 tsp.	2	.5
CREAM OF WHEAT, cereal			
(Nabisco):			
Regular	1 T.	40	8.8
Instant	1 T.	40	8.8
Mix'n Eat:			
Regular	1-oz. packet	100	21.0
Baked apple & cinnamon	1.25-oz. packet	130	30.0
Brown sugar	1.25-oz. packet	130	30.0
Maple & brown sugar	1.25-oz. packet	130	30.0
Strawberry	1.25-oz. packet	140	29.0
Quick	1 T.	40	8.8
CREME DE BANANA			
LIQUEUR (Mr. Boston):			
Regular, 27% alcohol	1 fl. oz.	93	12.1
Connoisseur, 21% alcohol	1 fl. oz.	82	11.4
CREME DE CACAO:			
(Hiram Walker) (27% alcohol)	1 fl. oz.	104	15.0
(Mr. Boston) 27% alcohol:			
Brown	1 fl. oz.	102	14.3
White	1 fl. oz.	93	12.0
CREME DE CASSIS			
(Mr. Boston) 17½% alcohol	1 fl. oz.	85	14.1

Food	Measure	Cals.	Carbs.
CREME DE MENTHE:			
(De Kuyper)	1 fl. oz.	94	11.3
(Mr. Boston) 27% alcohol:			
Green	1 fl. oz.	109	16.0
White	1 fl. oz.	97	13.0
CREME DE NOYAUX			
(Mr. Boston) 27% alcohol	1 fl. oz.	99	13.5
CREPE, frozen:			
(Mrs. Paul's):			
Crab	5½-oz. pkg.	248	24.6
Shrimp	5½-oz. pkg.	252	23.8
(Stouffer's):			
Chicken with mushroom sauce	8¼-oz. pkg.	390	19.0
Ham & asparagus	6¼-oz. pkg.	325	21.0
Ham & swiss cheese with cheddar cheese sauce	7½-oz. pkg.	410	23.0
Spinach with cheddar cheese sauce	9½-oz. pkg.	415	30.0
CRISPIX, cereal (Kellogg's)	¾ cup (1 oz.)	110	25.0
CRISP RICE CEREAL:			
(Malt-O-Meal) *Crisp 'N Crackling Rice*	1 cup (1 oz.)	108	24.8
(Safeway)	1 cup	110	25.0
CRISPY CRITTERS, cereal (Post)	1 cup (1 oz.)	110	24.0
CRISPY WHEATS 'N RAISINS, cereal (General Mills)	¾ cup (1 oz.)	110	23.0
CROAKER (USDA):			
Atlantic:			
Raw, whole	1 lb. (weighed whole)	148	0.0
Raw, meat only	4 oz.	109	0.0
Baked	4 oz.	151	0.0
White, raw meat only	4 oz.	95	0.0
Yellowfin, raw, meat only	4 oz.	101	0.0

Food	Measure	Cals.	Carbs.
CROUTON:			
(Kellogg's) *Croutettes*	⅔ cup (.7 oz.)	70	14.0
(Mrs. Cubbison's):			
Cheese & garlic or seasoned	½ oz.	60	9.0
Onion & garlic	½ oz.	70	10.0
(Pepperidge Farm)	½ oz	70	9.0
CUCUMBER (USDA):			
Eaten with skin	8-oz. cucumber (weighed whole)	32	7.4
Pared	7½" × 2" pared (7.3 oz.)	29	6.6
Pared	3 slices (.9 oz.)	4	.5
CUMIN SEED (French's)	1 tsp.	7	.7
CUPCAKE:			
Home recipe (USDA):			
Without icing	1.4-oz. cupcake	146	22.4
With chocolate icing	1.8-oz. cupcake	184	29.7
With boiled white icing	1.8-oz. cupcake	176	30.9
With uncooked white icing	1.8-oz. cupcake	184	31.6
Packaged:			
(Dolly Madison) chocolate	1.6-oz. piece	170	29.0
(Hostess):			
Chocolate	1⅜-oz. piece	166	29.8
Orange	1½-oz. piece	151	26.8
(Tastykake):			
Buttercreme, iced:			
Regular	1 piece	250	42.0
Mini, iced	1 piece	110	15.0
Chocolate:			
Regular:			
Plain	1 piece	110	18.0
Creme, iced:			
Regular	1 piece	125	20.0
Mini	1 piece	55	9.0
Koffee Kake:			
Regular Creme:			
Regular	1 piece	80	35.0
Mini	1 piece	55	8.0
Low fat:			
Apple filled	1 piece	160	33.0
Lemon filled	1 piece	160	34.0

Food	Measure	Cals.	Carbs.
CURACAO LIQUEUR:			
(Bols)	1 fl. oz.	105	10.3
(Hiram Walker)	1 fl. oz.	96	11.8
CURRANT:			
Fresh (USDA):			
Black European:			
Whole	1 lb. (weighed with stems)	240	58.2
Stems removed	4 oz.	61	14.9
Red and white:			
Whole	1 lb. (weighed with stems)	220	53.2
Stems removed	1 cup (3.9 oz.)	55	13.3
Dried:			
(Del Monte) Zante	½ cup (2.4 oz.)	200	53.0
(Sun-Maid)	½ cup	220	53.0
CUSTARD:			
Home recipe (USDA)	½ cup (4.7 oz.)	152	14.7
Canned (Thank You Brand)			
egg	½ cup (4.6 oz.)	135	18.2
***C.W. POST,** cereal*	¼ cup (1 oz.)	128	21.4

D

Food	Measure	Cals.	Carbs.
DAIQUIRI MIX:			
Dry (Holland House)	.56-oz. pkg.	65	16.0
Liquid:			
(Bar-Tender's)	3½ fl. oz.	177	18.0
(Holland House):			
Regular	1 fl. oz.	36	9.0
Raspberry	1 fl. oz.	30	7.0
Strawberry	1 fl. oz.	31	7.0
*Frozen (Bacardi):			
Peach	4 fl. oz.	98	16.3
Raspberry	4 fl. oz.	97	15.9
Strawberry	4 fl. oz.	102	17.1

Food	Measure	Cals.	Carbs.
DAIRY QUEEN/BRAZIER:			
Banana split	13-oz. serving	510	96.0
Blizzard:			
Heath:			
Regular	14.3-oz. serving	820	119.0
Small	10.3-oz. serving	560	82.0
Strawberry:			
Regular	13½-oz. serving	740	92.0
Small	9.4-oz. serving	500	64.0
Breeze:			
Heath:			
Regular	13.4-oz. serving	680	113.0
Small	9.6-oz. serving	450	78.0
Strawberry:			
Regular	12½-oz. serving	590	90.0
Small	8.7-oz. serving	400	63.0
Brownie Delight, hot fudge	10.8-oz. serving	710	102.0
Buster Bar	5¼-oz. piece	450	41.0
Chicken sandwich, fillet:			
Breaded:			
Plain	6.7-oz. serving	430	37.0
With cheese	7.2-oz. serving	480	38.0
Grilled	6½-oz. serving	300	33.0
Dilly Bar	3-oz.	210	21.0
Double Delight	9-oz. serving	490	69.0
DQ Sandwich	2.1-oz.	140	24.0
Fish sandwich:			
Plain	6-oz. sandwich	370	39.0
With cheese	6½-oz. sandwich	420	40.0
Float	14-oz. serving	410	82.0
Freeze, vanilla	12-oz. serving	500	89.0
French fries:			
Regular	3½-oz. serving	300	40.0
Large	4½-oz. serving	390	52.0
Hamburger:			
Plain:			
Single	5-oz. burger	310	17.0
Double	7-oz. burger	460	29.0
Triple	9.6-oz. burger	710	33.0
With cheese:			
Single	5.7-oz. burger	410	33.0
Double	8.4-oz. burger	650	34.0
Triple	10.63-oz. burger	820	34.0
Homestyle Ultimate	9.7-oz. burger	700	30.0
Hot dog:			
Regular:			
Plain	3.5-oz. serving	280	22.0

Food	Measure	Cals.	Carbs.
With cheese	4-oz. serving	330	24.0
With chili	4½-oz. serving	320	26.0
DQ Hounder:			
Plain	1 serving	480	21.0
With cheese	1 serving	533	22.0
With chili	1 serving	575	25.0
Super:			
Plain	7-oz. serving	590	41.0
With cheese	6.9-oz. serving	580	45.0
With chili	7.7-oz. serving	570	47.0
Ice Cream Cone:			
Chocolate:			
Plain:			
Regular	5-oz. serving	230	36.0
Large	7½-oz. serving	350	54.0
Dipped:			
Regular	5½-oz. serving	330	40.0
Large	8¼-oz. serving	570	64.0
Queen's Choice	1 serving	326	40.0
Vanilla:			
Plain:			
Small	3-oz. serving	140	22.0
Regular	5-oz. serving	230	36.0
Large	71"-oz. serving	340	53.0
Queen's Choice	1 serving	320	40.0
Malt:			
Chocolate:			
Small	10¼-oz. serving	520	91.0
Regular	14¾-oz. serving	760	134.0
Large	20¾-oz. serving	1060	187.0
Queen, large	21-oz. serving	889	157.0
Vanilla, regular	14.7-oz. serving	610	106.0
Mr. Misty:			
Plain:			
Small	8¼-oz. serving	190	48.0
Regular	11.64-oz. serving	250	63.0
Large	15½-oz. serving	340	84.0
Float	14.5-oz. serving	390	74.0
Freeze	14.5-oz. serving	500	91.0
Onion rings	3-oz. serving	240	29.0
Peanut Butter Parfait	10¾-oz. serving	710	94.0
Salad, without dressing:			
Garden	10-oz. serving	200	7.0
Side	4.8-oz. serving	25	4.0
Salad dressing:			
Regular, 1000 Island	2 oz.	225	10.0
Dietic, French	2 oz.	90	11.0

Food	Measure	Cals.	Carbs.
Shake:			
Chocolate:			
Small	10¼-oz. serving	490	82.0
Regular	14-oz. serving	540	94.0
Large	20¾-oz. serving	990	168.0
Queen, large	21-oz. serving	831	140.0
Vanilla:			
Regular	14–oz. serving	520	88.0
Large	16.3-oz. serving	600	101.0
Sundae, chocolate:			
Small	3¾-oz. serving	190	33.0
Regular	6¼-oz. serving	310	56.0
Large	8¾-oz. serving	440	78.0
Tomato	½ oz.	4	1.0
Yogurt, frozen:			
Cone:			
Regular	5 oz.	180	38.0
Large	7½ oz.	260	56.0
Cup:			
Regular	5 oz.	170	35.0
Large	7 oz.	230	49.0
Sundae, strawberry	12½ oz.	200	43.0

DAMSON PLUM (See **PLUM**)

DANDELION GREENS, raw
(USDA).

Trimmed	1 lb.	204	41.7
Boiled, drained	½ cup (3.2 oz.)	30	5.8

DANISH (See **ROLL OR BUN**)

DATE, dry, domestic:
(USDA):

With pits	1 lb. (weighed with pits)	1081	287.7
Without pits	4 oz.	311	82.7
Without pits chopped	1 cup (6.1 oz.)	477	126.8
(Dromedary):			
Without pits	1 date	20	4.6
Without pits, chopped	¼ cup (1¼ oz.)	130	31.0

DENNY'S

Bacon	1 slice	48	.5
Bagel	1 serving	240	47.0
Bean, green	3-oz. serving	13	2.6

Food	Measure	Cals.	Carbs.
Biscuit	1 biscuit	217	35.0
Carrots	3-oz. serving	17	3.8
Catfish entree, seasoned	1 entree	317	44.4
Chicken:			
Fried, entree	4-piece serving	463	7.5
Grilled, entree	1 serving	192	2.5
Steak, fried, without gravy,			
entree	1 serving	252	16.0
Strips	4 pieces	290	21.0
Chili	4-oz. serving	170	15.0
Coleslaw	1 cup	120	8.5
Corn	3-oz. serving	65	15.0
Eggs:			
Benedict	1 serving	658	20.2
Omelet:			
Chili cheese	1 omelet	490	17.0
Denver	1 omelet	580	4.0
Mexican	1 omelet	540	14.0
Ultimate	1 omelet	577	7.7
Scrambled	1 serving	80	0.0
French toast	1 slice	364	23.0
Gravy, country	1-oz. serving	140	14.0
Ham slice	1 serving	155	.9
Hamburger:			
Bacon Swiss	1 serving	815	38.0
Dennyburger	1 serving	625	36.7
San Fran burger	1 serving (without lettuce, tomatoes & guacamole)	870	51.0
Works burger	1 serving	945	48.0
Liver entree, with bacon & onions	1 serving (2 slices)	334	10.0
Mozzarella strips	1 piece	88	7.3
Muffin:			
Blueberry	1 serving	310	42.0
English	1 serving	135	25.8
Onion rings	1 piece	85	9.0
Pancake	1 serving	135	26.0
Pea, green	3-oz. serving	40	7.0
Potato:			
Baked	1 serving	90	21.0
French fried	4-oz. serving	300	38.0
Hash browns	4-oz. serving	164	32.1
Mashed	4-oz. serving	75	14.0
Rice pilaf	⅓ cup	90	15.5
Roast beef entree	1 serving	965	41.0

Food	Measure	Cals.	Carbs.
Roll, cinnamon	1 serving	450	73.0
Salad:			
Chef	1 serving	490	12.9
Chicken, without shell	1 serving	205	4.0
Taco, without shell	1 serving	510	35.0
Tuna	1 serving	340	13.0
Salad dressing, ranch	1 T.	50	.6
Sandwich:			
BLT	1 sandwich	490	42.0
Cheese, grilled	1 sandwich	450	29.0
Chicken, grilled	1 serving	440	40.0
Patty melt	1 serving	760	27.0
Roast beef deluxe	1 serving	840	44.0
Shrimp, fried, entree	1 piece	45	7.0
Soup:			
Beef barley	1 bowl	80	10.9
Cheese	1 bowl	310	19.0
Chicken noodle	1 bowl	105	14.8
Chowder, clam	1 bowl	235	21.0
Potato	1 bowl	245	38.0
Spaghetti with meatballs, entree	1 serving	1000	119.0
Steak entree:			
Hamburger	1 serving	665	8.6
New York	1 serving	580	0.0
Top sirloin	1 serving	223	.7
Stir-fry entree	1 serving	325	5.0
Stuffing	½ cup	180	20.0
Tortilla shell, fried	1 serving	435	37.0
Turkey entree, no gravy	6-slice serving	505	40.0
Waffle	1 piece	261	35.0
DESSERT (See individual listings such as **APPLE BROWN BETTY; CAKE; FROZEN DESSERT; ICE CREAM; PRUNE WHIP; PUDDING TOFUTTI;** etc.)			
DEVIL DOG (Drake's)	1 piece	180	25.0
DILL SEED (French's)	1 tsp. (2.1 grams)	9	1.2
DINERSAURS, cereal (Ralston Purina)	1 cup (1 oz.)	110	25.0

Food	Measure	Cals.	Carbs.
DING DONGS (Hostess)	1 piece	170	21.0
DINNER, FROZEN (See individual listings such as **BEAN & FRANKFURTER DINNER; BEEF DINNER or ENTREE; LASAGNA,** frozen; etc.)			
DIP:			
Acapulco (Ortega):			
Plain	1 oz.	8	1.8
American cheese	1 oz.	60	1.1
Cheddar cheese	1 oz.	64	1.2
Monterey Jack cheese	1 oz.	59	1.4
Avocado (Kraft)	1 T.	25	1.5
Bacon horseradish (Sealtest)	1 T.	35	1.0
Bacon & onion (Kraft) premium	1 T.	30	1.0
Bean:			
(Chi-Chi's) _Fiesta_	1 oz.	30	4.0
(Eagle)	1 oz.	35	4.0
(Hain) hot	1T.	17	2.5
Bean, black:			
(Guiltless Gourmet)	1 oz.	23	4.0
(Tostitos) medium, fat free	1T.	15	3.0
Blue cheese:			
(Dean) tang	1 oz.	61	2.3
(Nalley's)	1 oz.	110	.9
Cheddar cheese:			
(Frito's)	1 oz.	45	3.0
(Guiltless Gourmet) queso, mild or spicy	1 oz.	20	5.0
Cheese (Chi-Chi's) _Fiesta_	1 oz.	40	3.0
Chili (La Victoria)	1 T.	5	1.0
Clam (Kraft)	1 T.	30	1.5
Enchilada, _Fritos_	1 oz.	37	3.9
Guacamole (Calavo)	1 oz.	55	3.5
Hot bean (Hain)	1 T.	17	2.5
Jalapeño (Wise)	1 T.	12	2.5
Nacho (Guiltless Gourmet)	1 T.	12	2.5
Onion (Hain) natural	1 T.	17	2.5
Picante sauce (Wise)	1 T.	6	1.5
Pinto bean (Guiltless Gourmet) any style	1 oz.	27	5.0
Taco (Thank You Brand)	1 T. (.8 oz.)	44	2.0

Food	Measure	Cals.	Carbs.
DIP 'UM SAUCE, canned (French's):			
BBQ	1 T.	22	5.0
Creamy mustard	1 T.	40	6.0
Hot mustard	1 T.	35	7.0
Sweet 'n Sour	1 T.	40	10.0
DISTILLED LIQUOR. The values below would apply to unflavored bourbon whiskey, brandy, Canadian whiskey, gin, Irish whiskey, rum, rye whiskey, Scotch whisky, tequila and vodka. The caloric content of distilled liquors depends on the percentage of alcohol. The proof is twice the alcohol percent and the following values apply to all brands (USDA):			
80 proof	1 fl. oz.	65	Tr.
86 proof	1 fl. oz.	70	Tr.
90 proof	1 fl. oz.	74	Tr.
94 proof	1 fl. oz.	77	Tr.
100 proof	1 fl. oz.	83	Tr.
D'LITES OF AMERICA:			
Cheese, light	1 slice	53	2.0
Chicken sandwich, fillet	1 serving	280	24.0
Chocolate D'Lite	1 serving	200	36.0
Fish fillet sandwich	1 serving	390	29.0
Ham & cheese sandwich	1 serving	280	26.0
Hamburger:			
Regular:			
Double D'Lite	1 serving	450	19.0
Jr. D'Lite	1 serving	200	19.0
¼-lb. D'Lite	1 serving	280	19.0
With cheese & bacon	1 serving	370	20.0
Potato:			
Baked:			
Regular	1 serving	230	50.0
With bacon & cheddar cheese	1 serving	490	52.0
With broccoli & cheddar cheese	1 serving	410	51.0
Mexican	1 serving	510	61.0

Food	Measure	Cals.	Carbs.
French fries:			
Regular order	1 serving	260	34.0
Large order	1 serving	320	42.0
Skins:			
Regular	1 serving	90	6.0
Mexi Skins	1 serving	99	6.0
Salad bar platter	1 serving	40	1.0
Salad dressing,			
mayonnaise, lite	1 T.	40	1.0
Tartar sauce, lite	1 T.	60	2.0
Vegetarian D'Lite sandwich	1 serving	270	20.0
DOUGHNUT (See also ***DUNKIN' DONUTS***):			
(USDA):			
Cake type	1.1-oz. piece	125	16.4
Yeast leavened	2-oz. piece	235	21.4
(Awrey's):			
Plain	1 piece	170	19.0
Crunch	1 piece	280	35.0
Sugared	1 piece	170	19.0
(Dolly Madison):			
Regular:			
Plain	1¼-oz. piece	140	17.0
Chocolate coated	1¼-oz. piece	150	18.0
Coconut crunch	1¼-oz. piece	140	20.0
Powdered sugar	1¼-oz. piece	140	19.0
Dunkin' Stix	1⅜-oz. piece	210	18.0
Gems:			
Chocolate coated	.5-oz. piece	65	7.0
Cinnamon sugar	.5-oz. piece	55	7.5
Coconut crunch	.5-oz. piece	60	8.0
Powdered sugar	.5-oz. piece	60	7.5
Jumbo:			
Plain	1.6-oz. piece	190	23.0
Cinnamon sugar	1.6-oz. piece	190	24.0
Sugar	1.7-oz. piece	210	27.0
Old fashioned:			
Cinnamon chip	2.2-oz. piece	280	32.0
Chocolate glazed	2.2-oz. piece	260	36.0
Chocolate iced	2.2-oz. piece	300	33.0
Glazed or orange crush	2.2-oz. piece	280	33.0
Powdered sugar	1.8-oz. piece	260	24.0
White iced	2.2-oz. piece	300	35.0
(Entenmann's):			
Crumb topped	1 piece	260	34.0
Devil's food crumb	1 piece	250	33.0

Food	Measure	Cals.	Carbs.
Rich, frosted	1 piece	400	37.0
(Hostess):			
Regular:			
Cinnamon, family pack	1 piece	120	14.0
Crumb	1 piece	160	16.0
Frosted	1 piece	190	20.0
Glazed, old fashioned	1 piece	250	33.0
Glazed whirl	1 piece	190	27.0
Honey Wheat	1 piece	250	32.0
Plain, old fashioned	1 piece	170	21.0
Donette Gems:			
Cinnamon	1 piece	60	7.0
Crumb or frosted	1 piece	80	8.0
(Tastykake):			
Cinnamon	1 piece	210	24.0
Glazed, orange	1 piece	220	33.0
Honey wheat:			
Regular	1 piece	230	33.0
Mini	1 piece	47	6.5
Powdered sugar, mini	1 piece	65	6.7
DRAMBUIE (Hiram Walker)			
(80 proof)	1 fl. oz.	110	11.0
DRUMSTICK, frozen:			
Ice Cream, in a cone:			
Topped with peanuts	1 piece	181	22.7
Topped with peanuts & cone			
bisque	1 piece	168	23.6
Ice Milk, in a cone:			
Topped with peanuts	1 piece	163	24.3
Topped with peanuts & cone			
bisque	1 piece	150	25.2
DUCK, raw (USDA):			
Domesticated:			
Ready-to-cook	1 lb. (weighed with bone)	1213	0.0
Meat only	4 oz.	187	0.0
Wild:			
Dressed	1 lb. (weighed dressed)	613	0.0
Meat only	4 oz.	156	0.0
DULCITO, frozen (Hormel):			
Apple	4-oz. serving	290	44.0
Cherry	4-oz. serving	300	48.0

Food	Measure	Cals.	Carbs.
DUNKIN' DONUTS:			
Bagel:			
Plain	1 bagel	240	47.0
Cinnamon-raisin	1 bagel	250	49.0
Egg	1 bagel	250	47.0
Onion	1 bagel	230	46.0
Cookie:			
Chocolate chunk:			
Plain	1 piece	200	25.0
With nuts	1 piece	210	23.0
Oatmeal pecan raisin	1 piece	200	28.0
Croissant:			
Plain	1 croissant	310	27.0
Almond	1 croissant	420	38.0
Chocolate	1 croissant	440	38.0
Cruller, french, glazed	1 cruller	140	16.0
Donut:			
Filled:			
Apple, cinnamon sugar	1 piece (2.8 oz.)	250	33.0
Bavarian, chocolate			
frosting	1 piece (2.8 oz.)	240	32.0
Blueberry	1 piece (2.4 oz.)	210	29.0
Boston Kreme	1 piece	240	30.0
Jelly	1 piece	220	31.0
Lemon	1 piece	260	33.0
Ring:			
Buttermilk, glazed	1 piece	290	37.0
Chocolate, glazed	1 piece	325	34.0
Yeast:			
Chocolate frosted	1 piece	200	25.0
Glazed	1 piece	200	26.0
Muffin:			
Apple & spice	1 muffin	300	50.0
Banana nut	1 muffin	310	49.0
Blueberry	1 muffin	280	45.0
Bran, with raisins	1 muffin	310	51.0
Corn	1 muffin	340	50.0
Cranberry nut	1 muffin	290	44.0
Oat bran	1 muffin	330	50.0

Food	Measure	Cals.	Carbs.

E

ECLAIR:
Home recipe (USDA), with
custard filling and chocolate

icing	4-oz. piece	271	26.3
Frozen:			
(Rich's) chocolate	2-oz. piece	196	25.5
(Weight Watchers) *Sweet*			
Celebrations	1 piece	150	26.0

***ECTO* COOLER DRINK,**

canned (Hi-C)	6 fl. oz.	95	23.3

EEL (USDA):

Raw, meat only	4 oz.	264	0.0
Smoked, meat only	4 oz.	374	0.0

EGG (USDA) (See also **EGG
SUBSTITUTE**):
Chicken:
Raw:

White only	1 large egg (1.2 oz.)	17	.3
White only	1 cup (9 oz.)	130	2.0
Yolk only	1 large egg (.6 oz.)	59	.1
Yolk only	1 cup (8.5 oz.)	835	1.4
Whole, small	1 egg (1.3 oz.)	60	.3
Whole, medium	1 egg (1.5 oz.)	71	.4
Whole, large	1 egg (1.8 oz.)	81	.4
Whole	1 cup (8.8 oz.)	409	2.3
Whole, extra large	1 egg (2. oz.)	94	.5
Whole, jumbo	1 egg (2.3 oz.)	105	.6
Cooked:			
Boiled	1 large egg (1.8 oz.)	81	.4
Fried in butter	1 large egg	99	.1

Food	Measure	Cals.	Carbs.
Omelet, mixed with milk and cooked in fat	1 large egg	107	1.5
Poached	1 large egg	78	.4
Scrambled, mixed with milk & cooked in fat	1 large egg	111	1.5
Scrambled, mixed with milk & cooked in fat	1 cup (7.8 oz.)	381	5.3
Dried:			
Whole	1 cup (3.8 oz.)	639	4.4
White, powder	1 oz.	105	1.6
Yolk	1 cup (3.4 oz.)	637	2.4
Duck, raw	1 egg (2.8 oz.)	153	.6
Goose, raw	1 egg (5.8 oz.)	303	2.1
Turkey, raw	1 egg (3.1 oz.)	150	1.5
EGG BREAKFAST, frozen:			
(Healthy Choice) omelet:			
Regular, with turkey sausage	4¾-oz. serving	210	30.0
Western	4¾-oz. serving	200	29.0
(Hormel) *Quick Meal*:			
On a biscuit & sausage	4½-oz. sandwich	350	30.0
On a muffin:			
With Canadian bacon & cheese	4½-oz. sandwich	250	29.0
With sausage & cheese	5.1-oz. sandwich	76	5.0
(Swanson) scrambled:			
Budget:			
with home fries	4.3-oz. meal	260	15.0
with silver dollar pancakes	4¼-oz. meal	180	20.0
Fiesta, with Canadian bacon, cheese, jalapeños & home fries	6½-oz. meal	390	18.0
Great Starts:			
With bacon & home fries	5¼-oz. meal	350	16.0
With sausage & hash browns	6¼-oz. meal.	430	19.0
(Weight Watchers) Handy, omelet with ham & cheese	1 meal	220	30.0
*EGG FOO YOUNG, dinner, canned:			
(Chun King) stir fry	5-oz. serving	138	9.1
(La Choy)	1 patty + ¼ cup sauce	164	19.2

Food	Measure	Cals.	Carbs.
EGGNOG, dairy:			
(Borden)	½ cup	160	16.0
(Crowley):			
Regular	½ cup	190	23.0
Light	½ cup	120	22.0
Nonfat	½ cup	130	25.0
(Johanna)	½ cup	195	22.4
EGGNOG COCKTAIL			
(Mr. Boston) 15% alcohol	3 fl. oz.	177	18.9
EGGPLANT:			
Raw (USDA) whole	1 lb. (weighed whole)	92	20.6
Boiled (USDA) drained, diced	1 cup (7.1 oz.)	38	8.2
Frozen:			
(Buitoni) parmigiana	5-oz. serving	168	17.6
(Celentano):			
Parmigiana	½ of 16-oz. pkg.	280	23.0
Rollatines	11-oz. pkg.	320	36.0
(Mrs. Paul's) parmesan	5-oz. serving	240	18.0
EGGPLANT APPETIZER			
(Progresso) Caponata	¼ cup	70	4.0
EGG ROLL, frozen:			
(Chun King):			
Regular:			
Chicken	3½ oz. piece	210	31.0
Meat & shrimp	3½-oz. piece	214	30.0
Shrimp	3½-oz. piece	189	30.0
Restaurant style, pork	3-oz. piece	172	23.0
(La Choy):			
Chicken	.5-oz. piece	30	4.0
Lobster	.5-oz. piece	27	4.3
Lobster	3-oz. piece	180	25.0
Meat & shrimp	.5-oz. piece	27	4.0
Shrimp	3-oz. piece	160	24.0
EGG ROLL DINNER OR ENTREE, frozen:			
(La Choy) entree:			
Almond chicken	2 pieces	450	43.0
Beef & broccoli	2 pieces	380	45.0
Spicy oriental chicken	2 pieces	300	32.0

Food	Measure	Cals.	Carbs.
Sweet & sour pork	2 pieces	430	56.0
(Van de Kamp's) Cantonese	10½-oz. serving	560	80.0
EGG ROLL WRAPPER			
(Nasoya)	1 piece	25	4.5
EGG SUBSTITUTE:			
Egg Magic (Featherweight)	½ of envelope	60	1.0
Scramblers (Morningstar Farms)	1 egg substitute	35	1.5
ELDERBERRY, fresh (USDA):			
Whole	1 lb. (weighed with stems)	307	69.9
Stems removed	4 oz.	82	18.6
EL POLLO LOCO RESTAURANT:			
Beans	4-oz. serving	100	16.0
Burrito:			
Bean, rice & cheese	9-oz. serving	530	86.0
Chicken:			
Regular	7-oz. serving	310	30.0
Classic	9½-oz. serving	560	66.0
Loco Grande	13.2-oz. serving	680	70.0
Spicy hot	10-oz. serving	570	66.0
Whole wheat	10½-oz. serving	510	67.0
Steak:			
Regular	6-oz. serving	450	31.0
Grilled	11-oz. serving	740	81.0
Vegetarian	6-oz. serving	340	54.0
Cheese, cheddar	1 oz.	90	3.0
Cheesecake	3½-oz. serving	310	30.0
Chicken:			
Breast	3-oz. serving	160	0.0
Leg	1¾-oz. serving	90	0.0
Thigh	2-oz. serving	180	0.0
Wing	1½-oz. serving	110	0.0
Cole slaw	2.8-oz. serving	80	5.0
Corn	3-oz. piece	110	20.0
Fajita meal:			
Chicken, with rice, beans, 3 tortillas, salsa, guacamole, cheese & sour cream	17½-oz. meal	780	120.0
Steak, including guacamole, cheese & sour cream	17½-oz. meal	1040	120.0

Food	Measure	Cals.	Carbs.
Guacamole	1 oz.	60	2.0
Pastry, churro	1½-oz. piece	140	4.0
Rice	2-oz. serving	110	19.0
Salad:			
Chicken, flame broiled	12-oz. serving	160	11.0
Potato	4-oz. serving	180	21.0
Side	9-oz. serving	50	10.0
Salad dressing:			
Regular:			
Blue cheese	1 oz.	80	14.0
French, deluxe	1 oz.	60	7.0
Ranch	1 oz.	75	4.0
Thousand Island	1 oz.	110	4.0
Dietetic, Italian	1 oz.	25	2.0
Salsa	2-oz. serving	10	3.0
Sour cream	1 oz.	60	1.0
Taco:			
Chicken	5 oz.	180	18.0
Steak	4½ oz.	250	18.0
Tortilla:			
Corn	1 tortilla	60	13.0
Flour	1 tortilla	90	15.0
ENCHANADA, frozen			
(Stouffer's) *Lean Cuisine:*			
Bean & beef	9¼-oz. meal	280	32.0
Chicken	9⅞-oz. meal	270	31.0
ENCHILADA OR			
ENCHILADA			
DINNER:			
Canned (Old El Paso) beef	1 enchilada	145	11.0
Frozen:			
Beef:			
(Banquet):			
Dinner	12-oz. dinner	500	72.0
Family Entree	2-lb. pkg.	1235	128.0
(Fred's Frozen Foods)			
Marquez	7½-oz. serving	304	23.5
(Healthy Choice)	13.4-oz. meal	370	65.0
(Old El Paso):			
Dinner, festive	11-oz. dinner	390	56.0
Entree	1 piece	210	16.0
(Patio)	13¼-oz. dinner	520	59.0
(Swanson)	13¾-oz. dinner	480	55.0

Food	Measure	Cals.	Carbs.
(Van de Kamp's):			
Dinner:			
Regular	12-oz. meal	390	45.0
Shredded	14¾-oz. meal	490	60.0
Entree:			
Regular	7½-oz. meal	250	20.0
Shredded	5½-oz. serving	180	15.0
(Weight Watchers) *Ultimate 200*, Ranchero	9.12-oz. meal	190	18.0
Cheese:			
(Banquet)	12-oz. dinner	550	71.0
(Old El Paso):			
Dinner, festive	11-oz. dinner	590	51.0
Entree	1 piece	250	24.0
(Patio)	12¼-oz. dinner	380	59.0
(Van de Kamp's):			
Dinner	12-oz. dinner	390	45.0
Entree	7½-oz. pkg.	250	20.0
(Weight Watchers) nacho	8.9-oz. meal	230	30.0
Chicken:			
(Healthy Choice)	13.4-oz. meal	320	58.0
(Old El Paso):			
Dinner, festive	11-oz. dinner	460	54.0
Entree:			
Regular	1 piece	226	20.0
With sour cream sauce	1 piece	280	18.0
(Weight Watchers) Suiza	9-oz. meal	230	25.0
ENCHILADA SAUCE:			
Canned:			
(El Molino) hot	1 T.	8	1.0
(La Victoria)	1 T.	5	1.0
(Old El Paso):			
Green chili	½ cup	36	7.2
Hot	½ cup	54	7.6
Mild	½ cup	50	7.2
(Rosarita)	3 oz.	19	4.0
Mix:			
*(Durkee)	½ cup	29	6.2
(French's)	1⅜-oz. pkg.	120	20.0
ENCHILADA SEASONING MIX (Lawry's)	1.6-oz. pkg.	152	29.9

Food	Measure	Cals.	Carbs.
ENDIVE, CURLY, raw (USDA):			
Untrimmed	1 lb. (weighed untrimmed)	80	16.4
Trimmed	½ lb.	45	9.3
Cut up or shredded	1 cup (2.5 oz.)	14	2.9
ENSURE, canned:			
Black walnut	8 fl. oz.	250	34.3
Chocolate:			
Regular	8 fl. oz.	250	33.8
With fiber	8 fl. oz.	260	37.8
Plus	8 fl. oz.	355	46.8
Coffee	8 fl. oz.	250	34.3
Egg nog	8 fl. oz.	250	34.3
Strawberry:			
Regular	8 fl. oz.	250	34.3
Plus	8 fl. oz.	355	47.3
Vanilla:			
Regular	8 fl. oz.	250	34.0
With fiber	8 fl. oz.	260	38.3
Plus	8 fl. oz.	355	47.3
ESCAROLE, raw (USDA):			
Untrimmed	1 lb. (weighed untrimmed)	80	16.4
Trimmed	½ lb.	46	9.2
Cut up or shredded	1 cup (2.5 oz.)	14	2.9
EULACHON OR SMELT, raw (USDA) meat only	4 oz.	134	0.0
EXPRESSO COFFEE LIQUEUR (Mr. Boston) 26½% alcohol	1 fl. oz.	104	15.0

F

Food	Measure	Cals.	Carbs.
FAJITA, frozen:			
(Healthy Choice):			
Beef	7-oz. meal	210	26.0
Chicken	7-oz. meal	200	25.0

Food	Measure	Cals.	Carbs.
(Weight Watchers):			
Beef	6¾-oz. meal	250	31.0
Chicken	6¾-oz. meal	210	24.0
FAJITA SEASONING			
MIX (Lawry's)	1.3-oz. pkg.	63	14.0
***FALAFEL MIX:**			
(Fantastic Foods)	3 oz.	129	20.0
(Near East)	1 patty	90	7.3
FARINA:			
(H-O) dry, regular	1 T. (.4 oz.)	40	8.5
Malt-O-Meal, dry:			
Regular	1 oz.	96	21.0
Quick cooking	1 oz.	100	22.2
*(Pillsbury) made with water			
and salt	⅔ cup	80	17.0
FAT, COOKING:			
(USDA):			
Lard	1 T. (.5 oz.)	115	0.0
Vegetable oil	1 T. (1.4 oz.)	106	0.0
Crisco:			
Regular	1 T. (.4 oz.)	110	0.0
Butter flavor	1 T. (.5 oz.)	126	0.0
(Mrs. Tucker's)	1 T.	120	0.0
(Rokeach) neutral nyafat	1 T.	99	0.0
Spry	1 T. (.4 oz.)	94	0.0
FENNEL SEED (French's)	1 tsp. (2.1 grams)	8	1.3
FETTUCINI			
Dry and fresh, refrigerated (See **PASTA DRY OR FRESH, REFRIGERATED**)			
Frozen:			
(Armour) *Dining Lite,* & broccoli	9-oz. meal	290	33.0
(Budget Gourmet)	10-oz. meal	290	34.0
(Green Giant) primavera	9½-oz. meal	230	26.0
(Healthy Choice):			
Afredo	8-oz. meal	240	39.0
Chicken	8½-oz. meal	240	29.0
(Stouffer's) Alfredo	10-oz. pkg.	480	38.0
(Weight Watchers) Alfredo:			

Food	Measure	Cals.	Carbs.
Regular	8-oz. meal	230	28.0
With broccoli, low fat	8-oz. meal	230	28.0
FIBER ONE, cereal			
(General Mills)	½ cup (1 oz.)	60	23.0
FIG:			
Fresh (USDA):			
Regular size	1 lb.	363	92.1
Small	1.3-oz. fig (1½"		
	dia.)	30	7.7
Candied (Bama)	1 T. (.7 oz.)	37	9.6
Canned, regular pack,			
solids & liq.:			
(USDA):			
Light syrup	4 oz.	74	19.1
Heavy syrup	3 figs & 2 T.		
	syrup (4 oz.)	96	24.9
Heavy syrup	½ cup (4.4 oz.)	106	27.5
Extra heavy syrup	4 oz.	117	30.3
(Del Monte) whole	½ cup (4.3 oz.)	100	28.0
(S&W) Kadota fancy, whole,			
in heavy syrup	½ cup	100	28.0
Canned, unsweetened or			
dietetic, solids & liq.:			
(USDA) water pack	4 oz.	54	14.1
(Diet Delight) Kadota	½ cup (4.4 oz.)	76	18.2
Dried (Sun-Maid):			
Calimyrna	½ cup (3.5 oz.)	250	58.0
Mission, regular or figlets	½ cup (3 oz.)	210	50.0
FIG JUICE (Sunsweet)	6 fl. oz.	120	30.0
FIGURINES (Pillsbury) all			
flavors	1 bar	100	10.0
FILBERT:			
(USDA):			
Whole	1 lb. (weighed in		
	shell)	1323	34.9
Shelled	1 oz.	180	4.7
(Fisher) oil dipped, salted	½ cup (2 oz.)	360	5.4
FILO PASTRY, frozen			
(Apollo)	1 oz.	80	18.0

FISH (See individual listings)

Food	Measure	Cals.	Carbs.
*FISH BOUILLON (Knorr)	8 fl. oz.	10	.4
FISH CAKE:			
Home recipe (USDA)	2 oz.	98	5.3
Frozen:			
(Captain's Choice)	2-oz. piece	130	14.0
(Mrs. Paul's) thins	1 piece	95	12.0
FISH & CHIPS, frozen:			
(Gorton's)	1 pkg.	1350	132.0
(Swanson):			
4-compartment dinner	10-oz. dinner	500	60.0
Homestyle Recipe	6½-oz. entree	340	37.0
(Van de Kamp's) batter			
dipped, french fried	7-oz. pkg.	440	35.0
FISH & CHIPS BATTER MIX			
(Golden Dipt)	1¼ oz.	120	27.0
FISH DINNER OR ENTREE,			
frozen (See also individual			
listings such as **COD**			
DINNER):			
(Banquet) platters	8¾-oz. dinner	450	33.0
(Kid Cuisine) nuggets	7-oz. meal	320	33.0
(Morton)	9¾-oz. dinner	370	46.0
(Stouffer's) *Lean Cuisine,* fillet:			
Divan	10⅜-oz. pkg.	210	13.0
Florentine	9⅝-oz. pkg.	220	13.0
(Weight Watchers) *Ultimate*			
200, oven baked	6.6-oz. meal	120	10.0
FISH FILLET, frozen:			
(Captain's Choice):			
Crisp & crunchy	1 fillet	155	14.0
Fried, battered	3-oz. piece	240	10.0
(Frionor) *Bunch O' Crunch,*			
breaded	1½-oz. piece	140	3.8
(Gorton's):			
Regular:			
Batter dipped, crispy	1 piece	250	18.0
Crunchy	1 piece	175	9.5
Potato crisp	1 piece	170	10.0
Light Recipe:			
Lightly breaded	1 piece	180	16.0
Tempura batter	1 piece	200	8.0

Food	Measure	Cals.	Carbs.
(Healthy Choice) breaded, 8 fillets	2½-oz. serving	120	11.0
(Mrs. Paul's):			
Batter dipped	1 fillet	165	14.0
Crispy crunchy	1 fillet	115	11.5
Crunchy batter	1 fillet	140	13.0
Light, in butter sauce	1 fillet	70	.5
FISH LOAF, home recipe (USDA)	4 oz.	141	8.3
FISH NUGGET, frozen:			
(Frionor) *Bunch O' Crunch*, breaded	.5-oz. piece	40	2.2
(Van de Kamp's) battered	1 piece	32	2.0
FISH SANDWICH, frozen:			
(Frionor) *Bunch O' Crunch*, microwave	5-oz. sandwich	320	31.0
(Hormel) *Quick Meal*	5.2-oz. serving	430	56.0
FISH STICKS, frozen:			
(Captain's Choice)	1 piece	76	7.0
(Frionor) *Bunch O' Crunch*, breaded	.7-oz. piece	58	3.5
(Gorton's):			
Crunchy, regular	1 piece	55	3.7
Potato crisp	1 piece	65	3.2
Value pack	1 piece	52	4.5
(Healthy Choice) breaded	1 piece	15	1.7
(Mrs. Paul's):			
Battered	1 piece	52	3.7
Crispy, crunchy, breaded	2.7 oz.	170	16.0
(Van de Kamp's):			
Battered	1 piece	40	3.0
Breaded:			
Regular	1 piece	50	3.7
Value Pack	1 piece	42	3.2
FLOUNDER:			
Raw (USDA):			
Whole	1 lb. (weighed whole)	118	0.0
Meat only	4 oz.	90	0.0
Baked (USDA)	4 oz.	229	0.0

Food	Measure	Cals.	Carbs.
Frozen:			
(Captain's Choice) fillet	3 oz.	99	0.0
(Frionor) *Norway Gourmet*	4-oz. piece	60	0.0
(Gorton's):			
Fishmarket Fresh	5 oz.	110	1.0
Microwave entree,			
stuffed	1 pkg.	350	21.0
(Mrs. Paul's) fillet:			
Crunchy batter	1 fillet	130	12.0
Light	1 fillet	240	20.0
FLOUR:			
(USDA):			
Buckwheat, dark, sifted	1 cup (3.5 oz.)	326	70.6
Buckwheat, light sifted	1 cup (3.5 oz.)	340	77.9
Cake:			
Unsifted, dipped	1 cup (4.2 oz.)	433	94.5
Unsifted, spooned	1 cup (3.9 oz.)	404	88.1
Carob or St. John's bread	1 oz.	51	22.9
Chestnut	1 oz.	103	21.6
Corn	1 cup (3.9 oz.)	405	84.5
Cottonseed	1 oz.	101	9.4
Fish, from whole fish	1 oz.	95	0.0
Lima bean	1 oz.	95	17.9
Potato	1 oz.	100	22.7
Rice, stirred spooned	1 cup (5.6 oz.)	574	125.6
Rye:			
Light:			
Unsifted, spooned	1 cup (3.6 oz.)	361	78.7
Sifted, spooned	1 cup (3.1 oz.)	314	68.6
Medium	1 oz.	99	21.1
Dark:			
Unstirred	1 cup (4.5 oz.)	419	87.2
Stirred	1 cup (4.5 oz.)	415	86.5
Soybean, defatted, stirred	1 cup (3.6 oz.)	329	38.5
Soybean, high fat	1 oz.	108	9.4
Sunflower seed, partially			
defatted	1 oz.	96	10.7
Wheat:			
All-purpose:			
Unsifted, dipped	1 cup (5 oz.)	521	108.8
Unsifted, spooned	1 cup (4.4 oz.)	459	95.9
Sifted, spooned	1 cup (4.1 oz.)	422	88.3
Bread:			
Unsifted, dipped	1 cup (4.8 oz.)	496	101.6
Unsifted, spooned	1 cup (4.3 oz.)	449	91.9
Sifted, spooned	1 cup (4.1 oz.)	427	87.4

Food	Measure	Cals.	Carbs.
Gluten:			
Unsifted, dipped	1 cup (5 oz.)	537	67.0
Sifted, spooned	1 cup (4.8 oz.)	514	64.2
Self-rising:			
Unsifted, dipped	1 cup (4.6 oz.)	458	96.5
Sifted, spooned	1 cup (3.7 oz.)	373	78.7
Whole wheat	1 oz.	94	20.1
(Aunt Jemima) self-rising	¼ cup (1 oz.)	109	23.6
Ballard:			
Self-rising	¼ cup	91	23.6
All-purpose	¼ cup (1 oz.)	100	21.8
Bisquick (Betty Crocker)	¼ cup (1 oz.)	120	18.5
(Drifted Snow)	¼ cup	100	21.8
(Elam's):			
Brown rice, whole grain, sodium & gluten free	¼ cup (1.2 oz.)	125	.2
Buckwheat, pure	¼ cup (1.4 oz.)	131	27.2
Pastry, whole wheat	¼ cup (1.2 oz.)	122	24.9
Rye, whole grain	¼ cup	118	24.2
Soy, roasted, defatted	¼ cup (1.1 oz.)	108	9.8
3-in-1 mix	1 oz.	99	20.0
White, with wheat germ	¼ cup (1 oz.)	101	20.7
Whole wheat	¼ cup (1.1 oz.)	111	21.7
Gold Medal:			
All purpose or unbleached	¼ cup (1 oz.)	100	21.8
Better For Bread	¼ cup	100	20.7
Self-rising	¼ cup	95	20.8
Whole wheat	¼ cup	98	19.5
Pillsbury's Best:			
All-purpose or rye and wheat Bohemian style	¼ cup	100	21.5
Bread or rye, medium	¼ cup	100	20.8
Self-rising	¼ cup	95	21.0
Shake & blend	1 T.	25	5.5
Whole wheat	¼ cup	100	21.0
(Quaker) corn:			
Masa Harina De Maiz	⅓ cup (1.34 oz.)	137	27.4
Masa Trigo	⅓ cup (1.3 oz.)	149	24.7
Red Band:			
All purpose or unbleached	¼ cup	97	21.2
Self-rising	¼ cup	95	20.8
Wondra	¼ cup	100	21.8

FOLLE BLANC WINE

Food	Measure	Cals.	Carbs.
(Louis M. Martini) 12.5% alcohol	3 fl. oz.	63	.2

Food	Measure	Cals.	Carbs.
FRANKEN*BERRY, cereal			
(General Mills)	1 cup (1 oz.)	110	24.0
FRANKFURTER, raw or cooked:			
(USDA), raw:			
Common type	1 frankfurter (10 per lb.)	140	.8
Meat	1 frankfurter (10 per lb.)	134	1.1
With cereal	1 frankfurter (10 per lb.)	112	.1
Cooked, common type	1 frankfurter (10 per lb.)	136	.7
(Ball Park) beef or beef, pork & chicken, lite	1 frankfurter	140	1.0
(Boar's Head):			
Beef:			
Regular:			
Natural casing	2-oz. frankfurter	160	1.0
Skinless	1.6-oz. frankfurter	120	0.0
Lite	1.6-oz. frankfurter	90	0.0
Meat, natural casing or skinless	2-oz. frankfurter	150	0.0
(Butterball) turkey	1 frankfurter	140	2.0
(Eckrich):			
Beef	1.2-oz. frankfurter	110	2.0
Beef	1.6-oz. frankfurter	150	3.0
Beef	2-oz. frankfurter	190	3.0
Cheese	2-oz. frankfurter	190	3.0
Meat	1.2-oz. frankfurter	120	2.0
Meat	1.6-oz. frankfurter	150	3.0
Meat	2.-oz. frankfurter	190	3.0
(Empire Kosher):			
Chicken	2-oz. frankfurter	106	1.0
Turkey	2-oz. frankfurter	107	1.0
(Health Valley) chicken	1 frankfurter	95	1.0
(Healthy Choice) turkey, pork & beef jumbo, low-fat	1 frankfurter	70	5.0

Food	Measure	Cals.	Carbs.
Hebrew National:			
Beef	1.7-oz. frankfurter	149	<1.0
Collagen	2.3-oz. frankfurter	202	<1.0
Lite, beef	1.7-oz. frankfurter	120	<1.0
Natural casing	2-oz. frankfurter	175	<1.0
(Hormel):			
Beef	1 frankfurter (12-oz. pkg.)	100	1.0
Beef	1 frankfurter (1 lb. pkg.)	140	1.0
Chili, *Frank 'n Stuff*	1 frankfurter	165	2.0
Meat	1 frankfurter (12-oz. pkg.)	110	1.0
Meat	1 frankfurter (1-lb. pkg.)	140	1.0
Range Brand	1 frankfurter	170	1.0
Wrangler, smoked:			
Beef	1 frankfurter	170	2.0
Cheese	1 frankfurter	180	1.0
(Louis Rich):			
Turkey	1.5-oz. frankfurter	95	1.0
Turkey	1.6-oz. frankfurter	100	1.0
Turkey	2.-oz. frankfurter	125	1.0
(Ohse):			
Beef	1-oz. frankfurter	85	1.0
Wiener:			
Regular	1-oz. frankfurter	90	1.0
Chicken, beef & pork	1-oz. frankfurter	85	1.0
(Oscar Mayer):			
Bacon & cheddar	1.6-oz. frankfurter	139	1.0
Beef:			
Regular	1.6-oz. frankfurter	143	1.1
Jumbo	2-oz. frankfurter	179	1.4
Big One	4-oz. frankfurter	357	2.7
Cheese	1.6-oz. frankfurter	144	1.0
Little Wiener	2" frankfurter	28	.2
Wiener	1.6-oz. frankfurter	144	1.1
Wiener	2-oz. frankfurter	180	1.4

Food	Measure	Cals.	Carbs.
(Safeway) beef or meat (Smok-A-Roma):	2-oz. frankfurter	170	1.0
Beef	2-oz. frankfurter	170	1.0
Meat	2-oz. frankfurter	140	1.0
FRANKFURTER SANDWICH, frozen:			
(Boar's Head) *Bagel Dog*	1 piece	310	DNA
(Hormel) *Quick Meal:*			
With cheese, *Cheesy Dog*	1 meal	310	29.0
Chili with cheese	1 piece	350	30.0
(Swanson) on a bun, *Fun Feast*	1 piece	350	47.0
FRANKFURTER WRAP, *Weiner Wrap*	1 piece	60	10.0
FRENCH TOAST, frozen:			
(Aunt Jemima):			
Original	1 piece	120	18.0
Cinnamon swirl	1 piece	120	18.0
(Downyflake)	1 piece	130	21.5
(Swanson) *Breakfast Blast:*			
Regular, mini	3-oz. serving	180	30.0
Slicks	3¾-oz. serving	280	44.0
FRENCH TOAST BREAK-FAST, frozen:			
(Aunt Jemima) Homestyle			
Regular	5.9-oz. meal	470	53.0
With sausages	5.3-oz. meal	390	35.0
(Swanson) *Great Starts:*			
Plain, with sausage	5½-oz. meal	410	36.0
Cinnamon swirl, with sausage	5½-oz. meal	440	38.0
FRITTERS:			
Home recipe (USDA):			
Clam	2" × 1¾" (1.4 oz.)	124	12.4
Corn	2" × 1½" (1.2 oz.)	132	13.9
Frozen (Mrs. Paul's) apple or corn	1 piece	120	17.5
FROG LEGS, raw (USDA):			
Bone-in	1 lb. (weighed with bone)	215	0.0

Food	Measure	Cals.	Carbs.
Meat only	4 oz.	83	0.0
FROOT LOOPS, cereal (Kellogg's)	1 cup (1 oz.)	110	25.0
FROSTED RICE, cereal (Ralston Purina)	1 cup (1 oz.)	110	26.0
FROSTEE (Borden):			
Chocolate flavored	1 cup	200	30.0
Strawberry flavored	1 cup	180	27.0
FROSTING (See **CAKE ICING**)			
FROZEN DESSERT (See ICE CREAM SUBSTITUTE OR IMITATION or **TOFUTTI**)			
FROZEN DINNER OR ENTREE (See individual listings such as **BEAN & FRANKFURTER DINNER; BEEF DINNER OR ENTREE; LASAGNA,** frozen; etc.)			
FRUIT (See individual listings such as **BANANA; FIG; KUMQUAT;** etc.)			
FRUIT, MIXED:			
Canned, solids & liq.:			
(Del Monte) Lite, chunky	½ cup	58	14.0
(Hunt's) *Snack Pack*	5-oz. container	120	31.0
Dried:			
(Sun-Maid/Sunsweet)	2 oz.	150	39.0
(Town House)	2 oz.	150	40.0
FRUIT BARS (General Mills) *Fruit Corners:* Regular:			
Cherry, grape or strawberry	1 bar	90	18.0

Food	Measure	Cals.	Carbs.
Orange pineapple or tropical	1 bar	90	17.0
Swirled	1 bar	90	18.0
FRUIT BITS, dried (Sun-Maid)	1 oz.	90	21.0
FRUIT 'N CHERRY JUICE (Tree Top):			
Canned	6 fl. oz.	80	21.0
*Frozen	6 fl. oz.	90	22.0
FRUIT 'N CITRUS JUICE (Tree Top):			
Canned	6 fl. oz.	100	24.0
*Frozen	6 fl. oz.	90	22.0
FRUIT COCKTAIL:			
Canned, regular pack, solids & liq.:			
(USDA):			
Light syrup	4 oz.	68	17.8
Heavy syrup	½ cup (4.5 oz.)	97	25.2
Extra syrup	4 oz.	104	26.9
(Hunt's)	½ cup (4 oz.)	90	23.0
(S&W):			
Juice pack	½ cup	90	21.0
Heavy syrup	½ cup	90	24.0
(Town House)	½ cup	90	24.0
Canned, dietetic or low calorie, solids & liq.:			
(Country Pure)	½ cup	50	14.0
(Diet Delight):			
Juice pack	½ cup (4.4 oz.)	50	14.0
Water pack	½ cup (4.3 oz.)	40	10.0
(Libby's) Lite, water pack	½ cup (4.4 oz.)	50	13.0
(S&W) *Nutradiet,* white or blue label	½ cup	40	10.0
FRUIT COMPOTE, canned (Rokeach)	½ cup (4 oz.)	120	31.0
FRUIT & CREAM BAR (Dole):			
Blueberry, peach or strawberry	1 bar	90	18.0
Chocolate-banana	1 bar	175	22.0

Food	Measure	Cals.	Carbs.
Chocolate-strawberry	1 bar	160	23.0
Raspberry	1 bar	90	19.0
FRUIT & FIBER, cereal (Post):			
Dates, raisins, walnuts with oat clusters	⅔ cup (1¼ oz.)	120	27.0
Tropical fruit with oat clusters	⅔ cup (1¼-oz.)	125	27.0
Whole wheat & bran flakes with peaches, raisins, almonds & oat clusters	⅔ cup (1¼ oz.)	121	266.0
FRUIT 'N GRAPE JUICE (Tree Top):			
Canned	6 fl. oz.	100	25.0
*Frozen	6 fl. oz.	110	27.0
FRUIT JUICE, canned (See individual listings such as *CRANAPPLE* JUICE DRINK; ORANGE-GRAPEFRUIT JUICE; PINEAPPLE JUICE; etc.)			
FRUIT 'N JUICE BAR: (Dole):			
Fresh Lites:			
Cherry, pineapple-orange & raspberry	1 bar	25	6.0
Lemon	1 bar	25	5.0
Fruit 'N Juice:			
Cherry or pineapple	1 bar	70	18.0
Peach passion fruit	1 bar	70	16.0
Piña colada	1 bar	80	15.0
Pineapple-orange-banana, raspberry or strawberry	1 bar	60	15.0
Sun Tops	1 bar	40	9.0
(Weight Watchers)	1.7-fl.-oz. bar	35	9.0
FRUIT & JUICE DRINK (Tree Top):			
Canned:			

Food	Measure	Cals.	Carbs.
Apple	6 fl. oz.	90	22.0
Berry	6 fl. oz.	80	21.0
Cherry	6 fl. oz.	100	24.0
Citrus	6 fl. oz.	90	22.0
Grape	6 fl. oz.	100	25.0
*Frozen:			
Apple	6 fl. oz.	90	23.0
Berry, cherry or citrus	6 fl. oz.	90	22.0
Grape	6 fl. oz.	110	27.0
FRUIT & NUT MIX (Estee)	1 piece	35	3.0
FRUIT PUNCH, canned:			
(Juicy Juice)	6 fl. oz.	100	23.0
(Snapple)	6 fl. oz.	90	21.7
FRUIT PUNCH DRINK:			
Canned:			
Bama (Borden)	8.45 fl.-oz. container	130	32.0
(Hi-C)	6 fl. oz.	96	23.7
(Lincoln) party	6 fl. oz.	90	23.0
(Minute Maid):			
Regular	8.45-fl.-oz. container	128	32.0
On the Go	10-fl.-oz. bottle	152	37.9
Chilled:			
(Minute Maid)	6 fl. oz.	91	22.7
(Sunkist)	8.45 fl. oz.	140	34.0
*Frozen (Minute Maid)	6 fl. oz.	91	22.7
*Mix:			
Regular (Funny Face)	8 fl. oz.	88	22.0
Dietetic, *Crystal Light* (General Foods)	8 fl. oz.	3	.1
FRUIT RINGS, cereal (Safeway)	1 oz.	110	26.0
FRUIT ROLLS:			
(Flavor Tree)	¾-oz. piece	80	18.0
Fruit Corners (General Mills):			
Apple, apricot, banana, cherry or grape	.5-oz. piece	50	12.0
Fruit punch	.5-oz. piece	60	12.0
(Sunkist)	.5-oz. piece	50	12.0

Food	Measure	Cals.	Carbs.
FRUIT SALAD:			
Canned, regular pack, solids & liq.:			
(USDA):			
Light syrup	4 oz.	67	17.6
Heavy syrup	½ cup (4.3 oz.)	85	22.0
Extra heavy syrup	4 oz.	102	26.5
(Dole) tropical, in light syrup	½ cup	70	17.0
(Libby's) heavy syrup	½ cup (4.4 oz.)	99	24.0
Canned, dietetic or low calorie, solids & liq.:			
(Diet Delight) juice pack	½ cup (4.4 oz.)	60	16.0
(S&W) *Nutradiet:*			
Juice pack, white label	½ cup	50	11.0
Water pack, blue label	½ cup	35	10.0
FRUIT SLUSH (Wyler's)	4 fl. oz.	157	39.3
FRUIT WRINKLES (General Mills) *Fruit Corners*	1 pouch	100	21.0
FRUITY YUMMY MUMMY, cereal (General Mills)	1 cup (1 oz.)	110	24.0
FUSILLI (See **PASTA, DRY OR FRESH, REFRIGERATED**)			

G

Food	Measure	Cals.	Carbs.
GARFIELD AND FRIENDS			
(General Mills):			
Pouch:			
1-2 Punch	.9-oz. pouch	100	21.0
Very strawberry	.9-oz. pouch	90	21.0
Roll	.5-oz. roll	50	12.0
GARLIC:			
Raw (USDA):			

Food	Measure	Cals.	Carbs.
Whole	2 oz. (weighed with skin)	68	15.4
Peeled	1 oz.	39	8.7
Flakes (Gilroy)	1 tsp.	13	2.6
Powder (French's)	1 tsp.	10	2.0
Salt (French's)	1 tsp.	4	1.0
Spread (Lawry's):			
Concentrate	1 T.	15	.2
Ready-to-use, bread spread	1 T.	94	2.0
GARLIC BREAD SPREAD			
(Lawry's)	½ tsp.	47	1.0
GARLIC PUREE			
(Progresso)	1 tsp.	4	Tr.
GARLIC SPREAD (Lawry's)			
concentrate	1 T.	15	Tr.
GATORADE (See **SPORTS DRINK**)			
GEFILTE FISH, canned:			
(Manischewitz):			
Fishlets	1 piece	8	4.4
Gefilte:			
Regular:			
12- or 24-oz. jar	3-oz. piece	53	4.4
4-lb. pkg.	2.7-oz. piece	48	4.4
Homestyle:			
12- or 24-oz. jar	3-oz. piece	55	6.2
4-lb. jar	2.7-oz. piece	50	6.2
Sweet:			
12- or 24-oz. jar	3-oz. piece	65	8.7
4-lb. jar	2.7-oz. piece	59	8.7
Whitefish & pike:			
Regular:			
12- or 24-oz. jar	3-oz. piece	49	4.8
4-lb. jar	2.7-oz. piece	44	4.8
Sweet:			
12- or 24-oz. jar	3-oz. piece	64	8.8
4-lb. jar	2.7-oz. piece	58	8.8
(Rokeach):			
Natural broth:			
12-oz. jar	2-oz. piece	46	3.0
24-oz. jar	2.6-oz. piece	60	4.0
Old Vienna:			

Food	Measure	Cals.	Carbs.
Regular:			
12-oz. jar	2-oz. piece	52	4.0
24-oz. jar	2.6-oz. piece	68	5.0
Jellied, whitefish & pike:			
12-oz. jar	2-oz. piece	54	4.0
24-oz. jar	2.6-oz. piece	70	5.0
Redi-Jell:			
12-oz. jar	2-oz. piece	46	3.0
24-oz. jar	2.6-oz. piece	60	4.0
Whitefish & pike, jellied broth:			
12-oz. jar	2-oz. piece	46	3.0
24-oz. jar	2.6-oz. piece	60	4.0
GELATIN, unflavored, dry:			
(USDA)	7-gram envelope	23	0.0
Carmel Kosher	7-gram envelope	30	0.0
(Knox)	1 envelope	25	0.0
GELATIN, DRINKING			
(Knox) orange	1 envelope	40	4.0
GELATIN BAR, frozen (Jell-O) all flavors	1 bar	35	8.0
GELATIN DESSERT:			
Canned, dietetic (Dia-Mel; Louis Sherry)	4-oz. container	2	Tr.
*Powder:			
Regular:			
Carmel Kosher, all flavors	½ cup (4 oz.)	80	20.0
(Jell-O) all flavors	½ cup (4.9 oz.)	83	18.6
(Royal) all flavors	½ cup (4.9 oz.)	80	19.0
Dietetic:			
Carmel Kosher, all flavors	½ cup	8	0.0
(D-Zerta) all flavors	½ cup (4.3 oz.)	7	.1
(Estee) all flavors	½ cup (4.2 oz.)	8	Tr.
(Featherweight):			
Regular	½ cup	10	1.0
Artificially sweetened	½ cup	10	0.0
(Jell-O) sugar free:			
Cherry	½ cup (4.3 oz.)	12	.1
Lime	½ cup	9	.1
Orange, raspberry or strawberry	½ cup	8	.1
(Louis Sherry)	½ cup	8	Tr.
(Royal)	½ cup	12	0.0

Food	Measure	Cals.	Carbs.
GIN, unflavored (See **DISTILLED LIQUOR**)			
GIN, SLOE:			
(DeKuyper)	1 fl. oz.	70	5.2
(Mr. Boston)	1 fl. oz.	68	4.7
GINGER, powdered (French's)	1 tsp.	6	1.2
GINGERBREAD:			
Home recipe (USDA)	1.9-oz piece (2" × 2" × 2")	174	28.6
Mix:			
*(Betty Crocker):			
Regular	⅑ of pkg.	220	35.0
No cholesterol recipe	⅑ of pkg.	210	35.0
(Dromedary)	2" × 2" square (¹⁄₁₆ of pkg.)	100	19.0
(Pillsbury)	3" square (⅑ of cake)	190	36.0
GOLDEN GRAHAMS, cereal (General Mills)	¾ cup (1 oz.)	110	24.0
GOOBER GRAPE (Smucker's)	1 T.	90	9.0
GOOD HUMOR (See **ICE CREAM**)			
GOOSE, domesticated (USDA):			
Raw	1 lb. (weighed ready-to-cook)	1172	0.0
Roasted:			
Meat & skin	4 oz.	500	0.0
Meat only	4 oz.	264	0.0
GOOSEBERRY (USDA):			
Fresh	1 lb.	177	44.0
Fresh	1 cup (5.3 oz.)	58	14.6
Canned, water pack, solids & liq.	4 oz.	29	7.5
GOOSE GIZZARD, raw (USDA)	4 oz.	158	0.0

Food	Measure	Cals.	Carbs.
GRAHAM CRACKER (See **CRACKERS, PUFFS & CHIPS,** Graham)			
GRANOLA BAR:			
Nature Valley:			
Cinnamon or oats & honey	.8-oz. bar	120	17.0
Oat bran honey graham	.8-oz. bar	110	16.0
Peanut butter	.8-oz. bar	120	15.0
(Hershey's) chocolate covered:			
Chocolate chip	1.2-oz. piece	170	22.0
Cocoa creme	1.2-oz. piece	180	22.0
Cookies & creme	1.2-oz. piece	170	23.0
Peanut butter	1.2-oz. piece	180	19.0
GRANOLA CEREAL:			
Nature Valley:			
Cinnamon & raisin, fruit & nut or toasted oat	⅓ cup (1 oz.)	130	19.0
Coconut & honey	⅓ cup (1 oz.)	150	18.0
Sun Country (Kretschmer):			
With almonds	¼ cup (1 oz.)	138	19.3
Honey almond	1 oz.	130	19.0
With raisins	¼ cup (1 oz.)	133	19.9
With raisins & dates	¼ cup (1 oz.)	130	20.0
GRANOLA SNACK:			
Kudos (M&M/Mars):			
Chocolate chip	1.25-oz. pkg.	180	21.0
Nutty fudge	1.3-oz. pkg.	190	19.0
Peanut butter	1.3-oz. pkg.	190	17.0
Nature Valley:			
Cinnamon or honey nut	1 pouch	140	19.0
Oats & honey	1 pouch	140	18.0
Peanut butter	1 pouch	140	17.0
GRAPE:			
Fresh:			
American type (slip skin), Concord, Delaware, Niagara, Catawba and Scuppernong:			
(USDA)	½ lb. (weighed with stem, skin & seeds)	98	22.4
(USDA)	½ cup (2.7 oz.)	33	7.5

Food	Measure	Cals.	Carbs.
(USDA)	3½" × 3" bunch (3.5 oz.)	43	9.9
European type (adherent skin), Malaga, Muscat, Thompson seedless, Emperor & Flame Tokay:			
(USDA)	½ lb. (weighed with stem & seeds)	139	34.9
(USDA) whole	20 grapes (¾" dia.)	52	13.5
(USDA) whole	½ cup (.3 oz.)	56	14.5
(USDA) halves	½ cup (.3 oz.)	56	14.4
Canned, solids & liq., (USDA) Thompson seedless, heavy syrup	4 oz.	87	22.7
Canned, dietetic pack, solids & liq.:			
(USDA) Thompson seedless, water pack	4 oz.	58	15.4
(Featherweight) water pack, seedless	½ cup	60	13.0
GRAPEADE:			
Canned (Snapple)	8 fl. oz.	120	10.0
Chilled or frozen (Minute Maid)	6 fl. oz.	94	23.4
GRAPE-APPLE DRINK, canned (Mott's)	9.5-fl. oz. container	158	40.0
GRAPE DRINK:			
Canned:			
(Borden) *Bama*	8.45-fl.-oz. container	120	29.0
(Hi-C)	6 fl. oz.	96	23.7
(Johanna Farms) *Ssips*	8.45-fl-oz. container	130	32.0
(Lincoln)	6 fl. oz.	90	23.0
(Welchade)	6 fl. oz.	90	23.0
Chilled (Sunkist)	8.45 fl. oz.	140	33.0
*Mix:			
Regular (Funny Face)	8 fl. oz.	88	22.0
Dietetic (Sunkist)	8 fl. oz.	6	2.0
GRAPE JAM (Smucker's)	1 T. (.7 oz.)	53	13.7

Food	Measure	Cals.	Carbs.
GRAPE JELLY:			
Sweetened:			
(Borden) *Bama*	1 T.	45	12.0
(Empress)	1 T.	52	13.5
(Smucker's):			
Regular	1 T. (.5 oz.)	54	12.0
Goober Grape	1 T.	90	9.0
Dietetic:			
(Diet Delight)	1 T. (.6 oz.)	12	3.0
(Estee)	1 T.	6	0.0
(Slenderella)	1 T.	21	6.0
(Weight Watchers)	1 T.	24	6.0
GRAPE JUICE:			
Canned, unsweetened:			
(USDA)	½ cup (4.4 oz.)	83	20.9
(Ardmore Farms)	6 fl. oz.	99	24.9
(Borden) *Sippin' Pak*	8.45-fl.-oz. container	130	32.0
(Johanna Farms) *Tree Ripe*	8.45-fl.-oz. container	164	40.0
(Minute Maid)	8.45-fl. oz. container	150	37.4
(Town House)	6 fl. oz.	120	30.0
(Tree Top) sparkling	6 fl. oz.	120	29.0
*Frozen:			
(Minute Maid)	6 fl. oz.	99	13.3
(Welch's)	6 fl. oz.	100	25.0
GRAPE JUICE DRINK, chilled:			
(Sunkist)	8.45 fl. oz.	140	33.0
(Welch's)	6 fl. oz.	110	27.0
GRAPE NUTS, cereal (Post):			
Regular	¼ cup (1 oz.)	105	23.0
Flakes	⅞ cup (1 oz.)	111	23.1
Raisin	¼ cup (1 oz.)	102	23.0
GRAPE PRESERVE OR JAM, sweetened (Welch's)	1 T.	52	13.5
GRAPE-RASPBERRY JUICE DRINK, canned (Boku)	8 fl. oz.	120	29.0
GRAPE-STRAWBERRY DRINK, canned (Mistic)	8 fl. oz.	110	31.0

Food	Measure	Cals.	Carbs.
GRAPEFRUIT:			
Fresh (USDA):			
White:			
Seeded type	1 lb. (weighed with seeds & skin)	86	22.4
Seedless type	1 lb. (weighed with skin)	87	22.6
Seeded type	½ med. grapefruit (3¾" dia., 8.5 oz.)	54	14.1
Pink and red:			
Seeded type	1 lb. (weighed with seeds & skin)	87	22.6
Seedless type	1 lb. (weighed with skin)	93	24.1
Seeded type	½ med. grapefruit (3¾" dia., 8.5 oz.)	46	12.0
Canned, syrup pack (Del Monte) solids & liq.	½ cup	74	17.5
Canned, unsweetened or dietetic pack, solids & liq.:			
(USDA) water pack	½ cup (4.2 oz.)	36	9.1
(Del Monte) sections	½ cup	46	10.5
(Diet Delight) sections, juice pack	½ cup (4.3 oz.)	45	11.0
(Featherweight) sections, juice pack	½ of 8-oz. can	40	9.0
(S&W) *Nutradiet,* sections	½ cup	40	9.0
GRAPEFRUIT DRINK, canned (Lincoln)	6 fl. oz.	100	25.0
GRAPEFRUIT JUICE:			
Fresh (USDA) pink, red or white	½ cup (4.3 oz.)	46	11.3
Canned, sweetened:			
(Ardmore Farms)	6 fl. oz.	78	18.1
(Johanna Farms)	6 fl. oz.	76	18.0
(Libby's)	6 fl.oz.	70	17.0
(Minute Maid) On the Go	10-fl oz. bottle	130	30.7
(Mott's)	9.5-fl. oz. can	118	29.0
Canned, unsweetened:			
(Libby's)	6 fl. oz.	75	18.0

Food	Measure	Cals.	Carbs.
(Ocean Spray)	6 fl. oz.	70	16.2
(Town House)	6 fl. oz.	70	15.0
(Tree Top)	6 fl. oz.	80	19.0
Chilled (Sunkist)	6 fl. oz.	72	17.0
*Frozen (Minute Maid)	6 fl. oz.	83	19.7
GRAPEFRUIT JUICE COCKTAIL, canned (Ocean Spray) pink	6 fl. oz.	80	20.0
GRAPEFRUIT-ORANGE JUICE COCKTAIL, canned, (Ardmore Farms)	6 fl. oz.	78	19.1
GRAPEFRUIT PEEL, CANDIED (USDA)	1 oz.	90	22.9
GRAVY, canned:			
Regular:			
Au jus (Franco-American)	2-oz. serving	10	2.0
Beef (Franco-American)	2-oz. serving	25	4.0
Brown (La Choy)	2-oz. serving	140	40.4
Chicken (Franco-American):			
Regular	2-oz. serving	45	3.0
Giblet	2-oz. serving	30	3.0
Cream (Franco-American)	2-oz. serving	35	4.0
Mushroom (Franco-American)	2-oz. serving	25	3.0
Pork (Franco-American)	2-oz. serving	40	3.0
Turkey:			
(Franco-American)	2-oz. serving	30	3.0
(Howard Johnson's) giblet	½ cup	55	5.5
Dietetic (Estee):			
Brown	¼ cup	14	3.0
Chicken & herb	¼ cup	20	4.0
GRAVYMASTER	1 tsp. (.2 oz.)	12	2.4
GRAVY MIX:			
Regular:			
Au jus:			
*(French's) *Gravy Makins*	½ cup	20	4.0
*(Lawry's)	½ cup	42	5.5
Brown:			
*(French's) *Gravy Makins*	½ cup	40	8.0
*(Knorr) classic	2 fl. oz.	25	3.1
*(Lawry's)	½ cup	47	18.2

Food	Measure	Cals.	Carbs.
*(Pillsbury)	½ cup	30	6.0
Chicken:			
*(French's) *Gravy Makins*	½ cup	50	8.0
(McCormick)	.85-oz. pkg.	82	13.4
*(Pillsbury)	½ cup	50	8.0
Homestyle:			
*(French's) *Gravy Makins*	½ cup	40	8.0
*(Pillsbury)	½ cup	30	6.0
Mushroom *(French's) *Gravy Makins*	½ cup	40	6.0
Onion:			
*(French's) *Gravy Makins*	½ cup	50	8.0
*(McCormick)	.85-oz. pkg.	72	9.8
Pork:			
(Durkee):			
*Regular	½ cup	35	7.0
Roastin' Bag	1.5-oz. pkg.	130	26.0
*(French's) *Gravy Makins*	½ cup	40	8.0
Pot roast (Durkee) *Roastin' Bag,* regular or onion	1.5-oz. pkg.	125	25.0
*Swiss steak (Durkee)	½ cup	22	5.4
Turkey:			
*(Durkee)	½ cup	47	7.0
*(French's) *Gravy Makins*	½ cup	50	8.0
*Dietetic (Estee):			
Brown	½ cup	28	6.0
Chicken, & herbs	½ cup	40	8.0

GRAVY WITH MEAT OR TURKEY, frozen (Banquet):
Cookin' Bag:

Food	Measure	Cals.	Carbs.
Mushroom gravy & charbroiled beef patty	5-oz. pkg.	210	8.0
& salisbury steak	5-oz. pkg.	190	8.0
& sliced beef	4-oz. pkg.	100	5.0
& sliced turkey	5-oz. pkg.	100	5.0

Family Entree:

Food	Measure	Cals.	Carbs.
Onion gravy & beef patties	¼ of 32-oz. pkg.	300	14.0
& salisbury steak	¼ of 32-oz. pkg.	300	12.0
& sliced beef	¼ of 32-oz. pkg.	160	8.0
& sliced turkey	¼ of 32-oz. pkg.	150	8.0

GREENS, MIXED, canned, solids & liq.:

Food	Measure	Cals.	Carbs.
(Allen's)	½ cup (4 oz.)	25	3.0
(Sunshine)	½ cup (4.1 oz.)	20	2.7

Food	Measure	Cals.	Carbs.
GRENADINE (Rose's)			
non-alcoholic	1 T.	45	11.0
GROUPER, raw (USDA):			
Whole	1 lb. (weighed whole)	170	0.0
Meat only	4 oz.	99	0.0
GUACAMOLE SEASONING MIX (Lawry's)	.7-oz. pkg.	60	12.6
GUANABANA PUNCH, canned (Knudsen & Sons) *Rain Forest*	8 fl. oz.	125	29.0
GUAVA, COMMON, fresh (USDA):			
Whole	1 lb. (weighed untrimmed)	273	66.0
Whole	1 guava (2.8 oz.)	48	11.7
Flesh only	4 oz.	70	17.0
GUAVA, STRAWBERRY, fresh (USDA):			
Whole	1 lb. (weighed untrimmed)	289	70.2
Flesh only	4 oz.	74	17.9
GUAVA-CRANBERRY JUICE, canned (Santa Cruz Natural) organic	8 fl. oz.	130	30.0
GUAVA FRUIT DRINK, canned, *Mauna La'i*	6 fl. oz.	100	25.0
GUAVA JAM (Smucker's)	1 T.	53	13.5
GUAVA JELLY (Smucker's)	1 T.	53	13.5
GUAVA JUICE (Welch's) *Orchard Tropicals*:			
Bottled	6 fl. oz.	100	25.0
*Frozen	6 fl. oz.	100	25.0
GUAVA NECTAR (Libby's)	6 fl. oz.	70	17.0

Food	Measure	Cals.	Carbs.
GUAVA-PASSION FRUIT			
DRINK, canned, *Mauna La'i*	6 fl. oz.	100	25.0
GUINEA HEN, raw (USDA):			
Ready-to-cook	1 lb. (weighed)	594	0.0
Meat & skin	4 oz.	179	0.0
*GYRO MIX (Casbah)	1 patty (2 oz.)	145	12.0

H

HADDOCK:			
Raw (USDA) meat only	4 oz.	90	0.0
Fried, breaded (USDA)	4" × 3" × ½" fillet (3.5 oz.)	165	5.8
Smoked (USDA)	4-oz. serving	117	0.0
Frozen:			
(Captain's Choice) fillet	3-oz. piece	95	0.0
(Frionor) *Norway Gourmet*	4-oz. fillet	70	0.0
(Gorton's):			
Fishmarket Fresh	4 oz.	90	0.0
Microwave entree, in lemon butter	1 pkg.	360	19.0
(Mrs. Paul's):			
Crunchy batter	1 fillet	95	11.0
Light	1 fillet	110	7.5
HALIBUT:			
Raw (USDA):			
Whole	1 lb. (weighed whole)	144	0.0
Meat only	4 oz.	84	0.0
Broiled (USDA)	4" × 3" × ½" steak (4.4 oz.)	214	0.0
Smoked (USDA)	4 oz.	254	0.0
Frozen (Van de Kamp's) batter dipped, french fried	½ of 8-oz. pkg.	260	18.0

Food	Measure	Cals.	Carbs.
HAM (See also **PORK**):			
Canned:			
(Hormel):			
Black Label (3- or 5-lb. size)	4 oz.	140	0.0
Chopped	3 oz. (8-lb. ham)	240	1.0
Chunk	6¾-oz. serving	310	0.0
Curemaster, smoked	4 oz.	140	1.0
EXL	4 oz.	120	0.0
Holiday Glaze	4 oz. (3-lb. ham)	140	2.9
Patties	1 patty	180	0.0
(Oscar Mayer) *Jubilee,* extra lean, cooked	1-oz. serving	31	.1
(Swift) *Premium*	1¾-oz. slice	111	.3
Deviled:			
(Hormel)	1 T.	35	0.0
(Libby's)	1 T. (.5 oz.)	43	0.0
(Underwood)	1 T. (.5 oz.)	49	Tr.
Packaged:			
(Boar's Head):			
Boiled, branded deluxe	1 oz.	30	1.0
Deluxe, Deli-Trition, low cholesterol	1 oz.	30	1.0
Maple glazed, honey coated	1 oz.	30	1.5
Smoked, regular or Virginian style	1 oz.	30	1.0
(Carl Buddig) smoked	1-oz. slice	50	Tr.
(Eckrich):			
Chopped	1 oz.	45	1.0
Cooked or imported, Danish	1.2-oz. slice	30	1.2
Loaf	1 oz.	70	1.0
(Healthy Deli):			
Baked, Virginia style:			
Regular	1 oz.	34	1.6
Less salt	1 oz.	32	1.4
Black Forest	1 oz.	32	0.4
Boiled	1 oz.	33	0.2
Deluxe	1 oz.	31	1.1
Honey Valley	1 oz.	31	1.2
Jalapeño	1 oz.	25	0.8
Lessalt	1 oz.	32	1.4
Taverne	1 oz.	31	0.3
(Hormel):			
Black peppered, *Light & Lean*	1 slice	25	0.0

Food	Measure	Cals.	Carbs.
Chopped	1 slice	44	0.0
Cooked, *Light & Lean*	1 slice	25	0.0
Glazed, *Light & Lean*	1 slice	25	0.0
Red peppered, *Light & Lean*	1 slice	25	0.0
Smoked, cooked, *Light & Lean*	1 slice	25	0.0
(Ohse):			
Chopped	1 oz.	65	1.0
Cooked	1 oz.	30	1.0
Smoked, regular	1 oz.	45	1.0
Turkey ham	1 oz.	30	2.0
(Oscar Mayer):			
Chopped	1-oz. slice	64	.9
Cooked, smoked	1-oz. slice	34	0.0
Jubilee boneless:			
Sliced	8-oz. slice	232	0.0
Steak	2-oz. steak	59	0.1
(Smok-A-Roma):			
Chopped	1-oz. slice	55	1.0
Cooked or honey	1-oz. slice	30	1.0
HAM & ASPARAGUS AU GRATIN, frozen (The Budget Gourmet) *Light & Healthy*	8.7-oz. meal	290	26.0
HAM & CHEESE:			
Canned (Hormel):			
Loaf	3 oz.	260	1.0
Patty	1 patty	190	0.0
Packaged:			
(Eckrich) loaf	1-oz. serving	60	1.0
(Hormel) loaf	1-oz. slice	65	0.0
(Ohse) loaf	1 oz.	65	2.0
(Oscar Mayer) spread	1 oz.	66	.6
HAM DINNER OR ENTREE:			
Canned (Hormel) *Micro Cup,* with scalloped potatoes	7½-oz. serving	260	21.0
Frozen:			
(Armour) *Dinner Classics*	10¾-oz. meal	270	36.0
(Banquet)	10-oz. meal	400	43.0
(Budget Gourmet) *Light & Healthy,* au gratin	8.7 oz. meal	300	26.0
(Morton)	10-oz. meal	290	49.0
(Stouffer's) & asparagus bake	9½-oz. meal	520	32.0

Food	Measure	Cals.	Carbs.
(Swanson) & scalloped potatoes	9-oz. meal	300	25.0
HAM & CHEESE BREAKFAST (Weight Watchers) *Ultimate 200*, on a bagel	3 oz.	210	28.0
HAM & CHEESE POCKET SANDWICH, frozen:			
(Croissant Pockets)	1 piece	360	39.0
(Hot Pockets)	4½-oz. serving	350	36.0
(Weight Watchers) *Ultimate 200*	4-oz. serving	200	24.0
HAM PATTY, canned (Hormel):			
Plain	1 patty	190	0.0
With cheese	1 patty	190	0.0
HAM SALAD, canned (Carnation)	¼ of 7½-oz. can (1.9 oz.)	110	4.0
HAM SALAD SPREAD (Oscar Mayer)	1 oz.	59	3.6
HAMBURGER (See **BEEF,** Ground; see also *MCDONALD'S; BURGER KING; DAIRY QUEEN; WHITE CASTLE;* etc.)			
*HAMBURGER MIX: **Hamburger Helper* (General Mills):			
Beef noodle	⅕ of pkg.	330	29.0
Beef romanoff	⅕ ot pkg.	350	31.0
Cheeseburger macaroni	⅕ of pkg.	370	28.0
Chili with beans	¼ of pkg.	350	25.0
Chili tomato	⅕ of pkg.	330	31.0
Hash	⅕ of pkg.	320	27.0
Lasagna	⅕ of pkg.	340	33.0
Pizza dish	⅕ of pkg.	360	37.0
Potatoes au gratin	⅕ of pkg.	320	28.0
Potato stroganoff	⅕ of pkg.	320	28.0
Rice oriental	⅕ of pkg.	340	38.0
Spaghetti	⅕ of pkg.	340	32.0
Stew	⅕ of pkg.	300	25.0

Food	Measure	Cals.	Carbs.
Tamale bake	⅕ of pkg.	380	39.0
Make a Better Burger (Lipton)			
mildly seasoned or onion	⅕ of pkg.	30	5.0
HAMBURGER SEASONING MIX:			
*(Durkee)	1 cup	663	7.5
(French's)	1-oz. pkg.	100	20.0
HARDEE'S:			
Big Cookie	2 oz. piece	280	40.0
Big Country Breakfast:			
Bacon	1 serving	820	60.0
Ham	8.85-oz. meal	620	51.0
Sausage	1 serving	1000	62.0
Biscuit:			
Bacon	3.3-oz. serving	360	34.0
Bacon & egg	1 serving	530	44.0
Bacon, egg & cheese	1 serving	610	45.0
Country ham:			
Plain	1 serving	430	45.0
& egg	4.9-oz. serving	400	35.0
Ham:			
Plain	3.7-oz. serving	400	47.0
With egg & cheese	1 serving	540	45.0
Rise 'N Shine:			
Plain	1 serving	390	44.0
Canadian bacon	5.7-oz. serving	470	35.0
Sausage:			
Plain	4.2-oz. serving	510	44.0
With egg	5.3-oz. serving	600	44.0
Steak:			
Plain	1 serving	580	56.0
With egg	6.3-oz. serving	550	47.0
Cheeseburger:			
Plain	1 serving	390	29.0
Bacon	1 serving	530	29.0
Big Hardee	1 serving	690	34.0
Quarter-pound	1 serving	420	31.0
Chicken fillet sandwich	6.1-oz. sandwich	420	46.0
Chicken, fried:			
Breast	5.2-oz. serving	370	29.0
Leg	2.4-oz. serving	170	15.0
Thigh	4.3-oz. serving	330	30.0
Wing	2.3-oz. serving	200	23.0
Chicken, grilled, sandwich	6.8-oz. sandwich	290	30.0
Cool Twist:			

Food	Measure	Cals.	Carbs.
Cone:			
Chocolate	4.2-oz. serving	180	35.0
Vanilla	4.2-oz. serving	170	34.0
Vanilla/chocolate	4.2-oz. serving	180	34.0
Sundae:			
Hot fudge	5.9-oz. serving	320	45.0
Strawberry	5.9-oz. serving	210	43.0
Fisherman's Fillet, sandwich	7.5-oz. sandwich	450	45.0
Hamburger:			
Plain	3.9-oz. serving	340	30.0
Big Hardee	7.6-oz. serving	590	33.0
Margarine/butter blend	.2-oz. serving	35	0.0
Muffin:			
Blueberry	1 muffin	400	56.0
Oat bran raisin	1 muffin	410	59.0
Pancakes, three:			
Plain	4.8-oz. serving	280	56.0
With sausage patty	6.2-oz. serving	430	56.0
With bacon strips	5.3-oz. serving	350	56.0
Potato:			
Crispy Curls	3-oz. serving	300	36.0
French fries:			
Small	3.3-oz. order	240	33.0
Large	6.1-oz. order	430	59.0
Hash Rounds	2.8-oz. serving	230	24.0
Mashed:			
Regular	4 oz. serving	70	14.0
Large	12 oz. serving	220	48.0
Omelet, ultimate	1 serving	530	45.0
Peach cobbler	6-oz. serving	310	60.0
Roast beef sandwich:			
Regular	1 serving	270	28.0
Big Roast Beef	1 serving	410	28.0
Salad:			
Chicken, grilled	1 serving	150	11.0
Garden	9.3-oz. serving	220	11.0
Side	3.9-oz. serving	25	4.0
Salad dressing:			
Regular:			
Blue cheese	2 oz.	210	10.0
House	2 oz.	290	6.0
Thousand Island	2 oz.	250	9.0
Dietetic:			
French	2 oz.	130	21.0
Italian	2 oz.	90	5.0
Shake:			
Chocolate	1 serving	370	67.0

Food	Measure	Cals.	Carbs.
Strawberry	1 serving	420	83.0
Vanilla	1 serving	350	65.0
HAWS, SCARLET, raw (USDA):			
Whole	1 lb. (weighed with core)	316	75.5
Flesh & skin	4 oz.	99	23.6
HEADCHEESE:			
(USDA)	1 oz.	76	.3
(Oscar Mayer)	1 oz.	55	0.0
HEART OF PALM (See **SWAMP CABBAGE**)			
HEARTWISE, cereal (Kellogg's)	⅔ cup (1 oz.)	90	23.0
HERRING:			
Raw (USDA):			
Lake (See **LAKE HERRING**)			
Atlantic:			
Whole	1 lb. (weighed whole)	407	0.0
Meat only	4 oz.	200	0.0
Pacific, meat only	4 oz.	111	0.0
Canned:			
(USDA) in tomato sauce, solids & liq.	4-oz. serving	200	4.2
(Vita):			
Bismarck, drained	5-oz. jar	273	6.9
In cream sauce, drained	8-oz. jar	397	18.1
Matjis, drained	8-oz. jar	304	26.2
In wine sauce, drained	8-oz. jar	401	16.6
Pickled (USDA) Bismarck type	4-oz. serving	253	0.0
Salted or brined (USDA)	4-oz. serving	247	0.0
Smoked (USDA):			
Bloaters	4-oz. serving	222	0.0
Hard	4-oz. serving	340	0.0
Kippered	4-oz. serving	239	0.0
HIBISCUS COOLER, canned (Knudsen & Sons)	8 fl. oz.	95	24.0

Food	Measure	Cals.	Carbs.
HICKORY NUT (USDA):			
Whole	1 lb. (weighed in shell)	1068	20.3
Shelled	4 oz.	763	14.5
HOMINY, canned, solids & liq. (Allen's) golden or white	½ cup	80	16.0
HOMINY GRITS:			
Dry:			
(USDA):			
Degermed	1 oz.	103	22.1
Degermed	½ cup (2.8 oz.)	282	60.9
(Albers) quick, degermed	1½ oz.	150	33.0
(Aunt Jemima)	3 T. (1 oz.)	101	22.4
(Pocono) creamy	1 oz.	101	23.6
(Quaker):			
Regular or quick	1 T. (.33 oz.)	34	7.5
Instant:			
Regular	.8-oz. packet	79	17.7
With imitation bacon bits	1-oz. packet	101	21.6
With artificial cheese flavor	1-oz. packet	104	21.6
With imitation ham bits	1-oz. packet	99	21.3
(3-Minute Brand) quick, enriched	⅙ cup (1 oz.)	98	22.2
Cooked (USDA) degermed	⅔ cup (5.6 oz.)	84	18.0
HONEY, strained:			
(USDA)	½ cup (5.7 oz.)	494	134.1
(USDA)	1 T. (.7 oz.)	61	16.5
(Golden Blossom)	1 T.	60	16.0
HONEY BUNCHES OF OATS, cereal (Post):			
With almonds	⅔ cup (1 oz.)	115	22.0
Honey roasted	⅔ cup (1 oz.)	111	23.0
HONEYCOMB, cereal (Post) crunch	1⅓ cups (1 oz.)	110	26.0
HONEYDEW, fresh (USDA):			
Whole	1 lb. (weighed whole)	94	22.0

Food	Measure	Cals.	Carbs.
Wedge	2" × 7" wedge (5.3 oz.)	31	7.2
Flesh only	4 oz.	37	8.7
Flesh only, diced	1 cup (5.9 oz.)	55	12.9
HONEY SMACKS, cereal (Kellogg's)	⅜ cup (1 oz.)	110	25.0
HORSERADISH:			
Raw, pared (USDA)	1 oz.	25	5.6
Prepared (Gold's)	1 tsp.	4	Tr.
HOT BITES, frozen (Banquet):			
Cheese, mozzarella nuggets	¼ of 10½-oz. pkg.	240	16.0
Chicken:			
Regular:			
Breast patties	¼ of 10½-oz. pkg.	210	13.0
Breast tenders:			
Regular	¼ of 10½-oz. pkg.	150	12.0
Southern fried	¼ of 10½-oz. pkg.	160	13.0
Drum snackers	¼ of 10½-oz. pkg.	220	13.0
Nuggets:			
Plain	¼ of 10½-oz. pkg.	210	11.0
Cheddar	¼ of 10½-oz. pkg.	250	11.0
Hot & spicy	¼ of 10½-oz. pkg.	250	10.0
Sticks	¼ of 10½-oz. pkg.	220	11.0
Microwave:			
Breast pattie:			
Regular, & bun	4-oz. pkg.	310	32.0
Southern fried, & biscuit	4-oz. pkg.	320	37.0
Breast tenders	4-oz. pkg.	260	24.0
Nuggets, with sweet & sour sauce	4½-oz. pkg.	360	22.0
HOT DOG (See **FRANKFURTER**)			
HOT WHEELS, cereal (Ralston Purina)	1 cup (1 oz.)	110	24.0
HULA COOLER DRINK, canned (Hi-C)	6 fl. oz.	97	23.9

Food	Measure	Cals.	Carbs.
HULA PUNCH DRINK, canned (Hi-C)	6 fl. oz.	87	21.4
HUMMUS MIX (Casbah) dry	1 oz.	110	10.0
HYACINTH BEAN (USDA): Young bean, raw: Whole	1 lb. (weighed untrimmed)	140	29.1
Trimmed	4 oz.	40	8.3
Dry seeds	4 oz.	383	69.2

I

Food	Measure	Cals.	Carbs.
ICE CREAM (Listed below by flavor or type. See also **ICE CREAM BAR, ICE CREAM SANDWICH** or **ICE CREAM SUBSTITUTE OR IMITATION:** Almond (Good Humor)	4 fl. oz.	350	29.4
Almond amaretto (Baskin-Robbins)	4 fl. oz.	280	26.0
Almond fudge (Baskin-Robbins) Jamocha	1 scoop	270	30.0
Almond praline (Edy's Grand)	½ cup	150	19.0
Apple strudel (Lucerne)	½ cup	140	16.0
Banana (Ben & Jerry's) *Chunky Monkey*	½ cup	280	29.0
Banana split (Edy's Grand)	½ cup	170	19.0
Blackberry pecan (Lucerne)	½ cup	150	20.0
Black walnut (Lucerne) regular	½ cup	150	16.0
Bon Bons (Carnation) Chocolate	1 piece	34	3.1
Vanilla	1 piece	33	2.8
Brownie, double fudge (Edy's Grand)	½ cup	170	20.0
Brownie Overload Triple (Häagen-Dazs) Exträas	½ cup	330	28.0
Butter almond (Breyers)	½ cup	170	15.0
Butter crunch (Sealtest)	½ cup	150	18.0

Food	Measure	Cals.	Carbs.
Butter pecan:			
(Ben & Jerry's)	½ cup	310	20.0
(Breyers)	½ cup	180	15.0
(Edy's Grand)	½ cup	160	17.0
(Fruson Glädjé)	½ cup	280	16.0
(Good Humor)	½ cup	150	14.0
(Häagen-Dazs)	½ cup	290	29.0
(Lucerne) gourmet	½ cup	190	16.0
(Sealtest)	½ cup	160	16.0
Caramel nut sundae (Häagen-Dazs)	½ cup	310	26.0
Cherry (Ben & Jerry's) *Cherry Garcia*	½ cup	240	25.0.
Cherry Blossom (Lucerne)	½ cup	140	16.0
Cherry chocolate chip (Edy's Grand)	½ cup	150	18.0
Cherry vanilla (Breyers)	½ cup	150	17.0
Chocolate:			
(Baskin-Robbins)	1 scoop	270	32.0
(Ben & Jerry's) deep, dark	½ cup	260	32.0
(Breyers)	½ cup	160	20.0
(Edy's Grand)	½ cup	160	16.0
(Frusen Glädjé)	½ cup	240	17.0
(Häagen-Dazs):			
Regular	½ cup	270	24.0
Deep	½ cup	290	26.0
(Lucerne) regular	½ cup	140	16.0
(Sealtest)	½ cup	140	18.0
Chocolate caramel nut (Basken-Robbins) light	½ cup	130	19.0
Chocolate chip:			
(Baskin-Robbins)	1 scoop	260	27.0
(Breyers)	½ cup	170	18.0
(Edy 'n Grand)	½ cup	160	18.0
(Häagen-Dazs)	½ cup	270	23.0
(Lucerne) regular or mint	½ cup	150	17.0
Chocolate chip chocolate (Häagen-Dazs)	½ cup	290	28.0
Chocolate chocolate chip:			
(Edy's Grand)	½ cup	160	17.0
(Frusen Glädjé)	½ cup	270	21.0
(Häagen Dazs)	½ cup	290	28.0
Chocolate chunk (Ben & Jerry's) *New York Super Fudge Chunk*	½ cup	290	28.0
Chocolate fudge:			
(Ben & Jerry's):			
Brownie	½ cup	250	31.0

Food	Measure	Cals.	Carbs.
Double	½ cup	280	35.0
(Häagen-Dazs) deep	½ cup	290	26.0
Chocolate marble (Lucerne)	½ cup	140	19.0
Chocolate marshmallow:			
(Lucerne)	½ cup	140	20.0
(Sealtest) sundae	½ cup	150	21.0
Chocolate peanut butter cookie			
dough (Ben & Jerry's)	½ cup	300	32.0
Chocolate raspberry truffle			
(Baskin-Robbins)	1 scoop	310	35.0
Chocolate truffle (Lucerne)	½ cup	170	24.0
Coconut almond fudge			
(Lucerne)	½ cup	150	16.0
Coconut almond fudge chip			
(Ben & Jerry's)	½ cup	320	24.0
Coffee:			
(Baskin-Robbins)			
Expresso & Cream	½ cup	120	15.0
(Ben & Jerry's) *Aztec*			
Harvest Coffee	½ cup	230	22.0
(Breyers)	½ cup	150	16.0
(Edy's Grand)	½ cup	140	15.0
(Häagen-Dazs)	½ cup	270	23.0
(Lucerne) regular	½ cup	140	16.0
(Sealtest)	½ cup	140	16.0
Coffee almond fudge (Ben &			
Jerry's)	½ cup	290	24.0
Coffee toffee crunch (Ben &			
Jerry's	½ cup	280	28.0
Cookie dough:			
(Edy's Grand)	½ cup	170	21.0
(Häagen-Dazs) dynamo	½ cup	300	31.0
Cookies & cream:			
(Breyers)	½ cup	170	19.0
(Edy's Grand)	½ cup	160	18.0
(Häagen-Dazs)	½ cup	280	26.0
Danish nut roll (Lucerne)	½ cup	145	16.0
Egg nog (Lucerne) regular	½ cup	140	16.0
Fudge marble (Edy's Grand)	½ cup	150	18.0
Fudge royale (Sealtest)	½ cup	140	19.0
Heath candy crunch (Edy's			
Grand)	½ cup	160	18.0
Heavenly hash:			
(Lucerne)	½ cup	150	18.0
(Sealtest)	½ cup	150	19.0
Macadamia brittle (Häagen-			
Dazs)	½ cup	280	25.0

Food	Measure	Cals.	Carbs.
Maple nut (Lucerne)	½ cup	150	16.0
Maple walnut (Häagen-Dazs)	½ cup	310	18.0
Mint with chocolate cookie (Ben & Jerry's)	½ cup	260	27.0
Mocha almond fudge:			
(Breyers)	½ cup	190	20.0
(Edy's Grand)	½ cup	160	17.0
Mocha fudge (Ben & Jerry's)	½ cup	270	30.0
Neapolitan (Lucerne)	½ cup	140	16.0
Peach:			
(Breyers)	½ cup	140	19.0
(Häagen-Dazs)	½ cup	210	15.0
(Lucerne)	½ cup	140	16.0
Peach pie, southern (Lucerne)	½ cup	130	17.0
Peanut butter (Lucerne)	½ cup	145	17.0
Peanut buttercup:			
(Ben & Jerry's)	½ cup	370	30.0
(Edy's Grand)	½ cup	170	16.0
Peanut butter sundae (Lucerne):			
Regular	½ cup	140	16.0
Nut	½ cup	140	16.0
Peppermint stick (Lucerne)	½ cup	150	17.0
Pralines & cream (Baskin-Robbins)	1 scoop	280	36.0
Ranch pecan (Lucerne)	½ cup	160	15.0
Rocky road:			
(Baskin-Robbins)	1 scoop	300	39.0
(Edy's Grand)	½ cup	170	18.0
Rum raisin (Häagen-Dazs)	½ cup	250	21.0
Strawberry:			
(Baskin-Robbins) very berry	1 scoop	220	30.0
(Breyers)	½ cup	130	16.0
(Edy's Grand) real	½ cup	130	16.0
(Frusen Glädjé)	½ cup	230	20.0
(Häagen-Dazs)	½ cup	250	23.0
(Lucerne) gourmet	½ cup	140	17.0
(Sealtest)	½ cup	130	18.0
Strawberry cheesecake (Lucerne) gourmet	½ cup	155	18.0
Swiss chocolate candy almond (Frusen Glädjé)	½ cup	270	18.0
Toffee (Ben & Jerry's) English toffee crunch	½ cup	310	30.0
Vanilla:			
(Baskin-Robbins)			
Regular	1 scoop	240	24.0

Food	Measure	Cals.	Carbs.
French	1 scoop	280	25.0
(Ben & Jerry's)	½ cup	230	21.0
(Breyers)	½ cup	150	15.0
(Eagle Brand) homestyle	½ cup	150	16.0
(Edy's Grand):			
Regular	½ cup	160	14.0
French	½ cup	160	16.0
(Frusen Glädjé)	½ cup	230	16.0
(Good Humor)	3-fl.-oz. cup	95	11.5
(Häagen-Dazs)	½ cup	260	23.0
(Land O'Lakes)	½ cup	140	16.0
(Lucerne):			
Regular	½ cup	140	16.0
French	½ cup	150	16.0
(Sealtest)	½ cup	140	16.0
Vanilla caramel fudge (Ben & Jerry's)	½ cup	280	33.0
Vanilla crunch (Ben & Jerry's) *Wavey Gravey*	½ cup	330	29.0
Vanilla fudge (Häagen-Dazs)	½ cup	270	26.0
Vanilla fudge twirl (Breyers)	½ cup	160	19.0
Vanilla-swiss almond (Frusen Glädjé)	½ cup	290	24.0
White Russian (Ben & Jerry's)	½ cup	240	23.0
ICE CREAM BAR:			
(Dove):			
Almond	1 bar	350	32.0
Chocolate:			
Dark chocolate coating	1 bar	350	34.0
Milk chocolate coating	1 bar	340	35.0
Crunchy cookies	1 bar	330	34.0
Fudge, peanut	1 bar	350	32.0
Vanilla:			
Dark chocolate coating	1 bar	340	33.0
Milk chocolate coating	1 bar	340	33.0
(Eskimo Pie):			
Chocolate fudge	1¾-fl.-oz. bar	60	14.0
Chocolate fudge	3-fl.oz. bar	110	24.0
Pie:			
Regular	3-fl.-oz. bar	170	16.0
Chocolate	3-fl.-oz. bar	170	15.0
Vanilla	3-fl.oz. bar	170	14.0
Vanilla:			
Dark chocolate coating:			
Regular	1 bar	180	16.0
Sugar-freedom	1 bar	140	13.0

Food	Measure	Cals.	Carbs.
Milk chocolate coating:			
Regular	1 bar	190	18.0
Sugar-freedom:			
& almonds	1 bar	140	12.0
& crisp rice	1 bar	150	12.0
(Good Humor):			
Chip candy crunch	3-fl.-oz. bar	255	21.2
Chocolate eclair	3-fl.-oz. bar	188	22.6
Chocolate fudge cake	6.3-fl.-oz. bar	214	18.1
Strawberry shortcake	3-fl.-oz. bar	176	23.8
Vanilla with chocolate-flavor coating	3-fl.-oz. bar	198	16.8
(Häagen-Dazs):			
Chocolate with dark chocolate coating	1 bar	390	32.0
Crunch bar:			
Caramel almond	1 bar	240	17.0
Chocolate peanut butter	1 bar	270	16.0
Coffee almond	1 bar	360	28.0
Vanilla crisp	4 fl.-oz. bar	220	16.0
Fudge	1 bar	210	19.0
Fudge peanut butter chocolate chip	1 bar	390	29.0
Vanilla:			
Dark chocolate coating	4-fl.-oz. bar	390	32.0
Milk chocolate coating:			
Plain	4-fl.oz. bar	360	26.0
Almond	4-fl. oz. bar	370	27.0
Caramel brittle	4-fl.-oz. bar	370	32.0
(Klondike):			
Chocolate	5-fl.-oz. bar	270	23.0
Vanilla, with chocolate flavor coating, lite	1 bar	110	14.0
(Mars) almond	1 bar	210	19.0
(Milky Way):			
Chocolate, milk chocolate coating	1 bar	190	21.0
Vanilla, dark chocolate coating	1 bar	190	22.0
(Nestlé):			
Chocolate, with milk chocolate coating	3-fl.-oz. bar	210	19.0
Milk chocolate, with almonds & milk chocolate coating	3.7-fl.-oz. bar	350	28.0
Vanilla:			

Food	Measure	Cals.	Carbs.
Alpine Premium, with white chocolate coating	3.7-fl.-oz. bar	350	25.0
Crunch, with chocolate coating & crisp rice:			
Regular	3-fl.-oz. bar	180	15.0
Lite	1 bar	120	16.0
ICE CREAM CONE, cone only:			
(Baskin-Robbins):			
Sugar	1 piece	60	11.0
Waffle	1 piece	140	28.0
(Comet) sugar	1 piece (.35 oz.)	40	9.0
(Keebler) sugar	1 cone	45	11.0
ICE CREAM CONES, cereal (General Mills)	¾ cup (1 oz.)	110	23.0
ICE CREAM CUP, cup only (Comet):			
Regular	1 cup	20	4.0
Chocolate	1 cup	25	5.0
*****ICE CREAM MIX** (Salada) any flavor	1 cup	310	31.0
ICE CREAM SANDWICH:			
(Eskimo Pie) *Sugar-freedom*, vanilla	1 piece	170	26.0
(Good Humor):			
Chocolate chip cookie:			
Large	4-fl.-oz. piece	246	35.1
Small	2.7-fl.-oz. piece	204	30.1
Vanilla	2½-fl.-oz. piece	165	26.9
(Klondike) vanilla:			
Regular	5-fl.-oz. piece	230	33.0
Lite	1 piece	100	18.0
ICE CREAM & SHERBET (See **SHERBET OR SORBET & ICE CREAM**)			
ICE CREAM SUBSTITUTE OR IMITATION (See also *TOFUTTI*):			
Almond praline (Edy's Grand) light	½ cup	110	16.0

Food	Measure	Cals.	Carbs.
Brownie chunk fudge (Simple Pleasures)	½ cup	110	24.0
Butter pecan (Edy's Grand)	½ cup	120	16.0
Butter pecan crunch (Healthy Choice)	½ cup	140	26.0
Caramel brickle (Simple Pleasures)	½ cup	100	22.0
Chocolate:			
(Edy's) sugar free	½ cup	90	13.0
(Healthy Choice)	½ cup	95	14.0
(Simple Pleasures) dutch	½ cup	100	18.0
(Weight Watchers):			
Regular	½ cup	80	19.0
Swirl	½ cup	90	22.0
Chocolate chip:			
(Edy's):			
Grand, light	½ cup	110	15.0
Sugar free	½ cup	100	14.0
(Healthy Choice):			
Regular	½ cup	130	24.0
Mint	½ cup	140	25.0
French silk (Edy's Grand)	½ cup	120	18.0
Fudge (Edy's Grand)	½ cup	110	15.0
Fudge marble (Edy's Grand) mint or mocha, sugar free	½ cup	110	17.0
Neapolitan:			
(Healthy Choice)	½ cup	120	22.0
(Weight Watchers)	½ cup	80	19.0
Rocky road (Edy's Grand)	½ cup	110	17.0
Strawberry:			
(Edy's):			
Fat free	½ cup	90	20.0
Sugar free	½ cup	90	13.0
(Simple Pleasures)	½ cup	120	22.0
Vanilla:			
(Edy's):			
Fat free	½ cup	90	20.0
Grand, light	½ cup	100	15.0
(Healthy Choice)	½ cup	120	21.0
(Simple Pleasures)	½ cup	100	17.0
(Weight Watchers)	½ cup	80	20.0
ICE MILK:			
(USDA):			
Hardened	1 cup (4.6 oz.)	199	29.3
Soft-serve	1 cup (6.3 oz.)	266	39.2
(Borden):			

Food	Measure	Cals.	Carbs.
Chocolate	½ cup	100	18.0
Strawberry or vanilla	½ cup	90	17.0
(Dean):			
Count Calorie, 2.1% fat	1 cup (4.8 oz.)	155	17.1
5% fat	1 cup (4.9 oz.)	227	35.0
(Edy's) low fat:			
Almond praline	½ cup	110	22.0
Cookies n' cream	½ cup	110	20.0
Mocha almond fudge	½ cup	110	20.0
Vanilla	½ cup	100	18.0
(Land O' Lakes) vanilla	4 fl. oz.	110	17.0
(Lucerne):			
Regular:			
Caramel nut	½ cup	105	19.0
Chocolate:			
Regular or marble	½ cup	110	19.0
Chip	½ cup	100	18.0
Pecan crunch or vanilla	½ cup	100	18.0
Rocky road	½ cup	110	19.0
Strawberry	½ cup	95	18.0
Triple treat	½ cup	100	19.0
Light:			
Chocolate	½ cup	120	20.0
Vanilla	½ cup	110	19.0
(Weight Watchers) *Grand Collection*:			
Chocolate:			
Regular or fudge	½ cup	110	18.0
Chip or swirl	½ cup	120	19.0
Fudge marble	½ cup	120	19.0
Neapolitan	½ cup	110	18.0
Pecan pralines 'n creme	½ cup	120	20.0
Strawberries 'n creme	½ cup	120	21.0
Vanilla	½ cup	100	16.0
ICE TEASERS (Nestlé)	8 fl. oz.	6	1.0

ICING (See **CAKE ICING**)

INSTANT BREAKFAST (See
individual brand name or
company listings)

IRISH WHISKEY (See
DISTILLED LIQUOR)

Food	Measure	Cals.	Carbs.

J

JACKFRUIT, fresh (USDA):

Food	Measure	Cals.	Carbs.
Whole	1 lb. (weighed with seeds & skin)	124	32.5
Flesh only	4 oz.	111	28.8

JACK-IN-THE-BOX **RESTAURANT:**

Food	Measure	Cals.	Carbs.
Breakfast Jack sandwich	4.4-oz. serving	300	30.0
Breadstick, sesame	.6-oz. serving	70	12.0
Burger:			
Regular	3.6-oz. serving	280	31.0
Cheeseburger:			
Regular	4-oz. serving	315	33.0
Bacon	8.1-oz. serving	710	40.0
Double	5¼-oz. serving	450	35.0
Outlaw Burger	1 serving	720	56.0
Ultimate	9.9-oz. serving	1030	30.0
Jumbo Jack:			
Regular	7.8-oz. serving	560	42.0
With cheese	8.5-oz. serving	650	42.0
Cheesecake	3.5-oz. serving	360	44.0
Chicken sandwich:			
Fillet, grilled	7.4-oz. serving	431	36.0
Spicy crispy	1 serving	560	55.0
Supreme	8.6-oz. serving	641	47.0
Chicken strips	1 piece	72	4.5
Chicken teriyaki bowl	1 serving	580	115.0
Chicken wings	1.2-oz. piece	141	13.0
Coffee, black	8 fl. oz.	2	.5
Egg roll	1 piece	147	18.4
Fajita sandwich, pita:			
Beef	6.2-oz. serving	333	27.0
Chicken	1 serving	292	29.0
Fish supreme sandwich	7.7-oz. sandwich	590	49.0
French fries:			
Regular	3.8-oz. order	351	45.0
Small	2.4-oz. order	219	28.0

Food	Measure	Cals.	Carbs.
Jumbo	4.3-oz. order	396	51.0
Jelly, grape	.5-oz. serving	38	9.0
Ketchup	1 serving	10	2.0
Mayonnaise	1 serving	152	.5
Milk, 2%	8 fl. oz.	122	12.0
Milk shake:			
Chocolate	10-oz. serving	390	74.0
Strawberry	10-oz. serving	330	60.0
Vanilla	10-oz. serving	350	62.0
Mustard	1 serving	8	.7
Onion rings	3.8-oz. serving	382	39.0
Orange juice	6.5-oz. serving	80	20.0
Pancake platter	1 serving	400	590
Salad:			
Chicken, garden	1 serving	200	8.0
Side	3.9-oz. salad	70	3.0
Salad dressing:			
Regular:			
Blue cheese	2½-oz. serving	210	11.0
Buttermilk	2½-oz. serving	290	6.0
1000 Island	2½-oz. serving	250	10.0
Dietetic or low calorie,			
French	2½-oz. serving	25	2.0
Sauce:			
A-1	1.8-oz. serving	35	9.0
BBQ	.9-oz. serving	39	9.4
Guacamole	.9-oz. serving	55	1.8
Mayo-mustard	.8-oz. serving	124	2.0
Mayo-onion	.8-oz. serving	143	1.0
Salsa	.9-oz. serving	8	2.0
Seafood cocktail	1-oz. serving	32	6.8
Sweet & sour	1-oz. serving	40	11.0
Sausage crescent sandwich	5.5-oz. serving	670	39.0
Soft drink:			
Sweetened:			
Coca-Cola Classic	16 fl. oz.	192	48.0
Dr Pepper	16 fl. oz.	192	49.0
Root beer, *Ramblin'*	16 fl. oz.	235	61.0
Sprite	16 fl. oz.	192	48.0
Dietetic, *Coca-Cola*	16 fl. oz.	Tr.	.3
Supreme crescent sandwich	5.1-oz. serving	570	39.0
Syrup, pancake	1.5-oz. serving	121	30.0
Taco:			
Regular	2.9-oz. serving	191	16.0
Super	4.8-oz. serving	288	21.0
Tea, iced, plain	12 fl. oz.	3	.8
Turnover, apple	3.9-oz. piece	354	40.0

Food	Measure	Cals.	Carbs.
JACK MACKEREL, raw (USDA) meat only	4 oz.	162	0.0
JAM, sweetened (See also individual listings by flavor) (USDA)	1 T. (.7 oz.)	54	14.0
JELL-O PUDDING POPS:			
Chocolate, chocolate-caramel swirl, chocolate with chocolate chips & vanilla with chocolate chips	1 bar	80	13.0
Chocolate covered chocolate & vanilla	1 bar	130	14.0
Chocolate-vanilla swirl & vanilla	1 bar	70	12.0
JELLY, sweetened (See also individual flavors) (Crosse & Blackwell) all flavors	1 T.	51	12.8
JERUSALEM ARTICHOKE (USDA):			
Unpared	1 lb. (weighed with skin)	207	52.3
Pared	4 oz.	75	18.9
JOHANNISBERG RIESLING WINE (Louis M. Martini)	3 fl. oz.	59	1.3
JUICE (See individual listings)			
JUJUBE OR CHINESE DATE (USDA):			
Fresh, whole	1 lb. (weighed with seeds)	443	116.4
Fresh, flesh only	4 oz.	119	31.3
Dried, whole	1 lb. (weighed with seeds)	1159	297.1
Dried, flesh only	4 oz.	325	83.5
JUST RIGHT, cereal (Kellogg's):			
with fiber nuggets	⅔ cup (1 oz.)	100	24.0
with fruit & nuts	¾ cup (1.3 oz.)	140	30.0

Food	Measure	Cals.	Carbs.

K

KABOOM, cereal (General Mills)	1 cup (1 oz.)	110	23.0
KALE:			
Raw (USDA) leaves only	1 lb. (weighed untrimmed)	154	26.1
Boiled, leaves only (USDA)	4 oz.	44	6.9
Canned (Allen's) chopped, solids & liq.	½ cup (4.1 oz.)	25	2.0
Frozen, chopped:			
(Bel-Air)	3.3 oz.	25	5.0
(Birds Eye)	⅓ of 10-oz. pkg.	31	4.6
(Frosty Acres)	3.3-oz. serving	25	5.0
(McKenzie)	⅓ of 10-oz. pkg.	30	5.0
KARO SYRUP (See **SYRUP**)			
KAUAI PUNCH, canned (Santa Cruz Natural organic	8 fl. oz.	120	28.0
KENMEI, cereal (Kellogg's):			
Plain	¾ cup (1 oz.)	110	24.0
Almond & raisin	¾ cup (1.4 oz.)	150	31.0
KENNY ROGERS ROASTERS:			
Beans, honey baked	5-oz. serving	152	DNA
Chicken, roasted:			
Whole:			
With skin	1 whole chicken (edible portion)	978	DNA
Without skin	1 whole chicken (edible portion	639	DNA
½ chicken:			
With skin	½ chicken	489	DNA
Without skin	½ chicken	300	DNA
¼ chicken:			
With skin:			
Dark meat	¼ chicken	239	DNA

Food	Measure	Cals.	Carbs.
White meat	¼ chicken	250	DNA
Without skin:			
Dark meat	¼ chicken	182	DNA
White meat	¼ chicken	147	DNA
Chicken pot pie	12½-oz. serving	816	DNA
Chicken sandwich pita:			
BBQ	7.35-oz. sandwich	356	DNA
Caesar	9¼-oz. sandwich	566	DNA
Roasted	10.8-oz. sandwich	593	DNA
Cole slaw	5-oz. serving	225	DNA
Corn on the cob	2¼-oz. serving	68	DNA
Macaroni & cheese	5½-oz. serving	197	DNA
Muffin, corn	1.8-oz. muffin	113	DNA
Potatoes:			
Garlic parsley	6½-oz. serving	341	DNA
Mashed, with gravy	8-oz. serving	149	DNA
Rice pilaf	5-oz. serving	173	DNA
Salad:			
Chicken caesar	9.4-oz. serving	587	DNA
Chicken, roasted	16.9-oz. serving	355	DNA
Pasta	5-oz. serving	272	DNA
Potato	7-oz. serving	390	DNA
Side	4.7-oz. serving	23	DNA
Tomato-cucumber	6-oz. serving	174	DNA
Salad dressing:			
Regular:			
Blue cheese	2½-oz. serving	370	DNA
Buttermilk ranch	2½-oz. serving	430	DNA
Caesar	2½-oz. serving	340	DNA
Dijon honey mustard	2½-oz. serving	320	DNA
Honey french	2½-oz. serving	350	DNA
Thousand island	2½-oz. serving	330	DNA
Dietetic, Italian, fat free	2½-oz. serving	35	DNA
Soup, chicken noodle:			
Bowl	10-oz. serving	171	DNA
Cup	6-oz. serving	111	DNA
Vegetables, steamed	4½-oz. serving	48	DNA
KFC (KENTUCKY FRIED CHICKEN)			
Biscuit, buttermilk	2.3-oz. serving	235	28.0
Chicken:			
Original Recipe:			
Breast:			

Food	Measure	Cals.	Carbs.
Center	3.6-oz. piece	260	8.8
Side	1 piece	275	10.0
Drumstick	1 piece	152	3.0
Thigh	1 piece	287	8.0
Wing	1 piece	172	5.0
Extra Tasty Crispy:			
Breast:			
Center	4.8-oz. piece	344	15.0
Side	1 piece	343	15.0
Drumstick	2.4-oz. piece	205	7.0
Thigh	1 piece	414	15.0
Wing	1 piece	255	9.3
Hot & Spicy:			
Breast:			
Center	4.3-oz. piece	382	16.0
Side	4.1-oz. piece	398	18.0
Drumstick	2½-oz. piece	207	10.0
Thigh	1 piece	412	16.0
Wing	2.2-oz. piece	244	9.0
Hot wings	.8-oz. piece	78	3.0
Rotisserie Gold:			
With skin:			
Dark meat quarter	5.1-oz. serving	333	1.0
White meat quarter with wing	6.2-oz. serving	335	1.0
Skin free:			
Dark meat quarter	4.1-oz. serving	217	0.0
White meat quarter with wing	4.1-oz. serving	199	0.0
Skinfree Crispy:			
Breast:			
Center	1 piece	295	11.0
Side	1 piece	293	11.0
Drumstick	1 piece	154	8.0
Thigh	1 piece	255	9.0
Chicken Littles	1.7-oz. sandwich	169	13.8
Chicken nugget, *Kentucky Nuggets*	1 piece	46	2.2
Chicken sandwich, *Colonel's*	1 sandwich	482	39.0
Coleslaw	3.2-oz. serving	114	13.2
Corn on the cob	5.3-oz. serving	222	27.0
Hot wings	1 piece	78	3.0
Potatoes:			
French fries	2.7-oz. regular order	244	31.0
Crispy	2½-oz. serving	210	24.0
Mashed & gravy	4.2-oz. serving	71	15.0

Food	Measure	Cals.	Carbs.
Rice, garden	3.8-oz. serving	75	15.0
Roll, sourdough	1.7-oz. piece	128	24.0
Salad:			
Garden	3.1-oz. serving	16	3.0
Macaroni	3.8-oz. serving	248	20.0
Pasta	3.8-oz. serving	135	14.0
Potato	4.4-oz. serving	180	18.0
Vegetable medley	4-oz. serving	126	21.0
Salad dressing:			
Italian	1 oz.	15	2.0
Ranch	1 oz.	170	1.0
Sauce:			
Barbecue	1-oz. serving	35	7.1
Honey	.5-oz. serving	49	12.1
Mustard	1-oz. serving	36	6.0
Sweet & sour	1-oz. serving	58	13.0

KETCHUP (See **CATSUP**)

KIDNEY (USDA):
Beef, braised	4 oz.	286	.9
Calf, raw	4 oz.	128	.1
Lamb, raw	4 oz.	119	1.0

KIELBASA (See **SAUSAGE,** Polish-style)

KINGFISH, raw (USDA):
Whole	1 lb. (weighed whole)	210	0.0
Meat only	4 oz.	119	0.0

KIPPER SNACKS (King David Brand) Norwegian
	3¼-oz. can	195	0.0

KIWIFRUIT (Calavo)
	1 fruit (5-oz. edible portion)	45	9.0

KIWI NECTAR, canned (Knudsen & Sons)
	8 fl. oz.	60	14.0

KIWI-STRAWBERRY JUICE DRINK, canned:
(Mistic)	8 fl. oz.	110	31.0
(Snapple)	8 fl. oz.	130	33.0

KIX, cereal (General Mills)
	1½ cups (1 oz.)	110	24.0

Food	Measure	Cals.	Carbs.
KNOCKWURST (See **SAUSAGE**)			
KOFFEE KAKE (Tastykake):			
Regular	2½-oz. serving	270	45.0
Cupcakes (See **CUPCAKE**)			
KOHLRABI (USDA):			
Raw:			
Whole	1 lb. (weighed with skin, without leaves)	96	21.9
Diced	1 cup (4.8 oz.)	40	9.1
Boiled:			
Drained	4 oz.	27	6.0
Drained	1 cup (5.5 oz.)	37	8.2
KOO KOOS (Dolly Madison)	1½-oz. piece	190	25.0
KOOL-AID (General Foods):			
Canned, *Kool Aid Koolers*:			
Cherry or mountainberry punch	8.45 fl. oz.	142	37.6
Grape	8.45 fl. oz.	136	35.5
Great Bluedini	8.45 fl. oz.	110	29.0
Mountain Berry Punch	8.45 fl. oz.	140	37.0
Orange	8.45 fl. oz.	115	30.1
Rainbow punch or strawberry	8.45 fl. oz	135	35.6
Sharkleberry Fin	8.45 fl. oz.	140	36.8
Tropical punch	8.45 fl. oz.	132	34.9
*Mix:			
Unsweetened, sugar to be added	8 fl. oz.	98	25.0
Pre-sweetened:			
Regular:			
Grape	8 fl. oz.	80	21.0
Orange, surfin berry punch	8 fl. oz.	79	20.0
Sunshine punch	8 fl. oz.	83	21.0
Dietetic:			
Rainbow punch	8 fl. oz.	4	Tr.
Raspberry	8 fl. oz.	2	Tr.
All others	8 fl. oz.	3	Tr.
KRIMPETS (Tastykake):			
Butterscotch	1 piece	100	19.0
Jelly	1 piece	90	19.0

Food	Measure	Cals.	Carbs.
KRISPIES, cereal (Kellogg's):			
Plain	1 cup (1 oz.)	110	25.0
Frosted	¾ cup (1 oz.)	110	26.0
Fruity marshmallow	1¼ cups (1.3 oz.)	140	32.0
KUMQUAT, fresh (USDA):			
Whole	1 lb. (weighed with seeds)	274	72.1
Flesh & skin	4 oz.	74	19.4

L

Food	Measure	Cals.	Carbs.
LAKE HERRING (See also **HERRING**), raw (USDA):			
Whole	1 lb.	226	0.0
Meat only	4 oz.	109	0.0
LAKE TROUT, raw (USDA):			
Whole	1 lb. (weighed whole)	404	0.0
Meat only	4 oz.	191	0.0
LAKE TROUT OR SISCOWET (See also **TROUT**), raw (USDA):			
Less than 6.5 lb.:			
Whole	1 lb. (weighed whole)	404	0.0
Meat only	4 oz.	273	0.0
More than 6.5 lb.:			
Whole	1 lb. (weighed whole)	856	0.0
Meat only	4 oz.	594	0.0
LAMB, choice grade (USDA):			
Chop, broiled:			
Loin. One 5-oz. chop (weighed before cooking with bone) will give you:			
Lean & fat	2.8 oz.	280	0.0
Lean only	2.3 oz.	122	0.0

Food	Measure	Cals.	Carbs.
Rib. One 5-oz. chop (weighed before cooking with bone) with give you:			
Lean & fat	2.9 oz.	334	0.0
Lean only	2 oz.	118	0.0
Fat, separable, cooked	1 oz.	201	0.0
Leg:			
Raw, lean & fat	1 lb. (weighed with bone)	845	0.0
Roasted, lean & fat	4 oz.	316	0.0
Roasted, lean only	4 oz.	211	0.0
Shoulder:			
Raw, lean & fat	1 lb. (weighed with bone)	1092	0.0
Roasted, lean & fat	4 oz.	383	0.0
Roasted, lean only	4 oz.	232	0.0
LAMB'S QUARTERS (USDA):			
Raw, trimmed	1 lb.	195	33.1
Boiled, drained	4 oz.	36	5.7
LARD:			
(USDA) pork	1 cup (6.2 oz.)	1849	0.0
(USDA)	1 T. (.5 oz.)	117	0.0
LASAGNA:			
Dry or fresh, refrigerated (See **PASTA, DRY OR FRESH, REFRIGERATED**)			
Canned:			
(Chef Boyardee)	7½-oz. serving	230	31.0
(Hormel):			
Micro Cup	7½ oz.	250	25.0
Top Shelf, Italian	10 oz.	350	30.0
(Libby's) Diner	7¾ oz.	200	29.0
(Top Shelf) vegetable	12-oz. serving	240	39.0
(Ultra Slim Fast):			
With meat sauce	12-oz. serving	330	38.0
Vegetable	12-oz. serving	240	39.0
Freeze-dried (Mountain House)	1 cup	240	24.0
Frozen:			
(Armour) *Dining Lite:*			
Cheese	9-oz. meal	260	36.0
Meat sauce	9-oz. meal	240	36.0

Food	Measure	Cals.	Carbs.
(Banquet) *Family Entree* with meat sauce	28-oz. pkg.	1080	120.0
(Budget Gourmet):			
Cheese, three	10-oz. serving	400	38.0
With meat sauce, *Light and Healthy*	9.4-oz. serving	290	30.0
Sausage, Italian	10-oz. serving	420	38.0
Vegetable, *Light and Healthy*	10½-oz. serving	290	36.0
(Buitoni):			
Alforno	8-oz. meal	327	31.8
Cheese, sorrentino	8-oz. serving	286	37.4
Individual portion	9-oz. serving	342	30.9
With meat sauce	5-oz. serving	212	23.4
(Celentano):			
Regular	½ of 16-oz. pkg.	370	32.0
Regular	¼ of 25-oz. pkg.	300	25.0
Great Choice, low fat	10-oz. serving	260	42.0
Primavera	11-oz. pkg.	330	34.0
(Healthy Choice) with meat sauce	10-oz. meal	260	37.0
(Le Menu) healthy style, entree:			
Garden vegetable	10½-oz. meal	260	35.0
With meat sauce	10-oz. meal	290	36.0
(Mrs. Paul's) seafood, light	9½-oz. meal	290	39.0
(Stouffer's):			
Regular:			
Plain	10½-oz. meal	360	33.0
Vegetable	10½-oz. meal	420	23.0
Lean Cuisine:			
With meat sauce	10¼-oz. meal	270	24.0
Tuna, with spinach noodles & vegetables	9¾-oz. meal	240	29.0
Zucchini	11-oz. meal	260	34.0
(Swanson) *Homestyle Recipe*, with meat sauce	10½-oz. meal	400	39.0
(Weight Watchers):			
Regular:			
Original	10¼-oz. meal	270	29.0
Cheese, Italian	11-oz. meal	290	29.0
Garden	11-oz. meal	260	30.0
Smart Ones, florentine	11-oz. meal	220	34.0
Mix (Golden Grain) Stir-N-Serv	⅕ of pkg.	150	28.0

LATKES, frozen (Empire Kosher):

Food	Measure	Cals.	Carbs.
Mini	3 oz.	190	20.0
Rounds	2½ oz.	120	20.0
Triangles	3 oz.	140	12.0
LEEKS, raw (USDA):			
Whole	1 lb. (weighed untrimmed)	123	26.4
Trimmed	4 oz.	59	12.7
LEMON, fresh (USDA):			
Whole	2⅛" lemon (109 grams)	22	11.7
Peeled	2⅛" lemon (74 grams)	20	6.1
LEMONADE:			
Canned, regular pack:			
(Ardmore Farms)	6 fl. oz.	89	22.5
(Arizona):			
Regular	8 fl. oz.	100	27.0
Pink	8 fl. oz.	110	28.0
Country Time	6 fl. oz.	69	17.2
(Hi-C)	6 fl. oz.	77	19.3
(Johanna Farms) Ssips	8.45-fl.-oz. container	85	21.0
(Knudsen & Sons):			
Natural	8 fl. oz.	100	26.0
Cherry	8 fl. oz.	105	31.0
Cranberry	8 fl. oz.	115	29.0
Raspberry	8 fl. oz.	110	28.0
Kool-Aid Koolers	8.45-fl.-oz. container	120	31.5
(Mistic) tropical pink	8 fl. oz.	110	30.0
(Santa Cruz Natural):			
Regular, sparkling	8 fl. oz.	85	20.0
Cherry, dark, sweet	8 fl. oz.	60	20.0
Cranberry	8 fl. oz.	100	24.0
Raspberry, regular	8 fl. oz.	60	20.0
(Snapple) pink	8 fl. oz.	110	26.0
Canned, dietetic (Snapple) pink	8 fl. oz.	13	3.0
Chilled (Minute Maid) regular or pink	6 fl. oz.	81	21.3
*Frozen:			
Country Time, regular or pink	6 fl. oz.	68	18.0
Minute Maid	6 fl. oz.	77	20.1

Food	Measure	Cals.	Carbs.
(Sunkist)	6 fl. oz.	92	24.2
*Mix:			
Regular:			
Country Time, regular			
or pink	6 fl. oz.	68	20.6
(4C)	8 fl. oz.	80	20.0
(Funny Face)	8 fl. oz.	88	22.0
Kool-Aid, regular or pink:			
Sugar to be added	6 fl. oz.	73	18.8
Pre-sweetened with			
sugar	6 fl. oz.	65	16.3
Lemon Tree (Lipton)	6 fl. oz.	68	16.5
(Minute Maid)	6 fl. oz.	80	20.0
(Wyler's):			
Regular	8 fl. oz.	91	19.6
Wild strawberry	8 fl. oz.	80	20.7
Dietetic:			
Crystal Light	6 fl. oz.	4	.2
Kool-Aid	6 fl. oz.	3	.2
LEMONADE BAR (Sunkist)	3 fl. oz. bar	68	17.6
LEMONADE-CHERRY JUICE			
DRINK, canned (Boku)	8 fl. oz.	120	29.0
LEMONADE-LIMEADE			
DRINK, canned (Mistic)	8 fl. oz.	110	28.0
*LEMONADE PUNCH, mix			
Country Time, regular	8 fl. oz.	82	20.0
LEMON JUICE:			
Fresh (USDA)	1 T. (.5 oz.)	4	1.2
Plastic container, *ReaLemon*	1 T. (.5 oz.)	3	.5
*Frozen (Sunkist)			
unsweetened	1 fl. oz.	7	2.0
*LEMON-LIMEADE DRINK,			
MIX:			
Regular:			
(Minute Maid)	6 fl. oz.	80	20.0
Country Time	6 fl. oz.	65	16.2
Dietetic, *Crystal Light*	6 fl. oz.	4	.2
LEMON PEEL, CANDIED			
(USDA)	1 oz.	90	22.9

Food	Measure	Cals.	Carbs.
LEMON & PEPPER			
SEASONING:			
(Lawry's)	1 tsp.	6	1.2
(McCormick)	1 tsp.	7	.8
LENTIL:			
Whole:			
Dry:			
(USDA)	½ lb.	771	136.3
(USDA)	1 cup (6.7 oz.)	649	114.8
(Sinsheimer)	1 oz.	95	17.0
Cooked (USDA) drained	½ cup (3.6 oz.)	107	19.5
Split (USDA) dry	½ lb.	782	140.2
LENTIL MEAL, canned			
(Health Valley)			
Fast Menu, with vegetables,			
fat free	5 oz.	80	12.0
LENTIL PILAF MIX:			
(Casbah)	1 oz.	100	19.0
*(Near East)	1 cup	210	37.0
LETTUCE (USDA):			
Bibb, untrimmed	1 lb.	47	8.4
Bibb, untrimmed	7.8-oz. head		
	(4" dia.)	23	4.1
Boston, untrimmed	1 lb.	47	8.4
Boston, untrimmed	7.8-oz. head		
	(4" dia.)	23	4.1
Butterhead varieties (See Bibb;			
Boston)			
Cos (See Romaine)			
Dark green (See Romaine)			
Grand Rapids	1 lb. (weighed		
	untrimmed)	52	10.2
Great Lakes	1 lb. (weighed		
	untrimmed)	56	12.5
Great Lakes, trimmed	1 lb. head		
	(4¾" dia.)	59	13.2
Iceberg:			
Untrimmed	1 lb.	56	12.5
Trimmed	1 lb. head		
	(4¾" dia.)	59	13.2
Leaves	1 cup (2.3 oz.)	9	1.9
Chopped	1 cup (2 oz.)	8	1.7
Chunks	1 cup (2.6 oz.)	10	2.1

Food	Measure	Cals.	Carbs.
Looseleaf varieties (See Salad Bowl)			
New York	1 lb. (weighed untrimmed)	56	12.5
New York	1 lb. head (4¾" dia.)	59	13.2
Romaine:			
Untrimmed	1 lb.	52	10.2
Trimmed, shredded & broken into pieces	½ cup	4	.8
Salad Bowl	1 lb. (weighed untrimmed)	52	10.2
Salad Bowl	2 large leaves (1.8 oz.)	9	1.8
Simpson	1 lb. (weighed untrimmed)	52	10.2
Simpson	2 large leaves (1.8 oz.)	9	1.8
White Paris (See Romaine)			
LIFE, cereal (Quaker) regular or cinnamon	⅔ cup (1 oz.)	105	19.7
LIME, fresh (USDA) peeled fruit	2" dia. lime (1.8 oz.)	15	4.9
***LIMEADE,** frozen (Minute Maid)	6 fl. oz.	71	19.2
LIME JUICE, *ReaLime*	1 T.	2	.5
LINGCOD, raw (USDA):			
Whole	1 lb. (weighed whole)	130	0.0
Meat only	34 oz.	95	0.0
LINGUINI:			
Dry or fresh, refrigerated (See **PASTA, DRY OR FRESH, REFRIGERATED**)			
Canned (Top Shelf) with clam sauce	1 serving	330	30.0
Frozen:			
(Banquet) *Healthy Balance,* with meat sauce)	11½-oz. meal	290	49.0

Food	Measure	Cals.	Carbs.
(Budget Gourmet) with shrimp	10-oz. meal	330	33.0
(Healthy Choice) with shrimp	9½-oz. meal	230	40.0
(Mrs. Paul's) with shrimp & clams	10-oz. meal	240	36.0
(Stouffer's) *Lean Cuisine*, with clam sauce	9⅝-oz. meal	210	27.0

LIQUEUR (See individual kinds such as **CREME DE BANANA; PEACH LIQUEUR;** etc.)

LIQUOR (See **DISTILLED LIQUOR**)

LITCHI NUT (USDA):

Fresh:			
Whole	4 oz. (weighed in shell with seeds)	44	11.2
Flesh only	4 oz.	73	18.6
Dried:			
Whole	4 oz. (weighed in shell with seeds)	145	36.9
Flesh	2 oz.	157	40.1

LITTLE CAESAR'S:

Crazy Bread	1 piece	98	18.0
Crazy Sauce	1 serving	63	11.0
Pizza:			
Baby Pan! Pan!	1 pizza	525	53.0
Pizza!Pizza!:			
Round:			
Cheese:			
Small	1 slice	138	14.0
Medium	1 slice	154	16.0
Large	1 slice	169	18.0
Cheese & pepperoni:			
Small	1 slice	151	14.0
Medium	1 slice	168	16.0
Large	1 slice	185	18.0
Square:			
Cheese:			
Small	1 slice	188	22.0
Medium	1 slice	185	22.0
Large	1 slice	188	22.0
Cheese & pepperoni			

Food	Measure	Cals.	Carbs.
Small	1 slice	204	22.0
Medium	1 slice	201	22.0
Large	1 slice	204	22.0
Salad:			
Antipasto, small	1 salad	96	8.0
Greek, small	1 salad	85	6.0
Tossed, small	1 salad	37	7.0
Sandwiches:			
Ham & cheese	1 sandwich	520	55.0
Italian submarine	1 sandwich	590	55.0
Tuna melt	1 sandwich	700	58.0
Turkey	1 sandwich	450	49.0
Veggie	1 sandwich	620	58.0
LIVER:			
Beef:			
(USDA):			
Raw	1 lb.	635	24.0
Fried	4 oz.	260	6.0
(Swift) packaged, True-Tender, sliced, cooked	⅕ of 1-lb. pkg.	141	3.1
Calf (USDA):			
Raw	1 lb.	635	18.6
Fried	4 oz.	296	4.5
Chicken:			
Raw	1 lb.	585	13.2
Simmered	4 oz.	187	3.5
Goose, raw (USDA)	1 lb.	826	24.5
Hog (USDA):			
Raw	1 lb.	594	11.8
Fried	4 oz.	273	2.8
Lamb (USDA):			
Raw	1 lb.	617	13
LIVERWURST SPREAD, canned:			
(Hormel)	1 oz.	70	0.0
(Underwood)	2.4 oz.	220	3.0
LOBSTER:			
Raw (USDA):			
Whole	1 lb. (weighed whole	107	.6
Meat only	4 oz.	103	.6
Cooked, meat only (USDA)	4 oz.	108	.3
Canned (USDA) meat only	4 oz.	108	.3

Food	Measure	Cals.	Carbs.
Frozen, South African rock lobster	2-oz. tail	65	.1
LOBSTER NEWBURG:			
Home recipe (USDA)	4 oz.	220	5.8
Frozen (Stouffer's)	6½ oz.	380	9.0
LOBSTER PASTE, canned (USDA)	1 oz.	51	.4
LOBSTER SALAD, home recipe (USDA)	4 oz.	125	2.6
LOGANBERRY (USDA):			
Fresh:			
Untrimmed	1 lb. (weighed with caps)	267	64.2
Trimmed	1 cup (5.1 oz.)	89	21.5
Canned, solids & liq.:			
Extra heavy syrup	4 oz.	101	25.2
Heavy syrup	4 oz.	101	25.2
Juice pack	4 oz.	61	14.4
Light syrup	4 oz.	79	19.5
Water pack	4 oz.	45	10.7
LONGAN (USDA):			
Fresh:			
Whole	1 lb. (weighed with shell & seeds)	147	38.0
Flesh only	4 oz.	69	17.9
Dried:			
Whole	1 lb. (weighed with shell & seeds)	467	120.8
Flesh only	4 oz.	324	83.9
LONG ISLAND TEA COCKTAIL (Mr. Boston) 12½% alcohol	3 fl. oz.	93	9.0
LONG JOHN SILVER'S:			
Bean, green	3½-oz. serving	20	3.0
Breadstick	1.2-oz. serving	110	18.0
Brownie, walnut	1 brownie (3.4 oz.)	440	54.0

Food	Measure	Cals.	Carbs.
Cake, pineapple cream cheese cake	3.2-oz. serving	310	34.0
Catfish:			
Dinner or entree, with fries, 3 hushpuppies & coleslaw	1 serving	860	90.0
Fillet	2.7-oz. piece	203	12.0
Catsup	.4-oz. packet	15	3.0
Chicken:			
Light herb	3½-oz. serving	120	<1.0
Planks, plain	2-oz. piece	120	11.0
Chicken dinner or entree:			
Kids Meal, two pieces chicken with fries & a hushpuppy	7.8-oz. serving	560	60.0
Planks:			
2 pieces, with fries, hushpuppies & coleslaw	6.9-oz. serving	490	50.0
3 pieces with fries, hushpuppies & coleslaw	14.1-oz. serving	890	101.0
4 pieces with fries & coleslaw	1 serving	940	94.0
With rice, green beans, coleslaw & a roll without margarine	15.9-oz. serving	590	82.0
Chicken sandwich, batter-dipped, without sauce	4½-oz. sandwich	280	39.0
Clam, breaded	4.7-oz. serving	526	48.0
Clam dinner or entree, with French fries, hushpuppies & coleslaw	12.7-oz. serving	990	114.0
Coleslaw	1 serving	140	20.0
Cookie:			
Chocolate chip	1.8-oz. serving	230	25.0
Oatmeal raisin	1.8-oz. serving	160	15.0
Corn on the cob	3.3-oz. serving	140	18.0
Fish:			
Baked, with sauce	5½-oz. serving	150	0.0
Batter-dipped	1 piece (3.1 oz.)	180	12.0
Crispy	1.8-oz. serving	122	8.0
Kitchen breaded	2-oz. serving	122	8.0
Lemon crumb	1 piece (1.6 oz.)	50	0.8
Paprika, light	1 piece (1.6 oz.)	40	Tr.
Scampi sauce	1 piece (1.7 oz.)	57	0.7
Fish & chicken dinner or entree:			

Food	Measure	Cals.	Carbs.
Regular, with fries, hushpuppies & coleslaw	15.2-oz. serving	950	102.0
Kids Meal, with fries & hushpuppies	8.9-oz. serving	620	61.0
Fish dinner or entree:			
Regular:			
Baked, with sauce, coleslaw & mixed vegetables	1 serving	385	19.0
Crispy, 3 pieces with fries, hushpuppies & coleslaw	13½-oz. serving	980	92.0
Fish & fries:			
2 pieces with fries	9.2-oz. serving	610	52.0
3 pieces with fries & 2 hushpuppies	1 serving	810	77.0
Fish & more, 1 piece, with fries, hushpuppies & coleslaw	14.4-oz. serving	890	92.0
Homestyle, 6 pieces with fries, 2 hushpuppies & coleslaw	1 serving	1260	124.0
Kitchen breaded with fries, hushpuppies & coleslaw:			
2 pieces	1 serving	818	76.0
3 pieces	1 serving	940	84.0
Lemon crumb, 2 pieces with rice & salad	11.8-oz. serving	290	40.0
Paprika, light, 2 pieces with rice & a small salad	10-oz. serving	300	45.0
Fish & shrimp dinner or entree, with fries, hushpuppies & coleslaw	17.2-oz. serving	1140	108.0
Fish sandwich, homestyle	1 serving	510	58.0
Fish sandwich platter with fries & coleslaw	1 serving	870	108.0
Fish, shrimp & chicken dinner or entree with fries, hushpuppies & coleslaw	18.1-oz. serving	1160	113.0
Fish, shrimp & clams dinner or entree, with fries, hushpuppies & coleslaw	18.1-oz. serving	1240	123.0
French fries	3-oz. serving	220	30.0
Hushpuppy	1 piece	70	10.0
Oyster, breaded	1 piece (.7 oz.)	60	6.0

Food	Measure	Cals.	Carbs.
Oyster dinner or entree, 6 pieces with fries & coleslaw	1 serving	789	78.0
Pie:			
Apple	4½-oz. serving	320	45.0
Cherry	4½-oz. serving	360	55.0
Lemon	4-oz. serving	340	60.0
Pecan	4-oz. serving	446	59.0
Pumpkin	4-oz. serving	251	34.0
Rice pilaf	6-oz. serving	210	43.0
Salad:			
Plain, without dressing	1.9-oz. serving	8	0.0
Garden, with crackers	1 serving	170	13.0
Ocean chef, with crackers	1 serving	250	19.0
Seafood:			
Plain	1 scoop	210	26.0
with crackers	1 serving	270	36.0
Without dressing or crackers	9.8-oz. serving	380	12.0
Shrimp, with crackers	1 serving	183	12.0
Salad dressing:			
Regular:			
Blue cheese	1½-oz. serving	225	3.0
Sea salad	1½-oz. serving	220	5.0
Thousand Island	1½-oz. serving	225	8.0
Dietetic, Italian	1½-oz. serving	20	3.0
Sauce:			
Honey mustard	1 oz.	45	14.0
Seafood	1 oz.	34	9.0
Sweet & sour	.42-oz.	20	5.0
Tartar	1 oz.	117	5.0
Scallop, battered	1 piece (.7 oz.)	53	4.0
Scallop dinner, with fries & coleslaw	1 serving	747	66.0
Seafood gumbo (made with cod)	7-oz. serving	120	4.0
Shrimp:			
Batter-dipped	.4-oz. piece	30	2.0
Breaded	4.7-oz. serving	388	33.0
Shrimp dinner or entree:			
Breaded, 21 pieces, with fries, hushpuppies & coleslaw	1 serving	1070	130.0
With scampi sauce	5.2-oz. serving	120	2.0
10 pieces with fries, hushpuppies & coleslaw	11.7-oz. serving	840	88.0

Food	Measure	Cals.	Carbs.
LOQUAT, fresh, flesh only (USDA)	2 oz.	27	7.0
LUCKY CHARMS, cereal (General Mills)	1 cup (1 oz.)	110	24.0
LUNCHEON MEAT (See also individual listings such as **BOLOGNA; HAM;** etc.):			
All meat (Oscar Mayer)	1-oz. slice	95	.7
Banquet loaf (Eckrich)	¾-oz. slice	50	1.0
Bar-B-Que Loaf:			
(Eckrich)	1-oz. slice	35	1.0
(Oscar Mayer)	1-oz. slice	46	1.7
Beef, jellied (Hormel) loaf	1 slice	45	0.0
Gourmet loaf (Eckrich):			
Regular	1-oz. slice	35	2.0
Smorgas Pac	¾-oz. slice	25	2.0
Ham & cheese (See **HAM & CHEESE**)			
Honey loaf:			
(Eckrich):			
Regular	1-oz. slice	40	3.0
Smorgas Pac	¾-oz. slice	30	2.0
Smorgas Pac	1-oz. slice	35	3.0
(Hormel)	1 slice	45	.5
(Oscar Mayer)	1-oz. slice	34	1.1
Iowa Brand (Hormel)	1 slice	45	0.0
Jalapeño loaf (Oscar Mayer)	1-oz. slice	72	2.4
Liver cheese (Oscar Mayer)	1.3-oz. slice	114	.5
Liver loaf (Hormel)	1 slice	80	6.5
Macaroni-cheese loaf (Eckrich)	1-oz. slice	70	3.0
Meat loaf (USDA)	1-oz. serving	57	.9
New England Brand sliced sausage:			
(Eckrich)	1-oz. slice	35	1.0
(Oscar Mayer)	.8-oz. slice	29	.4
Old fashioned loaf:			
(Eckrich):			
Regular	1-oz. slice	70	3.0
Smorgas Pac	¾-oz. slice	50	2.0
(Oscar Mayer)	1-oz. slice	62	2.3
Olive loaf:			
(Eckrich)	1-oz. slice	80	2.0
(Hormel)	1 slice	55	2.5
(Oscar Mayer)	1-oz. slice	60	3.1
Pastrami (See **PASTRAMI**)			

Food	Measure	Cals.	Carbs.
Peppered loaf:			
(Eckrich)	1-oz. slice	40	1.0
(Oscar Mayer)	1-oz. slice	39	1.3
Pickle loaf:			
(Eckrich):			
Regular	1-oz. slice	80	2.0
Smorgas Pac	¾-oz. slice	50	1.0
(Hormel) *Light & Lean*	1 slice	50	1.5
(Ohse)	1 oz.	60	2.0
Pickle & pimiento loaf (Oscar Mayer)	1-oz. slice	62	3.7
Picnic loaf (Oscar Mayer)	1-oz. slice	60	1.2
Prosciutto (Hormel)	1 oz.	90	0.0
Spiced (Hormel)	1 slice	75	.5

LUNCHEON MEAT COMBINATION MEALS,

Food	Measure	Cals.	Carbs.
packaged:			
(Eckrich) *Lunch Makers:*			
Ham, swiss cheese & crackers	1 piece each	40	2.0
Turkey, cheddar cheese & crackers	1 piece each	40	2.0
(Louis Rich) *Lunch Breaks:*			
Turkey & cheddar cheese	1 pkg.	410	23.0
Turkey & monterey jack cheese	1 pkg.	400	27.0
Turkey ham & swiss cheese	1 pkg.	380	25.0
Turkey salami & cheddar cheese	1 pkg.	430	25.0
(Oscar Mayer) *Lunchables:*			
Bologna, American cheese & crackers	4½-oz. pkg.	480	20.0
Chicken, Monterey jack cheese, crackers & pudding	6.2-oz. pkg.	380	32.0
Ham & crackers:			
With American cheese & pudding	6.2-oz. pkg.	410	33.0
With cheddar cheese	4½-oz. pkg.	370	18.0
With swiss cheese	4½-oz. pkg.	340	18.0
With swiss cheese & a cookie	4.2-oz. pkg.	380	29.0
Turkey:			
With cheddar cheese & crackers	4½-oz. pkg.	360	19.0

Food	Measure	Cals.	Carbs.
With cheddar cheese, crackers & trail mix	5-oz. pkg.	460	41.0
With Monterey jack cheese & wheat crackers	4½-oz. pkg.	360	18.0
LUNG, raw (USDA):			
Beef	1 lb.	435	0.0
Calf	1 lb.	481	0.0
Lamb	1 lb.	467	0.0

M

Food	Measure	Cals.	Carbs.
MACADAMIA NUT (Royal Hawaiian)	1 oz.	197	4.5
MACARONI:			
Cooked dry (USDA):			
8-10 minutes, firm	4-oz. serving	168	34.1
14-20 minutes, tender	4-oz. serving	126	26.0
MACARONI & BEEF:			
Canned (Franco-American)			
BeefyO's, in tomato sauce	7½-oz. can	220	30.0
Frozen:			
(Morton)	10-oz. meal	245	30.4
(Stouffer's):			
Regular, with tomatoes	11½-oz. meal	340	38.0
Lean Cuisine, in tomato sauce	10-oz. meal	250	35.0
(Swanson) 3-compartment	12-oz. dinner	370	48.0
(Weight Watchers)	9-oz. meal	220	31.0
MACARONI & CHEESE:			
Canned:			
(Chef Boyardee)	7½-oz. meal	180	27.0
(Franco-American)	7.3-oz. can	160	24.0
(Hormel) *Micro-Cup*	7½-oz. serving	189	26.0
(Libby's) diner	7½-oz. serving	360	27.0
Frozen:			
(Banquet):			

Food	Measure	Cals.	Carbs.
Casserole	8-oz. pkg.	350	36.0
Dinner	10-oz. dinner	420	36.0
Family Entree	2-lb. pkg.	1160	128.0
(Birds Eye):			
Classics	½ of 10-oz. pkg.	236	24.0
For One	5¾-oz. pkg.	304	27.0
(Budget Gourmet):			
Regular, with cheddar & parmesan cheese, Light & Healthy	10½-oz. meal	330	49.0
Side Dish	5¾-oz. meal	230	22.0
(Celentano) baked	½ of 12-oz. pkg.	290	29.0
(Green Giant) one serving	5½-oz. pkg.	230	28.0
(Healthy Choice) *Quick Meal*:			
Regular	9-oz. meal	280	45.0
Nacho cheese	9-oz. meal	280	44.0
(Kid Cuisine) *Mega Meal*	12.4-oz. meal	470	75.0
(Morton):			
Casserole	6½-oz. serving	290	30.0
Dinner	11-oz. dinner	278	45.8
Family Meal	2-lb. pkg.	1043	143.7
(Stouffer's)	6-oz. serving	250	22.0
(Swanson)			
3-compartment	12¼-oz. dinner	340	48.0
(Weight Watchers)	9-oz. meal	280	43.0
Mix:			
(Golden Grain) deluxe	¼ of 7¼-oz. pkg.	190	35.0
*(Kraft):			
Regular, plain or spiral	¼ of box	190	36.0
Velveeta	¼ of pkg.	270	32.0
*(Town House)	1 cup	370	51.0
MACARONI & CHEESE LOAF, packaged (Ohse)	1 oz.	60	4.0
MACARONI & CHEESE PIE, frozen (Swanson)	7-oz. pie	200	24.0
***MACARONI SALAD,** mix (Betty Crocker) creamy	⅙ of pkg.	200	20.0
MACE (French's)	1 tsp.	10	.8
MACKEREL (See also **SPANISH MACKEREL**) (USDA):			

Food	Measure	Cals.	Carbs.
Atlantic:			
Raw:			
Whole	1 lb. (weighed whole)	468	0.0
Meat only	4 oz.	217	0.0
Broiled with butter	8½" × 2½" × ½" fillet (3.7 oz.)	268	0.0
Canned, solids & liq.	4 oz.	208	0.0
Pacific:			
Raw:			
Dressed	1 lb. (weighed with bones & skin)	519	0.0
Meat only	4 oz.	180	0.0
Canned, solids & liq.	4 oz.	204	0.0
Salted	4 oz.	346	0.0
Smoked	4 oz.	248	0.0
MADEIRA WINE (Leacock)			
19% alcohol	3 fl. oz.	120	6.3
MAHI MAHI (Captain's Choice)			
frozen	3-oz. fillet	73	0.0
MALT, dry (USDA)	1 oz.	104	21.9
MALT COOLER (Bartles & Jaymes):			
Berry, peach or strawberry	12 fl. oz.	210	33.0
Black cherry	12 fl. oz.	200	32.0
Fuzzy navel	12 fl. oz.	230	39.0
Mai Tai	12 fl. oz.	240	40.0
Sangria, red	12 fl. oz.	200	31.0
Tropical	12 fl. oz.	230	37.0
MALTED MILK MIX (Carnation):			
Chocolate	3 heaping tsps. (.7 oz.)	85	18.0
Natural	3 heaping tsps. (.7 oz.)	88	15.8
MALT LIQUOR:			
Colt 45	12 fl. oz.	156	11.1
Elephant	12 fl. oz.	212	17.1
Kingsbury, no alcohol	12 fl. oz.	60	12.8
Mickey's	12 fl. oz.	156	11.1

Food	Measure	Cals.	Carbs.
Schlitz	12 fl. oz.	88	7.2
MALT-O-MEAL, cereal:			
Regular	1 T. (.3 oz.)	33	7.3
Chocolate-flavored	1 T. (.3 oz.)	33	7.0
MAMEY OR MAMMEE APPLE, fresh (USDA)	1 lb. (weighed with skin & seeds)	143	35.2
MANDARIN ORANGE (See **TANGERINE**)			
MANGO, fresh (USDA):			
Whole	1 lb. (weighed with seeds & skin)	201	51.1
Flesh only, diced or sliced	½ cup	54	13.8
MANGO DRINK, canned (Arizona) *Mucho Mango Cowboy Cocktail*	8 fl. oz.	100	27.0
MANGO MADNESS COCK-TAIL DRINK, canned (Snapple)	8 fl. oz.	110	29.0
MANGO NECTAR, canned (Libby's)	6 fl. oz.	110	26.0
MANHATTAN COCKTAIL (Mr. Boston) 20% alcohol	3 fl. oz.	123	12.3
MANICOTTI, DRY (See **PASTA, DRY OR FRESH, REFRIGERATED.**)			
MANICOTTI, frozen:			
(Budget Gourmet) cheese, with meat sauce	10-oz. serving	450	33.0
(Buitoni)	9-oz. serving	470	45.0
Plain	8-oz. serving	300	36.0
Cheese, with sauce	7-oz. serving	360	35.0
Low fat, *Great Choice*	10-oz. serving	250	41.0
(Healthy Choice) cheese	9¼-oz. meal	220	34.0
(Le Menu) 3-cheese	11¾-oz. dinner	390	44.0

Food	Measure	Cals.	Carbs.
(Weight Watchers) cheese	9¼-oz. dinner	260	31.0
MANWICH (Hunt's):			
Dry mix:			
Mix only	.25 oz	20	5.0
*Sandwich	1 serving	320	31.0
Extra thick & chunky:			
Sauce only	2½ oz.	60	15.0
*Sandwich	1 serving	330	36.0
Mexican:			
Sauce only	2½ oz.	35	9.0
*Sandwich	1 serving	310	30.0
MAPLE SYRUP (See **SYRUP,** Maple)			
MARGARINE, salted or unsalted:			
Regular:			
(USDA)	1 lb.	3266	1.8
(USDA)	1 cup (8 oz.)	1633	.9
(Autumn) soft or stick	1 T.	80	0.0
(Blue Bonnet) soft or stick	1 T. (.5 oz.)	90	0.0
(Chiffon):			
Soft	1 T.	90	0.0
Stick	1 T.	100	0.0
(Fleischmann's) soft or stick	1 T. (.5 oz.)	100	0.0
(Golden Mist)	1 T.	100	0.0
(Holiday)	1 T. (.5 oz.)	102	0.0
I Can't Believe It's Not Butter, any type	1 T. (.5 oz.)	90	0.0
(Imperial) soft or stick	1 T. (.5 oz.)	102	Tr.
(Land O' Lakes)	1 T.	100	0.0
(Mazola)	1 T.	100	0.0
(Parkay)	1 T.	100	0.0
(Promise) soft or stick	1 T.	90	Tr.
Imitation or dietetic:			
Country Morning:			
Regular:			
Stick	1 T.	100	0.0
Tub	1 T.	90	0.0
Light	1 T.	60	0.0
Imperial:			
Regular	1 T.	50	Tr.
Light	1 T.	60	Tr.
(Land O' Lakes):			
Tub, 64% soy oil spread	1 T.	75	0.0

Food	Measure	Cals.	Carbs.
Stick, sweet cream	1 T.	90	0.0
Mazola	1 T.	50	Tr.
(Weight Watchers):			
Regular	1 T.	60	0.0
Corn oil	1 T.	50	0.0
Whipped:			
(Blue Bonnet)	1 T. (9 grams)	70	0.0
(Chiffon)	1 T.	70	0.0
(Fleischmann's)	1 T.	70	0.0
(Imperial)	1 T. (9 grams)	45	0.0
(Parkay) cup	1 T.	67	Tr.

MARGARITA COCKTAIL
(Mr. Boston) 12½% alcohol:

Regular	3 fl. oz.	105	10.8
Strawberry	3 fl. oz.	138	18.9

MARGARITA COCKTAIL MIX:
Dry (Holland House):

Regular	.5-oz. pkg.	57	14.0
Strawberry	.6-oz. pkg.	66	16.0
*Frozen (Bacardi):			
Water only	4 fl. oz.	49	12.4
Made with liquor	4 fl. oz.	82	12.4
Liquid (Holland House):			
Regular	1 fl. oz.	27	6.0
Strawberry	1 fl. oz.	31	7.0

MARINADE MIX:

Chicken (Adolph's)	1-oz. packet	64	14.4
Meat:			
(Adolph's)	.8-oz. pkg.	38	8.5
(Durkee)	1-oz. pkg.	47	9.0
(French's)	1-oz. pkg.	80	16.0
(Kikkoman)	1-oz. pkg.	64	12.5

MARJORAM (French's)

	1 tsp. (1.2 grams)	4	.8

MARMALADE:
Sweetened:

(USDA)	1 T. (.7 oz.)	51	14.0
(Empress)	1 T.	52	13.5
(Keiller)	1 T.	60	15.0
(Knudsen & Sons)	1 T.	17	4.0

Food	Measure	Cals.	Carbs.
(Smucker's)	1 T. (.7 oz.)	54	12.0
Dietetic:			
(Estee; Louis Sherry)	1 T. (.6 oz.)	6	0.0
(Featherweight)	1 T.	16	4.0
(S&W) *Nutradiet,* red label	1 T.	12	3.0
MARSHMALLOW (See **CANDY, GENERIC** and **CANDY, COMMERCIAL**)			
MARSHMALLOW FLUFF	1 heaping tsp.	59	14.4
MARSHMALLOW KRISPIES, cereal (Kellogg's)	1¼ cups (1.3 oz.)	140	32.0
MARTINI COCKTAIL (Mr. Boston) 20% alcohol:			
Gin, extra dry	3 fl. oz.	99	Tr.
Vodka	3 fl. oz.	102	Tr.
MATZO:			
(Goodman's):			
Diet-10s	1 sq.	109	23.0
Unsalted	1 matzo (1 oz.)	109	23.0
(Horowitz-Margareten)			
unsalted	1 matzo	135	28.2
(Manischewitz):			
Regular:			
Plain	1 piece	110	24.0
American	1-oz. piece	115	22.0
Egg	1 piece	108	26.6
Egg & onion	1 piece	112	23.0
Miniature	1 piece	9	20.0
Tam Tams	1 piece	15	DNA
Wheat	1 piece	9	1.8
Dietetic:			
Tam Tams	1 piece	14	DNA
Thins	1 piece	91	19.0
MATZO MEAL (Manischewitz)	½ cup	267	DNA
MAYONNAISE:			
Real:			
(Bama)	1 T.	100	0.0
(Bennett's)	1 T.	110	1.0
(Luzianne) *Blue Plate*	1 T.	100	1.0

Food	Measure	Cals.	Carbs.
Hellmann's (Best Foods)	1 T. (.5 oz.)	100	.1
(Kraft)	1 T.	100	0.0
(Nu Made)	1 T.	100	0.0
(Rokeach)	1 T.	100	0.0
Imitation or dietetic:			
Hellmann's Lite (Best Foods)	1 T.	50	1.0
(Luzianne) *Blue Plate*	1 T.	50	1.0
(Estee)	1 T. (.5 oz.)	50	1.0
Heart Beat (GFA)	1 T.	40	1.0
(Nu Made)	1 T.	40	1.0
(Weight Watchers)	1 T.	50	1.0
MAYPO, cereal:			
30-second	¼ cup (.8 oz.)	89	16.4
Vermont style	¼ cup (1.1 oz.)	121	22.0
McDONALD'S:			
Apple pie	2.9-oz. serving	260	34.0
Bacon bits	.1 oz.	15	.1
Biscuit:			
Plain, with spread	2.6-oz. piece	260	31.9
With bacon, egg & cheese	5.4-oz. piece	450	33.3
With sausage	4.3-oz. piece	430	33.0
With sausage & egg	6.0-oz. piece	520	32.6
Chicken McNuggets (6 pieces)	1 serving (4 oz.)	300	16.5
Chicken McNuggets sauce:			
Barbecue	1-oz. serving	45	10.0
Honey	.4-oz. serving	45	11.5
Honey mustard	.5-oz. serving	50	3.0
Hot mustard	1-oz. serving	60	7.0
Sweet & sour	1.1-oz. serving	50	11.0
Chicken sandwich, *McChicken*	6.7-oz. serving	510	44.0
Cookies:			
Chocolate chip	1 package	330	41.9
McDonaldland	1 package	260	41.0
Danish:			
Apple	3.7-oz. piece	360	51.2
Cheese, iced	3.9-oz. piece	410	47.0
Cinnamon raisin	3.7-oz. piece	430	57.5
Raspberry	3.7-oz. piece	400	58.0
Egg McMuffin	1 serving	290	28.1
Egg, scrambled	1 serving	170	1.2
English muffin, with butter	1 muffin	140	26.7
Filet-O-Fish	1 sandwich	360	37.9
Hamburger:			
Plain:			
Regular	3.6-oz. serving	270	34.0

Food	Measure	Cals.	Carbs.
Big Mac	7.6-oz. serving	530	47.0
McLean Deluxe	7.3-oz. serving	350	38.0
Quarter Pounder	6.1-oz. serving	420	37.0
With cheese:			
Regular	4.1-oz. serving	320	35.0
McLean Deluxe	8.0-oz. serving	400	39.0
Quarter Pounder	6.8-oz. serving	530	38.0
Hot cakes with butter & syrup	1 serving	580	100.0
Milk shake, low fat:			
Chocolate	10.4 fl. oz.	340	64.0
Strawberry	10.4 fl. oz.	340	62.0
Vanilla	10.4 fl. oz.	340	63.0
Muffin, fat free, apple bran	2.5-oz. piece	170	38.0
Orange juice	6 fl. oz.	80	18.5
Potato:			
Fried	1 small order	210	26.6
Hash browns	1.9-oz. piece	130	14.9
Salad:			
Chef	11.0-oz. serving	210	9.0
Chicken, fajita	10-oz. serving	160	9.0
Garden	8.2-oz. serving	80	6.2
Side	5-oz. serving	45	4.0
Salad dressing:			
Regular:			
Bleu cheese	1 pkg.	190	8.0
Ranch	1 pkg.	230	10.0
1000 Island	1 pkg.	190	16.0
Dietetic:			
Ranch	1 pkg.	40	5.2
Vinaigrette	1 pkg.	50	9.0
Sausage	1.5-oz. piece	170	0.0
Sausage McMuffin:			
Plain	4-oz. piece	360	26.0
With egg	5.8-oz. piece	440	27.9
Soft drink:			
Sweetened:			
Coca-Cola, classic	12 fl. oz.	110	29.0
Coca-Cola, classic	16 fl. oz.	150	40.0
Coca-Cola, classic	21 fl. oz.	210	58.0
Orange drink (Hi-C)	12 fl. oz.	120	32.0
Orange drink (Hi-C)	16 fl. oz.	160	44.0
Orange drink (Hi-C)	21 fl. oz.	240	64.0
Sprite	12 fl. oz.	110	28.0
Sprite	16 fl. oz.	150	39.0
Sprite	21 fl. oz.	210	56.0
Dietetic, Diet Coke	12 fl. oz.	0	0.0
Vanilla soft-serve, with cone	3 fl. oz.	140	21.9

Food	Measure	Cals.	Carbs.
MEATBALL SEASONING MIX:			
*(Durkee) Italian	1 cup	619	4.5
(French's)	¼ of 1.5-oz. pkg.	35	7.0
MEATBALL STEW:			
Canned (Hormel) *Dinty Moore*	⅓ of 24-oz. can	240	15.0
Frozen (Stouffer's) *Lean Cuisine*	10-oz. meal	250	20.0
MEATBALL, SWEDISH, frozen:			
(Armour) *Dinner Classics*	11¼-oz. meal	360	32.0
(Budget Gourmet) with noodles	10-oz. meal	590	37.0
(Stouffer's) with parsley noodles	11-oz. meal	480	37.0
MEAT LOAF DINNER, frozen:			
(Armour) *Dinner Classics*	11¼-oz. dinner	360	32.0
(Banquet):			
Cookin' Bag	4-oz. meal	200	8.0
Dinner	11-oz. meal	440	27.0
(Healthy Choice) low fat & cholesterol	12-oz. meal	340	48.0
(Morton)	10-oz. dinner	310	26.0
(Stouffer's):			
Regular, homestyle	9⅞-oz. meal	370	250
Lean Cuisine, with macaroni & cheese	9⅜-oz. meal	280	26.0
(Swanson)	10¾-oz. dinner	360	41.0
MEAT LOAF SEASONING MIX:			
(Bell's)	4½-oz. serving	300	14.0
(Contadina)	3¾-oz. pkg.	360	72.4
MEAT TENDERIZER:			
Regular (Adolph's; McCormick)	1 tsp.	2	.5
Seasoned (McCormick)	1 tsp.	5	.8
MELBA TOAST, salted (Old London):			
Garlic, onion or white rounds	1 piece	10	1.8
Pumpernickel, rye, wheat or white	1 piece	17	3.4

Food	Measure	Cals.	Carbs.
Sesame, flat	1 piece	18	3.0
MELON (See individual kinds)			
MELON BALLS, in syrup, frozen (USDA)	½ cup (4.1 oz.)	72	18.2
MELONBERRY COCKTAIL, canned (Snapple)	8 fl. oz.	120	29.0
MENHADEN, Atlantic, canned (USDA) solids & liq.	4 oz.	195	0.0
MENUDO, canned (Old El Paso)	½ can	476	14.0
MERLOT WINE (Louis M. Martini) 12½% alcohol	3 fl. oz.	63	TR.
MEXICAN DINNER, frozen:			
(Banquet) dinner:			
Regular	12-oz. dinner	490	62.0
Combination	12-oz. dinner	520	72.0
(Budget Gourmet)	12.8-oz. meal	500	56.0
(Morton)	10-oz. dinner	300	44.0
(Patio):			
Regular	13¼-oz. meal	540	64.0
Fiesta	12¼-oz. meal	470	55.0
(Swanson):			
4-course	14¼-oz. dinner	490	62.0
Hungry Man	20¼-oz. dinner	820	88.0
MILK, CONDENSED, sweetened, canned:			
(USDA)	1 T. (.7 oz.)	61	10.4
(Carnation)	1 fl. oz.	123	20.8
(Borden) *Eagle Brand*	1 T. (.7 oz.)	60	10.4
(Milnot) *Dairy Sweet*	1 fl. oz. (1.3 oz.)	119	19.3
MILK, DRY:			
Whole (USDA) packed cup	1 cup (5.1 oz.)	728	55.4
*Nonfat, instant:			
(USDA)	8 fl. oz.	82	10.8
(Alba):			
Regular	8 fl. oz.	81	11.6
Chocolate flavor	8 fl. oz.	80	12.9

Food	Measure	Cals.	Carbs.
(Carnation)	8 fl. oz.	80	12.0
(Lucerne)	8 fl. oz.	80	12.0
MILK, EVAPORATED:			
Regular:			
(Carnation)	½ cup (4 fl. oz.)	170	12.2
(Lucerne)	½ cup	170	12.0
(Pet)	½ cup (4 fl. oz.)	170	12.0
Filled, *Dairymate*	½ cup	150	12.0
Low fat (Carnation)	½ cup	110	12.0
Skimmed:			
(Carnation)	½ cup	100	14.0
Pet 99	½ cup	100	14.0
MILK, FRESH:			
Buttermilk:			
(Friendship) lowfat	1 cup	120	12.0
(Johanna Farms)	1 cup	120	11.0
(Land O' Lakes)	8 fl. oz.	110	12.0
(Lucerne):			
Regular	8 fl. oz.	120	12.0
Bulgarian or old time	8 fl. oz.	150	11.0
Chocolate:			
(Borden) *Dutch Blend,* lowfat	1 cup	180	25.0
(Hershey's) lowfat	1 cup	190	29.0
(Johanna Farms):			
Regular	1 cup	200	26.0
Lowfat	1 cup	150	26.0
(Land O' Lakes) lowfat:			
½%	8 fl. oz.	150	26.0
with *Nutrasweet*	8 fl. oz.	110	14.0
(Lucerne) lowfat	1 cup	180	26.0
(Nestlé) *Quik*	1 cup	220	30.0
White:			
Whole (3.25% butterfat) (USDA)	1 cup	159	12.0
Lowfat:			
(Borden):			
1% milkfat	1 cup	100	11.0
2% milkfat, *Hi-Protein Brand*	1 cup	140	13.0
(Johanna Farms):			
1% lowfat, protein fortified	1 cup	110	13.0
2% lowfat, *Mighty Milk*	1 cup	140	13.0
(Land O' Lakes):			

Food	Measure	Cals.	Carbs.
1% milkfat	8 fl. oz.	100	12.0
2% milkfat	8 fl. oz.	120	11.0
(Lucerne):			
Acidophilus or 2-10	8 fl. oz.	140	13.0
½%, 1% or 1½% milkfat	8 fl. oz.	90	11.0
2% milkfat	8 fl. oz.	120	11.0
Skim:			
(Land O' Lakes)	8 fl. oz.	90	12.0
(Weight Watchers)	1 cup	90	13.0
MILK, GOAT (USDA) whole	1 cup	163	11.2
MILK, HUMAN (USDA)	1 oz. (by wt.)	22	2.7
MILK, LACTOSE-REDUCED (Lactaid):			
2% fat	1 cup	130	12.0
Skim	1 cup	80	13.0
MILK, SOY (See **SOYBEAN MILK**)			
MILNOT	½ cup	151	12.2
MINERAL WATER (See also **VICHY WATER**)	any quantity	0	0.0
MINI-WHEATS, cereal (Kellogg's):			
Regular	¼-oz. biscuit	25	6.0
Bite size	½ cup (1 oz.)	100	24.0
MINT, LEAVES, raw, trimmed (HEW/FAO)	½ oz.	4	.8
MIRACLE WHIP (See **SALAD DRESSING,** Mayonnaise-type)			
MOLASSES:			
Barbados (USDA)	1 T. (.7 oz.)	51	13.3
Blackstrap (USDA)	1 T. (.7 oz.)	40	10.4
Dark (Brer Rabbit)	1 T. (.7 oz.)	33	10.6
Light (USDA)	1 T. (.7 oz.)	48	12.4
Medium (USDA)	1 T.	44	11.4
Unsulphured (Grandma's)	1 T.	60	15.0

Food	Measure	Cals.	Carbs.
MONOSODIUM GLUTAMATE, MSG			
(Tone's)	1 tsp	0	0.0
MORNING FUNNIES, cereal			
(Ralston Purina)	1 cup (1 oz.)	110	25.0
MORTADELLA, sausage			
(USDA)	1 oz.	89	.2
MOUSSE:			
Frozen (Weight Watchers)			
Sweet Celebrations:			
Chocolate	2½-oz. serving	170	24.0
Praline pecan	½ of 5.4-oz. pkg.	190	27.0
*Mix:			
Regular (Knorr)			
Unflavored	½ cup	80	8.0
Chocolate:			
Dark	½ cup	90	10.0
Milk	½ cup	90	11.0
White	½ cup	80	10.0
Dietetic:			
(Estee):			
Amaretto	½ cup	70	10.0
Chocolate or orange	½ cup	70	9.0
Lite Whip (TKI Foods):			
Chocolate:			
Skim milk	½ cup	70	10.0
Whole milk	½ cup	80	10.0
Lemon:			
Skim milk	½ cup	60	9.0
Whole milk	½ cup	70	9.0
Vanilla:			
Skim milk	½ cup	50	7.0
Whole milk	½ cup	70	9.0
*(Weight Watchers):			
Cheesecake or raspberry	½ cup	60	12.0
Chocolate:			
Regular	½ cup	60	9.0
White	½ cup	60	6.0
MUESLI, cereal (Ralston Purina):			
Raisins, dates & almonds	½ cup (1.45 oz.)	140	32.0
Raisins, peaches & pecan or raisins, walnuts & cranberries	½ cup (1.45 oz.)	150	30.0

Food	Measure	Cals.	Carbs.
MÜESLIX, cereal (Kellogg's):			
Crispy blend	⅔ cup (1½ oz.)	160	33.0
Golden Crunch	½ cup (1.2 oz.)	120	25.0
MUFFIN (See also *DUNKIN' DONUTS*)			
Non-frozen:			
Plain (USDA) home recipe	1.4 oz. muffin	118	16.9
Apple:			
(Awrey's):			
Regular:			
Small	1½-oz. muffin	130	17.0
Large	2½-oz. muffin	220	30.0
Banana nut, Grande	4.2-oz. muffin	260	27.0
(Hostess) with banana walnut, mini	1 muffin	32	3.4
Apple spice (Health Valley) fat free	1 muffin	130	30.0
Apple streusel (Awrey's) *Grande*	4.2-oz. muffin	340	50.0
Banana (Health Valley) fat free	1 muffin	130	29.0
Banana nut (Tastykake)	1 piece	240	52.0
Blueberry:			
(USDA) home recipe	1.4-oz. muffin	112	16.8
(Awrey's)	1½-oz. muffin	130	18.0
(Entenmann's)	1 muffin	200	29.0
(Hostess) mini	1 muffin	48	5.8
(Tastykake)	4-oz. muffin	460	60.0
Blueberry-apple (Health Valley) fat free, twin pack	1 muffin	140	32.0
Bran (USDA) home recipe	1.4-oz. muffin	104	17.2
Carrot (Health Valley) fat-free, twin pack	1 muffin	130	30.0
Corn:			
(USDA) home recipe, prepared with whole-ground cornmeal	1.4-oz. muffin	115	17.0
(Awrey's):			
Small	1½-oz. muffin	130	20.0
Large	2½-oz. muffin	220	33.0
(Tastykake)	4-oz. muffin	440	60.0
Cranberry (Awrey's)	1½-oz. muffin	290	44.0
English:			
(Mrs. Wright's)	2-oz. muffin	130	27.0
(Pritikin)	2.3-oz. muffins	150	28.0

Food	Measure	Cals.	Carbs.
(Roman Meal):			
Regular	1 muffin	146	28.5
Wheathery	1 muffin	140	28.0
(Tastykake)	1 muffin	130	26.0
(Thomas'):			
Regular	2-oz. muffin	133	25.7
Honey wheat	1 muffin	129	24.0
Oat bran	1 muffin	116	26.0
Raisin	2.2-oz. muffin	153	30.4
Rye	1 muffin	120	27.0
Granola (Mrs. Wright's)	2.3-oz. muffin	150	29.0
Oat bran:			
(Awrey's)	2¾-oz. muffin	180	27.0
(Hostess)	1 muffin	160	21.0
Oat bran-almond-date			
(Health Valley) low fat	1 muffin	180	31.0
Oat bran, banana nut			
(Hostess)	1 muffin	140	20.0
Raisin bran (Awrey's)			
Regular	1½-oz. muffin	110	18.0
Large	2½-oz. muffin	190	30.0
Grande	4.2-oz. muffin	320	50.0
Raisin cinnamon (Mrs.			
Wright's)	2-3-oz. muffin	150	31.0
Raisin spice (Health Valley)			
fat free	1 muffin	140	32.0
Raspberry (Health Valley)			
fat free, twin pack	1 muffin	130	30.0
Rice-bran raisin (Health			
Valley)	1 muffin	215	35.0
Frozen:			
Apple spice:			
(Healthy Choice)	2½-oz. muffin	190	40.0
(Sara lee)	2½-oz. muffin	220	36.0
(Weight Watchers)			
microwave	2½-oz. muffin	160	29.0
Banana nut:			
(Healthy Choice)	2½-oz. muffin	180	32.0
(Weight Watchers)			
microwave	2½-oz. muffin	170	32.0
Blueberry:			
(Healthy Choice)	2½-oz. muffin	190	39.0
(Pepperidge Farm)	1 muffin	170	27.0
(Sara Lee):			
Regular	2½-oz. muffin	200	34.0
Free & Light	1 muffin	128	28.0
(Weight Watchers)			
microwave	2½-oz. muffin	170	32.0

Food	Measure	Cals.	Carbs.
Cheese streusel (Sara Lee)	2.1-oz. muffin	220	27.0
Chocolate chunk (Sara Lee)	2.1-oz. muffin	220	33.0
Cinnamon swirl (Pepperidge Farm)	1 muffin	190	30.0
Corn (Pepperidge Farm)	1 muffin	180	27.0
English (Pepperidge Farm):			
Regular	1 muffin	140	27.0
Cinnamon apple	1 muffin	140	27.0
Cinnamon chip	1 muffin	160	28.0
Cinnamon raisin	1 muffin	150	29.0
Sourdough	1 muffin	135	27.0
Honey bran:			
(Sara Lee) golden	2½-oz. muffin	250	31.0
(Weight Watchers)	2½-oz. muffin	160	32.0
Oat bran:			
(Pepperidge Farm) with apple	1 muffin	190	29.0
(Sara Lee):			
Plain	2½-oz. muffin	210	35.0
Apple	2½-oz. muffin	210	35.0
Raisin bran:			
(Pepperidge Farm) cholesterol free	1 muffin	170	30.0
(Sara Lee)	2½-oz. muffin	220	37.0
MUFFIN MIX:			
*Apple cinnamon (Betty Crocker):			
Regular	¹⁄₁₂ of pkg.	120	18.0
No cholesterol recipe	¹⁄₁₂ of pkg.	110	18.0
*Banana nut (Betty Crocker)	¹⁄₁₂ of pkg.	150	21.0
Blueberry:			
*(Betty Crocker) wild:			
Regular	1 muffin	120	18.0
No cholesterol recipe	1 muffin	110	18.0
(Duncan Hines):			
Bakery style	¹⁄₁₂ of pkg.	184	32.7
Wild	¹⁄₁₂ of pkg.	98	17.0
*Gold Medal	⅙ of pkg.	170	26.0
*Carrot nut (Betty Crocker)	¹⁄₁₂ of pkg.	150	22.0
*Chocolate chip (Betty Crocker)	¹⁄₁₂ of pkg.	150	22.0
Regular	¹⁄₁₂ of pkg.	150	22.0
No cholesterol recipe	¹⁄₁₂ of pkg.	140	22.0
*Cinnamon streusel (Betty Crocker)	¹⁄₁₀ of pkg.	200	27.0

Food	Measure	Cals.	Carbs.
Cinnamon swirl (Duncan Hines) bakery style	1 muffin	195	34.1
Corn:			
*(Dromedary)	1 muffin	120	20.0
*(Flako)	1 muffin	140	23.0
*Gold Medal	⅙ of pkg.	130	24.0
Cranberry orange nut (Duncan Hines) bakery style	¹⁄₁₂ of pkg.	184	27.1
*Honey bran, Gold Medal	⅙ of pkg.	170	25.0
*Oat, Gold Medal	⅙ of pkg.	150	23.0
Oat bran:			
*(Betty Crocker):			
Regular	⅛ of pkg.	190	25.0
No cholesterol recipe	⅛ of pkg.	180	25.0
(Duncan Hines):			
Blueberry	¹⁄₁₂ of pkg.	97	16.2
& honey	¹⁄₁₂ of pkg.	129	20.7
*Oatmeal raisin (Betty Crocker):			
Regular	¹⁄₁₂ of pkg.	140	22.0
No cholesterol recipe	¹⁄₁₂ of pkg.	130	22.0
Pecan nut (Duncan Hines) bakery style	¹⁄₁₂ of pkg.	211	27.3
MUSCATEL WINE (Gallo) 14% alcohol	3 fl. oz.	86	7.9
MUSHROOM:			
Raw (USDA):			
Whole	½ lb. (weighed untrimmed)	62	9.7
Trimmed, sliced	½ cup (1.2 oz.)	10	1.5
Canned (Green Giant) solids & liq., whole or sliced,	¼ cup	12	2.0
Frozen (Birds Eye)	⅓ of 8-oz. pkg.	19	4.0
MUSHROOM, CHINESE, dried (HEW/FAO):			
Dry	1 oz.	81	18.9
Soaked, drained	1 oz.	12	2.4
MUSKELLUNGE, raw (USDA):			
Whole	1 lb. (weighed whole)	242	0.0
Meat only	4 oz.	234	0.0

Food	Measure	Cals.	Carbs.
MUSKMELON (See **CANTALOUPE; CASABA; HONEYDEW;** etc.)			
MUSKRAT, roasted (USDA)	4 oz.	174	0.0
MUSSEL (USDA):			
Atlantic & Pacific, raw:			
In shell	1 lb. (weighed in shell)	153	7.2
Meat only	4 oz.	108	3.7
Pacific, canned, drained	4 oz.	129	1.7
MUSTARD:			
Powdered (dry) (French's)	1 tsp. (1.5 grams)	9	.3
Prepared:			
Brown (French's; Gulden's)	1 tsp.	5	.3
Chinese (Chun King)	1 tsp.	5	.3
Cream salad (French's)	1 tsp.	3	.3
Dijon, *Grey Poupon*	1 tsp. (.2 oz.)	6	Tr.
Horseradish (French's)	1 tsp. (.2 oz.)	5	.3
Medford (French's)	1 tsp.	5	.3
Onion (French's)	1 tsp.	8	1.6
Yellow (Gulden's)	1 tsp.	5	.4
MUSTARD GREENS:			
Raw (USDA) whole	1 lb. (weighed untrimmed)	98	17.8
Boiled (USDA) drained	1 cup (7.8 oz.)	51	8.8
Canned (Allen's) chopped, solids & liq.	½ cup (4.1 oz.)	20	2.0
Frozen, chopped:			
(Bel-Air)	3.3 oz.	20	3.0
(Birds Eye)	⅓ of 10-oz. pkg.	25	3.2
(Frosty Acres)	3.3-oz. serving	20	3.0
MUSTARD SPINACH (USDA):			
Raw	1 lb.	100	17.7
Boiled, drained, no added salt	4-oz. serving	18	3.2

Food	Measure	Cals.	Carbs.

N

NATHAN'S:

French fries	1 reg. order	550	60.0
Hamburger	4½-oz. sandwich	360	18.0
Hot dog	3.4-oz. serving	290	19.0

NATURAL CEREAL:
Familia:

Regular	½ cup (1.8 oz.)	187	34.8
With bran	½ cup (1.7 oz.)	166	29.0
With granola	½ cup (2.0 oz.)	257	37.2
No added salt	½ cup (1.8 oz.)	181	32.1

Heartland:

Plain, coconut or raisin	¼ cup (1 oz.)	130	18.0
Trail mix	¼ cup (1 oz.)	120	19.0

Nature Valley:

Cinnamon & raisin	⅓ cup (1 oz.)	120	20.0
Fruit & nut or toasted oat	⅓ cup (1 oz.)	130	19.0

NATURE SNACKS (Sun-Maid):

Carob Crunch	1 oz.	143	16.8
Carob Peanut	1¼ oz.	190	18.0
Carob Raisin or Yogurt Raisin	1¼ oz.	160	25.0
Nuts Galore	1 oz.	170	5.0
Raisin Crunch or Rocky Road	1 oz.	126	19.1
Sesame Nut Crunch	1 oz.	154	14.6
Tahitian Treat or Yogurt Crunch	1 oz.	123	19.4
Yogurt Peanut	1¼ oz.	200	18.0

NECTARINE, fresh (USDA):

Whole	1 lb. (weighed with pits)	267	71.4
Flesh only	4 oz.	73	19.4

NINTENDO CEREAL SYSTEM, cereal

(Ralston Purina)	1 cup (1 oz.)	110	25.0

Food	Measure	Cals.	Carbs.
NOODLE (See also **PASTA, DRY OR FRESH, REFRIGERATED** or **SPAGHETTI**). Plain noodle products are essentially the same in caloric value and carbohydrate content on the same weight basis. The longer they are cooked, the more water is absorbed and this affects the nutritive values. Also, the longer they are cooked, the amount of calories decreases somewhat. (USDA):			
Dry	1 oz.	110	20.4
Dry, 1½" strips	1 cup (2.6 oz.)	283	52.6
Cooked	1 oz.	35	6.6
NOODLE MIX (See also **PASTA & SAUCE, MIX**):			
(Lipton) & Sauce:			
Alfredo:			
Regular	¼ of pkg.	131	20.4
Carbonara	¼ of pkg.	126	20.2
Beef	¼ of pkg.	120	21.7
Butter	¼ of pkg.	142	21.7
Butter & herb	¼ of pkg.	136	21.8
Cheese	¼ of pkg.	136	23.9
Chicken	¼ of pkg.	125	21.8
Parmesan	¼ of pkg.	138	20.2
Sour cream & chive	¼ of pkg.	142	22.6
Stroganoff	¼ of pkg.	110	19.1
Noodle Roni (See also **PASTA & SAUCE MIX**)	⅕ of 6-oz. pkg.	130	21.0
(Ultra Slim Fast) with Alfredo sauce	8-oz. serving	240	47.0
NOODLES & BEEF:			
Canned (Heinz) in sauce	7½-oz. serving	170	17.0
Frozen (Banquet) *Family Entrees*:			
With gravy	8-oz. serving	200	22.0
& julienne beef with sauce	7-oz. serving	170	22.0
NOODLES & CHICKEN:			
Canned:			
(Heinz)	7½-oz. serving	160	19.0

Food	Measure	Cals.	Carbs.
(Hormel) *Dinty Moore, American Classics*	10-oz. serving	230	24.0
Frozen:			
(Banquet):			
Regular	10-oz. serving	350	42.0
Family Favorites	10-oz. serving	340	42.0
(Swanson)	10½-oz. serving	280	45.0
NOODLES, CHOW MEIN:			
(Chun King)	1 oz.	139	16.5
(La Choy)	½ cup (1 oz.)	150	16.0
NOODLES & FRANKFURTERS, canned (Van Camp's) *Noodle Weenee*	1 cup	245	33.0
NOODLES, RICE (La Choy)	1 oz.	130	21.0
NOODLES ROMANOFF, frozen			
(Stouffer's)	⅓ of 12-oz. pkg.	170	15.0
NOODLES & TUNA, canned:			
(Heinz)	7½-oz. serving	170	20.0
(Hormel) *Dinty Moore, American Classics,* casserole	10-oz. serving	240	28.0
NUT (See specific variety such as **CASHEW NUT; COCONUT; PEANUT;** etc.)			
NUT, MIXED:			
Dry roasted:			
(Flavor House) salted	1 oz.	172	5.4
(Planters)	1 oz.	160	7.0
Oil roasted (Planters) with or without peanuts	1 oz.	180	6.0
NUT & HONEY CRUNCH, cereal (Kellogg's)	⅔ cup (1 oz.)	110	24.0
NUT & HONEY CRUNCH Os, cereal (Kellogg's)	⅔ cup (1 oz.)	110	22.0
NUTMEG (French's)	1 tsp. (1.9 grams)	11	.9

Food	Measure	Cals.	Carbs.
NUTRIFIC, cereal			
(Kellogg's)	1 cup (1.3 oz.)	120	28.0
NUTRI-GRAIN, cereal			
(Kellogg's):			
Almond raisin	⅔ cup (1.4 oz.)	140	31.0
Raisin bran	1 cup (1.4 oz.)	130	31.0
Wheat	⅔ cup (1 oz.)	100	24.0

O

Food	Measure	Cals.	Carbs.
OATBAKE, cereal (Kellogg's)	⅓ (1 oz.)	110	21.0
OAT FLAKES, cereal (Post)	⅔ cup (1 oz.)	107	21.5
OATMEAL:			
Dry:			
Regular:			
(USDA)	½ cup (1.2 oz.)	140	44.5
(Elam's):			
Scotch style or stone			
ground	1 oz.	108	18.2
Steel cut, whole grain	¼ cup (1.6 oz.)	174	30.4
(H-O) old fashioned	1 T. (.14 oz.)	14	2.6
(Safeway)	1 oz.	100	18.0
(3-Minute Brand)	⅓ cup (1 oz.)	160	24.0
Instant:			
(H-O):			
Regular, boxed	1 T.	15	2.6
Regular, packets	1-oz. packet	105	17.9
With bran & spice	1½-oz. packet	157	29.0
Country apple & brown			
sugar	1.1-oz. packet	121	22.7
With maple & brown			
sugar flavor	1½-oz. packet	160	31.8
Sweet & mellow	1.4-oz. packet	149	28.7
Oatmeal Swirlers (General			
Mills):			
Apple cinnamon	1.7-oz. pkg.	160	24.0
Cherry or strawberry	1.7-oz. pkg.	150	32.0

Food	Measure	Cals.	Carbs.
Cinnamon spice or maple brown sugar	1.6-oz. pkg.	160	35.0
Milk chocolate	1.7-oz. pkg	170	37.0
(3-Minute Brand):			
Regular	1-oz.-pkg.	160	26.0
Apple cinnamon	1⅜-oz. pkg.	210	37.0
Cinnamon & spice	1½-oz. pkg.	240	41.0
Maple & brown sugar	1½-oz. pkg.	220	38.0
Total (General Mills):			
Regular	1.2-oz. pkg.	110	22.0
Apple cinnamon	1¼-oz. pkg.	150	32.0
Cinnamon raisin	1.8-oz. pkg.	170	38.0
Maple brown sugar	1.6-oz. pkg.	160	34.0
Cooked:			
Regular (USDA)	1 cup (8.5 oz.)	132	23.3
Quick:			
(Harvest Brand)	⅓ cup (1 oz.)	110	18.1
(H-O)	½ cup (1.2 oz.)	129	22.2
(Quaker)	⅓ cup (1 oz.)	109	18.5
(Ralston Purina)	⅓ cup (1 oz.)	110	18.0
(Safeway)	1 oz.	100	18.0
Total (General Mills)	1 oz.	90	18.0
OCTOPUS, raw (USDA) meat only	4 oz.	83	0.0
OIL, COD LIVER (Hain) any flavor	1 T.	120	0.
OIL, SALAD OR COOKING:			
(USDA) all kinds, including olive	1 T. (.5 oz.)	124	0.0
(USDA) all kinds, including olive	½ cup (3.9 oz.)	972	0.0
(Bertoli) olive	1 T.	120	0.0
(Calavo) avocado	1 T.	120	0.0
(Country Pure) canola	1 T.	120	0.0
Crisco; Fleischmann's; Mazola	1 T. (.5 oz.)	120	0.0
(Golden Thistle; Goya)	1 T. (.5 oz.)	130	0.0
Mrs. Tucker's, corn or soybean	1 T.	130	0.0
(Planters) peanut or popcorn	1 T.	130	0.0
Sunlite; Wesson	1 T.	120	0.0
OKRA:			
Raw (USDA) whole	1 lb. (weighed untrimmed)	140	29.6
Boiled (USDA) drained:			

Food	Measure	Cals.	Carbs.
Whole	½ cup (3.1 oz.)	26	5.3
Pods	8 pods (3 oz.)	25	5.1
Slices	½ cup (2.8 oz.)	23	4.8
Frozen:			
(Bel-Air):			
Cut	3.3 oz.	25	6.0
Whole	3.3 oz.	30	7.0
(Birds Eye)			
Whole, baby	⅓ of 10-oz. pkg.	36	6.7
Cut	⅓ of 10-oz. pkg.	30	5.7
(Frosty Acres):			
Cut	3.3-oz. serving	25	6.0
Whole	3.3-oz. serving	30	7.0
(McKenzie):			
Cut	3.3 oz.	30	6.0
Whole	3.3 oz.	35	7.0
(Ore-Ida) breaded	3 oz.	170	17.0
OLIVE:			
Greek style (USDA):			
With pits, drained	1 oz.	77	2.0
Pitted, drained	1 oz.	96	2.5
Green (USDA)	1 oz.	33	.4
Ripe, by variety (USDA):			
Ascalano, any size, pitted & drained	1 oz.	37	.7
Manzanilla, any size	1 oz.	37	.7
Mission	3 small or 2 large	18	.3
Mission, slices	½ cup (2.2 oz.)	26	6.1
Ripe, by size (Lindsay):			
Colossal	1 olive	9	.6
Extra large	1 olive	6	.3
Jumbo	1 olive	7	.5
Large	1 olive	6	.4
Medium	1 olive	3	.2
Super colossal	1 olive	11	.8
ONION (See also **ONION, GREEN; ONION, WELCH**):			
Raw (USDA):			
Whole	1 lb. (weighed untrimmed)	157	35.9
Whole	3.9-oz. onion (2½" dia.)	38	8.7
Chopped	½ cup (3 oz.)	33	7.5

Food	Measure	Cals.	Carbs.
Chopped	1 T. (.4 oz.)	4	1.0
Grated	1 T. (.5 oz.)	5	1.2
Slices	½ cup (2 oz.)	21	4.9
Boiled, drained (USDA):			
Whole	½ cup (3.7 oz.)	30	6.8
Whole, pearl onions	½ cup (3.2 oz.)	27	6.0
Halves or pieces	½ cup (3.2 oz.)	26	5.8
Canned, O & C (Durkee):			
Boiled	1-oz. serving	8	2.0
In cream sauce	1-oz. serving	143	17.0
Dehydrated:			
Flakes:			
(USDA)	1 tsp. (1.3 grams)	5	1.1
(Gilroy)	1 tsp.	5	1.2
Powder (Gilroy)	1 tsp.	9	2.0
French fried (Durkee), canned	¼ cup (13 grams)	80	5
Frozen:			
(Bel-Air) chopped	1 oz.	8	2.0
(Birds Eye):			
Chopped	1 oz.	8	2.0
Small, whole	¼ of 16-oz. pkg.	44	9.6
Small, with cream sauce	⅓ of 9-oz. pkg.	118	11.2
(Frosty Acres) chopped	1 oz.	8	2.0
(Mrs. Paul's) rings, breaded & fried	½ of 5-oz. pkg.	190	19.0
(Ore-Ida) chopped	2 oz.	20	4.0
ONION, COCKTAIL (Vlasic) lightly spiced	1 oz.	4	1.0
ONION, GREEN, raw (USDA):			
Whole	1 lb. (weighed untrimmed)	157	35.7
Bulb & entire top	1 oz.	10	2.3
Bulb without green top	3 small onions (.9 oz.)	11	2.6
Slices, bulb & white portion of top	½ cup (1.8 oz.)	22	5.2
Tops only	1 oz.	8	1.6
ONION, WELCH, raw (USDA):			
Whole	1 lb. (weighed untrimmed)	100	19.2
Trimmed	4 oz.	39	7.4

ONION BOUILLON:

Food	Measure	Cals.	Carbs.
(Herb-Ox):			
Cube	1 cube	10	1.3
Packet	1 packet	14	2.1
MBT	1 packet	16	2.0
(Wyler's)	1 tsp.	10	1.0
ONION SALT (French's)	1 tsp.	6	1.0
ONION SOUP (See **SOUP,** Onion)			
OPOSSUM (USDA) roasted, meat only	4 oz.	251	0.0
ORANGE, fresh (USDA):			
California Navel:			
Whole	1 lb. (weighed with rind & seeds)	157	39.3
Whole	6.3-oz. orange (2⅖" dia.)	62	15.5
Sections	1 cup (8.5 oz.)	123	30.6
California Valencia:			
Whole	1 lb. (weighed with rind & seeds)	174	42.2
Fruit, including peel	6.3-oz. orange (2⅝" dia.)	72	27.9
Sections	1 cup (8.6 oz.)	123	29.9
Florida, all varieties:			
Whole	1 lb. (weighed with rind & seeds)	158	40.3
Whole	7.4-oz. orange (3" dia.)	73	18.6
Sections	1 cup (8.5 oz.)	113	28.9
ORANGE, MANDARIN (See **TANGERINE**)			
ORANGE-BANANA FRUIT DRINK, canned (Boku)	6 fl. oz.	90	22.0
ORANGE-CRANBERRY JUICE, canned (Santa Cruz Natural)	8 fl. oz.	125	29.0

Food	Measure	Cals.	Carbs.
ORANGE DRINK:			
Canned:			
(Ardmore Farms)	6 fl. oz.	86	20.9
(Borden) *Bama*	8.45-fl.-oz. container	120	29.0
(Hi-C)	6 fl. oz.	95	23.3
(Johanna Farms) *Ssips*	8.45-fl.-oz. container	130	32.0
(Lincoln)	6 fl. oz.	90	23.0
*Mix:			
Regular:			
(Funny Face)	8 fl. oz.	88	22.0
(Town House)	6 fl. oz.	90	22.0
Dietetic:			
Crystal Light	6 fl. oz.	4	.4
(Sunkist)	8 fl. oz.	8	2.0
ORANGE EXTRACT (Virginia Dare) 79% alcohol	1 tsp.	22	0.0
ORANGE FRUIT JUICE BLEND, canned (Mott's)	9.5 fl. oz.	139	34.0
ORANGE-GRAPEFRUIT JUICE:			
Canned:			
(Del Monte):			
Sweetened	6 fl. oz.	91	21.1
Unsweetened	6 fl. oz.	79	18.3
(Libby's) unsweetened	6 fl. oz.	80	19.0
*Frozen (Minute Maid) unsweetened	6 fl. oz.	76	19.1
ORANGE JUICE:			
Fresh (USDA):			
California Navel	½ cup (4.4 oz.)	60	14.0
California Valencia	½ cup (4.4 oz.)	58	13.0
Florida, early or midseason	½ cup (4.4 oz.)	50	11.4
Florida Temple	½ cup (4.4 oz.)	67	16.0
Florida Valencia	½ cup (4.4 oz.)	56	13.0
Canned, unsweetened:			
(USDA)	½ cup (4.4 oz.)	60	13.9
(Ardmore Farms)	6 fl. oz.	84	20.1
(Borden) *Sippin' Pak*	8.45-fl.-oz. container	110	26.0
(Johanna Farms)	6 fl. oz.	84	19.5
(Land O' Lakes)	6 fl. oz.	90	22.0

Food	Measure	Cals.	Carbs.
(Ocean Spray)	6 fl. oz.	90	18.0
(Town House)	6 fl. oz.	82	21.0
(Tree Top)	6 fl. oz.	90	22.0
Canned, sweetened:			
(USDA)	6 fl. oz.	66	15.4
(Del Monte)	6 fl. oz.	76	17.4
Chilled:			
(Citrus Hill):			
Regular	6 fl. oz.	90	20.0
Lite	6 fl. oz.	60	14.0
(Minute Maid):			
Regular	6 fl. oz.	91	21.9
Calcium fortified	6 fl. oz.	93	21.9
Reduced acid	6 fl. oz.	89	21.9
(Sunkist)	6 fl. oz.	76	17.7
*Dehydrated crystals (USDA)	½ cup (4.4 oz.)	57	13.4
*Frozen:			
(USDA)	½ cup (4.4 oz.)	56	13.3
(Citrus Hill):			
Regular	6 fl. oz.	90	20.0
Lite	6 fl. oz.	60	14.0
(Minute Maid) regular	6 fl. oz.	91	21.9
(Sunkist)	6 fl. oz.	84	20.1
ORANGE JUICE BAR, frozen			
(Sunkist)	3-fl.-oz. bar	72	17.6
ORANGE JULIUS JUICE DRINKS:			
Orange	16 fl. oz.	265	66.0
Pina Colada	16 fl. oz.	300	71.0
Raspberry Cream supreme	16 fl. oz.	510	76.0
Strawberry	16 fl. oz.	340	82.0
Tropical Cream supreme	16 fl. oz.	510	67.0
ORANGE-PEACH FRUIT DRINK, canned (Boku)	6 fl. oz.	90	22.0
ORANGE PEEL, CANDIED (USDA)	1 oz.	90	22.9
ORANGE-PINEAPPLE-BANANA JUICE, canned (Land O' Lakes)	6 fl. oz.	100	24.0
ORANGE-PINEAPPLE DRINK, canned (Lincoln)	6 fl. oz.	90	23.0

Food	Measure	Cals.	Carbs.
ORANGE-PINEAPPLE JUICE, canned (Land O' Lakes)	6 fl. oz.	90	23.0
ORANGEADE, canned (Snapple)	8 fl. oz.	120	31.0
OREGANO (French's)	1 tsp.	6	1.0
OVEN FRY (General Foods):			
Chicken:			
Extra crispy	4.2-oz. pkg.	461	82.4
Homestyle flour	3.2-oz. pkg.	339	60.5
Pork, _Shake & Bake,_ extra crispy	4.2-oz. pkg.	482	83.1
OYSTER:			
Raw (USDA):			
Eastern, meat only	19–31 small or 13–19 med.	158	8.2
Pacific & Western, meat only	6–9 small or 4–6 med. (8.5 oz.)	218	15.4
Canned (Bumble Bee) shelled, whole, solids & liq.	1 cup (8.5 oz.)	218	15.4
Fried (USDA) dipped in milk, egg & breadcrumbs	4 oz.	271	21.1
OYSTER STEW (USDA):			
Home recipe:			
1 part oysters to 1 part milk by volume	1 cup (8.5 oz., 6–8 oysters)	245	14.2
1 part oysters to 2 parts milk by volume	1 cup (8.5 oz.)	233	10.8
1 part oysters to 3 parts milk by volume	1 cup (8.5 oz.)	206	11.3
Frozen:			
Prepared with equal volume milk	1 cup (8.5 oz.)	201	14.2
Prepared with equal volume water	1 cup (8.5 oz.)	122	8.2

Food	Measure	Cals.	Carbs.

P

PAC-MAN, cereal

(General Mills)	1 cup (1 oz.)	110	25.0

PANCAKE, frozen:
(Pillsbury) microwave:

Regular	1 pancake	80	15.7
Blueberry	1 pancake	83	16.3
Buttermilk	1 pancake	87	17.0
Harvest wheat	1 pancake	80	19.0

(Swanson) *Great Starts*:

With bacon	4½-oz. meal	400	43.0
& sausage	6-oz. meal	460	52.0
Silver dollar & sausage	3¾-oz. meal	310	37.0
Whole wheat, & lite links	5½-oz. meal	350	39.0
(Weight Watchers) buttermilk, microwave	2½-oz. serving	140	22.0

*PANCAKE BATTER,
frozen (Aunt Jemima):

Plain	4" pancake	70	14.1
Blueberry or buttermilk	4" pancake	68	13.8
Buttermilk	4" pancake	68	14.2

*PANCAKE & WAFFLE MIX:
Plain:
(Aunt Jemima):

Original	4" pancake	73	8.7
Complete	4" pancake	80	15.7

Bisquick Shake 'N Pour:

Regular	4" pancake	87	16.0
Complete	1 waffle	140	25.5
Fastshake (Little Crow)	½ container	266	50.0

(Mrs. Butterworth's):

Regular	4" pancakes	73	13.4
Complete	4" pancake	63	12.3

(Pillsbury) *Hungry Jack*:

Extra Lights, regular	4" pancake	70	10.0
Panshakes	4" pancake	83	14.3

Food	Measure	Cals.	Carbs.
*Apple cinnamon, *Bisquick Shake 'N Pour*	4" pancake	90	16.3
Blueberry (Pillsbury) *Hungry Jack*	4" pancake	107	9.7
Buttermilk:			
(Betty Crocker):			
Regular	4" pancake	93	13.0
Complete	4" pancake	70	13.7
(Mrs. Butterworth's)	4" pancake	63	12.3
(Pillsbury) *Hungry Jack:*			
Regular	4" pancake	80	9.7
Complete	4" pancake	63	13.0
Dietetic:			
(Estee)	3" pancake	33	7.0
(Featherweight) low sodium	4" pancake	43	8.0

PANCAKE & WAFFLE SYRUP
(See **SYRUP**, Pancake & Waffle)

PANCREAS, raw (USDA):

Beef, lean only	4 oz.	160	0.0
Calf	4 oz.	183	0.0
Hog or hog sweetbread	4 oz.	274	0.0

PAPAW, fresh (USDA):

Whole	1 lb. (weighed with rind & seeds)	289	57.2
Flesh only	4 oz.	96	19.1

PAPAYA, fresh (USDA):

Whole	1 lb. (weighed with skin & seeds)	119	30.4
Cubed	1 cup (6.4 oz.)	71	18.2

PAPAYA JUICE, canned:

(HEW/FAO)	4 oz.	77	19.6
(Knudsen & Sons)	4 fl. oz.	50	12.0

PAPAYA NECTAR, canned:

(Knudsen & Sons)	8 fl. oz.	100	26.0
(Libby's)	6 fl. oz.	110	28.0

PAPRIKA, domestic (French's) | 1 tsp. | 7 | 1.1 |

PARSLEY, fresh (USDA):

Food	Measure	Cals.	Carbs.
Whole	½ lb.	100	19.3
Chopped	1 T. (4 grams)	2	.3
PARSLEY FLAKES, dehydrated (French's)	1 tsp. (1.1 grams)	4	.6
PARSNIP (USDA):			
Raw, whole	1 lb. (weighed unprepared)	293	67.5
Boiled, drained, cut in pieces	½ cup (3.7 oz.)	70	15.8
PASSION FRUIT, fresh (USDA):			
Whole	1 lb. (weighed with shell)	212	50.0
Pulp & seeds	4 oz.	102	24.0
PASSION FRUIT JUICE, fresh (HEW/FAO)	4 oz.	50	11.5
PASTA, DRY OR FRESH, RE-FRIGERATED (See also individual listings such as **MANI-COTTI,** etc.) Plain spaghetti products are essentially the same in calorie value and car-bohydrate content on the same weight basis. The longer the cooking, the more water is ab-sorbed and this affects the nu-tritive and caloric value:			
Dry (Pritikin) whole wheat	1 oz.	110	18.0
Cooked dry (USDA):			
8–10 minutes, "Al Dente"	1 cup (5.1 oz.)	216	43.9
14–20 minutes, tender	1 cup (4.9 oz.)	155	32.2
Agnoletti (Contadina) fresh, refrigerated	3 oz.	270	38.0
Angel hair:			
Dry:			
(Creamette) wheat	2 oz.	210	42.0
(De Boles):			
Jerusalem artichoke, tomato & basil	2 oz.	210	41.0
Wheat	2 oz.	210	40.0
(Di Giorno)	2 oz.	166	31.3
Fresh, refrigerated (Contadina)	2 oz.	173	30.0

Food	Measure	Cals.	Carbs.
Bow tie or farfelle, dry:			
(De Cecco)	2 oz.	210	41.0
(Ronzoni)	2 oz.	210	42.0
Fettuccini:			
Dry:			
(De Cecco) egg, home style	2 oz.	210	40.0
(Ronzoni) egg, extra long	2 oz.	220	42.0
Fresh, refrigerated			
(Contadina)	2 oz.	173	30.0
Fusilli, dry (De Cecco) spinach			
or wheat	2 oz.	210	41.0
Lasagna dry:			
(Buitoni) precooked	1 sheet	48	8.9
(De Boles):			
Jerusalem artichoke	2 oz.	210	41.0
Whole wheat	2 oz.	210	40.0
(Creamette) 100% semolina	2 oz.	210	41.0
(De Cecco) 100% semolina	2 oz.	210	41.0
(Health Valley) whole wheat:			
Regular	2 oz.	170	40.0
With spinach	2 oz.	170	40.0
(Mueller's)	2 oz.	210	42.0
Linguini:			
Dry:			
(De Boles) Jerusalem			
artichoke	2 oz.	210	41.0
(De Cecco) wheat	2 oz.	210	41.0
(Ronzoni) wheat	2 oz.	210	42.0
Fresh, refrigerated (Di			
Giorno)	2 oz.	167	31.3
Penne Rigati, dry (De Cecco)	2 oz.	210	41.0
Rigatoni:			
Dry (De Cecco)	2 oz.	210	41.0
Fresh, refrigerated			
(Contadina)	2 oz.	174	29.6
Spaghetti, dry:			
(De Boles):			
Corn, no wheat	2 oz.	210	45.0
Jerusalem artichoke, plain			
or spinach	2 oz.	210	41.0
Whole wheat	2 oz.	210	40.0
(Health Valley):			
Amaranth	2 oz.	170	40.0
Oat bran	2 oz.	120	23.0
Whole wheat:			
Plain	2 oz.	170	40.0
Spinach	2 oz.	170	40.0

Food	Measure	Cals.	Carbs.
Tortellini, fresh, refrigerated:			
(Contadina):			
Cheese	3 oz.	260	39.0
Chicken & herb	⅓ pkg.	240	37.0
Sausage, Italian	3 oz.	260	37.0
Spinach:			
With cheese	3 oz.	260	38.0
With chicken &			
prosicutto	4½ oz.	340	53.0
(Di Giorno):			
Cheese	⅓ pkg.	270	41.0
Mozzarella-garlic	⅓ pkg.	260	35.0
Tricolor, dry (De Boles)			
primavera	2 oz.	200	41.0
Vermicelli, dry (Ronzoni)			
wheat	2 oz.	210	42.0
Ziti rigati, dry (Ronzoni)	2 oz.	210	42.0
PASTA, FROZEN (See individual listings such as **AGNOLETTI; LASAGNE; MANICOTTI;** etc.)			
PASTA ACCENTS, frozen			
(Green Giant):			
Creamy cheddar	⅙ of 16-oz. pkg.	100	12.0
Garden herb	⅙ of 16-oz. pkg.	80	11.0
Garlic or primavera	⅙ of 16-oz. pkg.	110	13.0
PASTA DINNER OR ENTREE:			
Canned:			
(Chef Boyardee):			
ABC's & 1, 2, 3's:			
In cheese-flavor sauce	7½-oz. serving	180	35.0
With mini meatballs	7½-oz. serving	260	32.0
Dinosaurs:			
In cheese-flavor sauce	7½-oz. serving	180	35.0
With meatballs	7½-oz. serving	240	32.0
Elbow macaroni in beef			
sauce	7½-oz. serving	210	29.0
Rings & meatballs	7½-oz. serving	220	33.0
Shell macaroni:			
In meat sauce	7½-oz. serving	210	32.0
In mushroom sauce	7½-oz. serving	230	28.0
Tic Tac Toes:			
In cheese-flavor sauce	7½-oz. serving	170	36.0
With mini meatballs	7½-oz. serving	250	30.0

Food	Measure	Cals.	Carbs.
Turtles:			
With meatballs	7½-oz. serving	210	30.0
In sauce	7½-oz. serving	160	32.0
Zesty, microwave main			
meal	10½-oz. serving	290	40.0
(Franco-American):			
Circus O's, in tomato &			
meat sauce	7⅜-oz. serving	170	32.0
Sporty O's:			
With meatballs in			
tomato sauce	7⅜-oz. serving	210	25.0
In tomato & cheese			
sauce	7½-oz. serving	170	33.0
In tomato & cheese			
sauce	7⅜-oz. can	170	33.0
Frozen:			
(Birds Eye):			
Continental	5-oz. serving	164	16.0
Marinara	5-oz. serving	115	21.0
Primavera	5-oz. serving	204	21.7
(Celentano) & cheese,			
baked	6-oz. serving	280	41.0
(Green Giant):			
Dijon	9½-oz. meal	260	21.0
Florentine	9½-oz. meal	230	27.0
Marinara	6-oz. meal	180	29.0
Parmesan	5½-oz. meal	170	24.0
(Lean Cuisine)	10-oz. serving	240	38.0
(Stouffer's):			
Carbonara	9¾-oz. meal	620	34.0
Casino	9¼-oz. meal	300	44.0
Mexicali	10-oz. meal	490	36.0
Oriental	9⅞-oz. meal	300	25.0
Primavera	10⅝-oz. meal	270	13.0
(Ultra Slim Fast) primavera	12-oz. serving	340	50.0
(Weight Watchers):			
Angel hair, *Smart Ones*	8.5-oz. serving	120	8.0
Primavera	8½-oz. meal	260	22.0
Rigati	11-oz. meal	290	30.0
PASTA FESUL MIX,			
(Casbah)	1.6-oz. pkg	150	10.0
PASTA SALAD, frozen			
(Birds Eye) Italian style	5-oz. serving	170	22.2
PASTA SALAD MIX:			

Food	Measure	Cals.	Carbs.
*(Betty Crocker) *Suddenly Salad:*			
Creamy macaroni	½ cup	200	21.0
Pasta, classic	½ cup	160	23.0
Pasta primavera	½ cup	190	20.0
Tortellini Italiano	½ cup	160	21.0
(Kraft):			
Garden primaveria	⅙ of pkg.	170	21.0
Italian, light	⅙ of pkg.	120	22.0
PASTA SAUCE (See also **TOMATO SAUCE**):			
Fresh, refrigerated:			
Alfredo:			
(Contadina):			
Regular	4 oz.	360	6.7
Light	4 oz.	180	8.4
(Di Giorno)	4 oz.	400	4.0
Bolognese (Contadinaa)	4 oz.	123	6.4
Carbonara (Di Giorno)	4 oz.	400	6.0
Clam (Contadina):			
Red	4 oz.	64	8.0
White	4 oz.	193	8.7
Four cheese:			
(Contadina)	4 oz.	313	5.3
(Di Giorno)	4 oz.	340	6.0
Marinara (Di Giorno)	4 oz.	88	9.6
Pesto:			
(Contadina)	4 oz.	600	10.3
(Di Giorno)	4 oz.	591	8.7
Canned, regular pack:			
Alfredo (Progresso):			
Regular	½ cup	340	6.0
Seafood	½ cup	220	5.0
Beef (Prego Plus) ground sirloin, with onion	4-oz. serving	160	20.0
Bolognese (Progresso)	½ cup	150	12.0
Cheese, three (Prego)	4 oz.	100	17.0
Chunky (Hunt's)	4 oz.	50	12.0
Chunk style (Town House)	4 oz.	80	14.0
Clam (Progresso):			
Red	½ cup	70	7.0
White:			
Regular	½ cup	110	1.0
Authentic pasta sauce	½ cup	130	4.0
Garden combinations (Prego) extra chunky	4 oz.	80	14.0

Food	Measure	Cals.	Carbs.
Garden Style (Ragú) chunky:			
Extra tomato, garlic & onion, green pepper & mushroom or mushroom & onion	¼ of 15½-oz. jar	80	14.0
Italian garden combination or sweet green & red bell pepper	¼ of 15½-oz. jar	80	12.0
Home style (Ragú):			
Plain or mushroom	4-oz. serving	70	12.0
Meat flavored	4-oz. serving	80	12.0
Lobster (Progresso) rock	½ cup	120	11.0
Marinara:			
(Prince)	4-oz. serving	80	12.4
(Progresso):			
Regular	½ cup	90	9.0
Authentic pasta sauce	½ cup	110	10.0
(Ragú)	4-oz. serving	120	12.0
Meat or meat flavored:			
(Hunt's)	4-oz. serving	70	12.0
(Prego)	4-oz serving	140	20.0
(Progresso)	½ cup	110	13.0
(Town House)	4 oz.	80	11.0
Meatless or plain:			
(Prego)	4-oz. serving	130	20.0
(Progresso)	½ cup	110	13.0
(Town House)	4 oz.	80	11.0
Mushroom:			
(Hunt's)	4-oz. serving	70	12.0
(Prego):			
Regular	4-oz. serving	130	20.0
Extra Chunky:			
Extra spice	4 oz.	100	17.0
& green pepper	4 oz.	100	14.0
& onion	4 oz.	100	13.0
& tomato	4 oz.	110	14.0
(Progresso)	½ cup	110	13.0
(Ragú):			
Regular	4-oz. serving	90	9.0
Extra Thick & zesty	4-oz. serving	110	13.0
Onion & garlic (Prego)	4 oz.	110	16.0
Primavera (Progresso) creamy	½ cup	190	8.0
Romano (Progresso)	½ cup	220	7.0
Sausage & green pepper (Prego)	4-oz. serving	160	19.0
Seafood (Progresso):			
Regular	½ cup	110	12.0

Food	Measure	Cals.	Carbs.
Authentic pasta sauce	½ cup	190	5.0
Sicilian (Progresso)	½ cup	30	2.0
Tomato & basil (Prego)	4 oz.	100	18.0
Tomato & onion (Prego)			
extra chunky	4 oz.	110	14.0
Traditional (Hunt's)	4 oz.	70	12.0
Canned, dietetic pack:			
(Estee)	4 oz.	60	13.0
(Furman's) low sodium	4 oz.	83	12.7
(Healthy Choice):			
Garlic & herb	4 oz.	50	10.0
Garlic & onion	4 oz.	40	10.0
Italian vegetable, chunky	4 oz.	40	9.0
Mushroom	4 oz.	45	10.0
Traditional	4 oz.	40	9.0
(Prego) plain, no salt added	4 oz.	110	11.0
(Pritikin):			
Original	4 oz.	60	14.0
Garden, chunky	4 oz.	50	11.0
(Weight Watchers):			
Meat flavored	4 oz.	50	9.0
Mushroom flavored	4 oz.	40	9.0
PASTA SAUCE MIX:			
*(Estee) prepared with			
margarine & skim milk	4 oz.	60	9.0
*(Featherweight) prepared with			
margarine & skim milk	4 oz.	60	11.0
(French's):			
*Regular:			
Italian style	⅝ cup	100	15.0
With mushrooms	⅝ cup	100	13.0
Pasta Toss:			
Cheese & garlic	2 tsp.	25	2.0
Italian	2 tsp.	25	2.0
Pesto	2 tsp.	20	1.0
(Lawry's):			
Alfredo	1 pkg.	226	19.2
With imported mushrooms	1 pkg.	143	26.0
Rich & thick	1 pkg.	147	28.1
*PASTA & SAUCE, MIX:			
(Lipton):			
Cheddar broccoli with fusilli	¼ of pkg.	135	23.9
Cheese supreme	¼ of pkg.	139	23.8
Garlic, creamy	¼ of pkg.	144	25.3
Mushroom & chicken	¼ of pkg.	124	23.4

Food	Measure	Cals.	Carbs.
Mushroom, creamy	¼ of pkg.	143	24.8
Oriental with fusilli	¼ of pkg.	130	25.5
Tomato, herb	¼ of pkg.	130	26.0
(*Pasta Roni*):			
Fettucini with cheese sauce	½ cup (¼ pkg.)	235	24.0
Penne with herb & butter sauce	2-oz. serving	430	39.0
Shells with white cheddar sauce	2½-oz. serving	390	DNA
PASTINA, DRY (USDA):			
Carrot	1 oz.	105	21.5
Egg	1 oz.	109	20.4
Spinach	1 oz.	104	21.2
PASTRAMI:			
(Boar's Head):			
Brisket, 1st cut	1 oz.	45	1.0
Round, extra lean	1 oz.	35	.5
(Butterball) turkey, *Slice 'n Serve*	1 oz.	35	5.0
(Carl Buddig) smoked, lean	1 oz.	40	1.0
(Healthy Deli) round	1 oz.	34	.8
(Hebrew National) 1st cut	1 oz.	44	<1.0
(Louis Rich) turkey:			
Deli Thin, 96% fat free	1 oz.	10	<1.0
Round, 96% fat free	1 oz.	35	<1.0
Thin sliced	1 oz.	11	.1
(Oscar Mayer)	.6-oz. slice	16	.1
PASTRY, FILO (See **FILO PASTRY**)			
PASTRY SHEET, PUFF, frozen (Pepperidge Farm)	1 sheet	1040	88.0
PASTRY SHELL, frozen:			
(Pepperidge Farm) regular	1 shell (1.7 oz.)	210	16.0
(Pet-Ritz)	3" shell	150	12.0
PÂTÉ:			
De foie gras (USDA)	1 T. (.5 oz.)	69	.7
Liver:			
(Hormel)	1 T.	35	.3
(Sell's)	½ of 4.8-oz. can	223	2.7
PEA, CHOWDER, frozen:			
(Birds Eye)	⅓ of 16-oz. pkg.	130	22.6

Food	Measure	Cals.	Carb.
(McKenzie)	3-oz. serving	130	23.0
(Southland)	⅕ of 16-oz. pkg.	130	23.0

PEA, GREEN:
Raw (USDA):

In pod	1 lb. (weighed in pod)	145	24.8
Shelled	1 lb.	381	65.3
Shelled	½ cup (2.4 oz.)	58	9.9
Boiled (USDA) drained	½ cup (2.9 oz.)	58	9.9

Canned, regular pack:
(USDA):
  Alaska, early or June:

Solids & liq.	½ cup (4.4 oz.)	82	15.5
Solids only	½ cup (3 oz.)	76	14.4

  Sweet:

Solids & liq.	½ cup (4.4 oz.)	71	12.9
Solids only	½ cup (3 oz.)	69	12.9
Drained liquid	4 oz.	25	4.9
(Green Giant)	½ cup	50	12.0
(Larsen) Freshlike	½ cup (4.4 oz.)	50	10.0

(Pathmark):

Little Gem	½ cup	70	12.0
No Frills	½ cup	60	12.5
(Town House)	½ cup	70	14.0

Canned, dietetic pack:
(USDA):
  Alaska, early or June:

Solids & liq.	4 oz.	62	11.1
Solids only	4 oz.	88	16.2

  Sweet:

Solids & liq.	4 oz.	53	9.5
Solids only	4 oz.	82	14.7
(Del Monte) no salt added, sweet, solids & liq.	½ cup (4.3 oz.)	60	11.0
(Diet Delight) solids & liq.	½ cup (4.3 oz.)	50	8.0
(Larsen) Fresh-Lite, no salt added	½ cup (4.4 oz.)	50	10.0
(Pathmark) no salt added	½ cup	50	10.0

Frozen:

(Bel-Air)	3.3 oz.	80	13.0

(Birds Eye):

Regular	⅓ of 10-oz. pkg.	78	13.3
In butter sauce	⅓ of 10-oz. pkg.	85	12.6
In cream sauce	⅓ of 8-oz. pkg.	84	14.3
Tiny, tender, deluxe	⅓ of 10-oz. pkg.	64	10.7

Food	Measure	Cals.	Carbs.
(Frosty Acres):			
Regular	3.3-oz. serving	80	13.0
Tiny	3.3-oz. serving	60	11.0
(Green Giant):			
Early June:			
Butter sauce, One			
Serving	4½-oz. pkg.	90	16.0
Harvest Fresh	½ cup (3 oz.)	60	13.0
Polybag	½ cup (2.7 oz.)	50	11.0
Sweet:			
Regular, *Harvest Fresh*			
or polybag	½ cup	50	11.0
Butter sauce	½ cup (4 oz.)	80	14.0
(Le Sueur) early, in			
butter sauce	⅓ of 10-oz. pkg.	67	11.7
(McKenzie):			
Regular	3.3 oz.	80	13.0
Tiny	3.3 oz.	60	10.0
PEA, MATURE SEED, dry			
(USDA):			
Whole	1 lb.	1542	272.5
Whole	1 cup	680	120.6
Split	1 lb.	1579	284.4
Split	1 cup (7.2 oz.)	706	127.3
Cooked, split, drained solids	½ cup (3.4 oz.)	112	20.2
PEA & CARROT:			
Canned, regular pack,			
solids & liq.:			
(Larsen) *Freshlike*	½ cup (4.6 oz.)	50	12.0
(S&W)	½ cup	50	9.0
(Veg-All)	½ cup	50	12.0
Canned, dietetic pack,			
solids & liq.:			
(Diet Delight)	½ cup (4.3 oz.)	40	6.0
(Larsen) *Freshlike,* no salt			
added	½ cup (4.6 oz.)	50	12.0
(Pathmark)	½ cup	60	18.0
Frozen:			
(Bel-Air)	3.3 oz.	60	11.0
(Birds Eye)	⅓ of 10-oz. pkg.	61	11.2
(Frosty Acres)	3.3-oz. serving	60	11.0
(McKenzie)	3.3-oz. serving	60	11.0
PEA & ONION:			
Canned (Larsen)	½ cup	60	12.0

Food	Measure	Cals.	Carbs.
Frozen (Birds Eye)	⅓ of 10-oz. pkg.	67	11.7
PEA POD:			
Raw (USDA) edible podded or Chinese	1 lb. (weighed untrimmed)	228	51.7
Boiled (USDA) drained	4 oz.	49	10.8
Frozen (La Choy)	6-oz. pkg.	70	12.0
PEA PUREE, canned (Larsen) no salt added	½ cup	50	10.0
PEACH:			
Fresh (USDA):			
Whole, without skin	1 lb. (weighed unpeeled)	150	38.3
Whole	4-oz. peach (2" dia.)	38	9.6
Diced	½ cup (4.7 oz.)	51	12.9
Sliced	½ cup (3 oz.)	31	8.2
Canned, regular pack, solids & liq.:			
(USDA):			
Extra heavy syrup	4 oz.	110	28.5
Heavy syrup	2 med. halves & 2 T. syrup (4.1 oz.)	91	23.5
Juice pack	4 oz.	51	13.2
Light syrup	4 oz.	66	17.1
(Del Monte):			
Cling:			
Halves or slices	½ cup (4 oz.)	80	22.0
Spiced	3½ oz.	80	20.0
Freestone	½ cup (4 oz.)	90	23.0
(Hunt's) halves or slices	4 oz.	80	23.0
(Town House)	½ cup	100	25.0
Canned, dietetic pack, solids & liq.:			
(Country Pure) halves or pieces	½ cup	50	14.0
(Del Monte) Lite:			
Cling	½ cup (4 oz.)	50	13.0
Freestone	½ cup (4 oz.)	60	13.0
(Diet Delight) Cling:			
Juice pack	½ cup (4.4 oz.)	50	14.0
Water pack	½ cup (4.3 oz.)	30	2.0
Dehydrated (USDA):			
Uncooked	1 oz.	96	24.9

Food	Measure	Cals.	Carbs.
Cooked, with added sugar, solids & liq.	½ cup (5.4 oz.)	184	47.6
Dried (USDA):			
Uncooked	½ cup	231	60.1
Cooked:			
Unsweetened	½ cup	111	28.9
Sweetened	½ cup (5.4 oz.)	181	46.8
Frozen (Birds Eye) quick thaw	5-oz. serving	141	34.1
PEACH, STRAINED, canned (Larsen) no salt added	½ cup	65	17.0
PEACH BUTTER (Smucker's)	1 T. (.7 oz.)	45	12.0
PEACH DRINK, canned (Hi-C)	6 fl. oz.	101	24.8
PEACH JUICE, canned (Smucker's)	8 fl. oz.	120	30.0
PEACH LIQUEUR (DeKupyer)	1 fl. oz.	82	8.3
PEACH NECTAR, canned (Ardmore Farms)	6 fl. oz.	90	23.4
PEACH PARFAIT, frozen (Pepperidge Farm) dessert light	4½-oz. serving	150	24.0
PEACH PRESERVE OR JAM:			
Sweetened (Smucker's)	1 T. (.7 oz.)	54	12.0
Dietetic (Dia-Mel)	1 T.	6	0.0
PEANUT:			
Raw (USDA):			
In shell	1 lb. (weighed in shell)	1868	61.6
With skins	1 oz.	160	5.3
Without skins	1 oz.	161	5.0
Roasted:			
(USDA):			
Whole	1 lb. (weighed in shell)	1769	62.6
Chopped	½ cup	404	13.0
Halves	½ cup	421	13.5
(Adams):			
Regular	1 oz.	170	5.0
Butter toffee	1 oz.	140	20.0

Food	Measure	Cals.	Carbs.
(Beer Nuts)	1 oz.	180	7.0
(Eagle):			
Fancy Virginia	1 oz.	180	6.0
Honey Roast	1 oz.	170	7.0
Lightly salted	1 oz.	170	5.0
(Fisher):			
In shell, salted	1 oz.	105	3.7
Shelled:			
Dry roasted, salted or unsalted	1 oz.	160	6.0
Oil roasted, salted	1 oz.	166	5.3
(Party Pride)	1 oz.	170	5.0
(Planters):			
Dry roasted	1 oz. (jar)	160	6.0
Oil roasted	¾-oz. bag	170	5.0
(Tom's):			
In shell	1 oz.	120	3.4
Shelled:			
Dry roasted	1 oz.	160	5.0
Hot flavored	1 oz.	170	4.0
Redskin or toasted	1 oz.	170	5.0
Spanish, roasted:			
(Adams)	1 oz.	170	5.0
(Frito-Lay's)	1 oz.	168	6.6
(Planters):			
Dry roasted	1 oz. (jar)	175	3.4
Oil roasted	1 oz. (can)	182	3.4
PEANUT BUTTER:			
Regular:			
(Algood) *Cap'n Kid*	1 T.	85	3.0
(Bama)	1 T.	100	3.0
(Estee) low sodium	1 T.	100	3.0
(Home Brands)	1 T.	105	2.5
Jif, creamy or extra crunchy	1 T.	93	2.7
(Peter Pan):			
Crunchy	1 T. (.6 oz.)	95	2.9
Smooth	1 T. (.6 oz.)	95	2.5
(Skippy) creamy or super chunk	1 T.	95	2.1
(Smucker's) Goober Grape	1 T.	90	9.0
Dietetic:			
(Adams) low sodium	1 T. (.6 oz.)	95	2.5
(Algood)	1 T.	95	3.0
(Estee)	1 T.	100	3.0
(Home Brands):			

Food	Measure	Cals.	Carbs.
Lightly salted or unsalted	1 T.	105	2.5
No sugar added	1 T.	90	3.0
(Smucker's) no salt added	1 T.	100	3.0
PEANUT BUTTER BOPPERS			
(General Mills):			
Cookie crunch or fudge chip	1 bar	170	15.0
Fudge graham	1 bar	160	15.0
Honey crisp	1 bar	160	14.0
Peanut crunch	1 bar	170	13.0
PEANUT BUTTER MORSELS:			
(Nestlé)	1 oz.	160	12.0
(Reese's)	1 oz.	153	21.3
PEAR:			
Fresh (USDA):			
Whole	1 lb. (weighed with stems & core)	252	63.2
Whole	6.4-oz. pear (3" 2½" dia.)	101	25.4
Quartered	1 cup (6.8 oz.)	117	29.4
Slices	½ cup (2.9 oz.)	50	12.5
Canned, regular pack, solids & liq.:			
(USDA):			
Extra heavy syrup	4 oz.	104	26.8
Heavy syrup	½ cup	87	22.3
Juice pack	4 oz.	52	13.4
Light syrup	4 oz.	69	17.7
(Hunt's) halves	4 oz.	90	22.0
(Town House) Bartlett, halves or sliced	½ cup	95	24.5
(Libby's) halves, heavy syrup	½ cup (4.5 oz.)	102	25.1
Canned, dietetic pack, solids & liq.:			
(Country Pure) halves or slices	½ cup	60	15.0
(Diet Delight):			
Juice pack	½ cup	60	16.0
Water pack	½ cup	35	9.0
(Libby's) water pack	½ cup	60	15.0
(S&W) *Nutradiet*, halves, quarters or slices, white or blue label	½ cup	35	10.0

Food	Measure	Cals.	Carbs.
Dried (Sun-Maid)	½ cup (3.5 oz.)	260	70.0
PEAR, CANDIED (USDA)	1 oz.	86	21.5
PEAR, STRAINED, canned (Larsen) no salt added	½ cup	65	17.0
PEAR-APPLE JUICE (Tree Top) canned or frozen	6 fl. oz.	90	23.0
PEAR-GRAPE JUICE (Tree Top) canned or frozen	6 fl. oz.	100	26.0
PEAR JUICE, canned:			
(Knudsen & Sons)	8 fl. oz.	110	28.0
(Santa Cruz Natural)	8 fl. oz.	135	32.0
PEAR NECTAR, canned:			
(Ardmore Farms)	6 fl. oz.	96	24.6
(Libby's)	6 fl. oz.	100	25.0
PEAR-PASSION FRUIT NECTAR, canned (Libby's)	6 fl. oz.	60	14.0
PEBBLES, cereal (Post):			
Cocoa	⅞ cup (1 oz.)	117	24.4
Fruity	⅞ cup (1 oz.)	116	24.5
PECAN:			
In shell (USDA)	1 lb. (weighed in shell)	1652	35.1
Shelled (USDA):			
Whole	1 lb.	3116	66.2
Chopped	½ cup (1.8 oz.)	357	7.6
Chopped	1 T. (7 grams)	48	1.0
Halves	12—14 halves (.5 oz.)	96	2.0
Halves	½ cup (1.9 oz.)	371	7.9
Oil dipped (Fisher) salted	¼ cup	410	8.9
Roasted, dry:			
(Fisher) salted	1 oz.	170	3.0
(Flavor House)	1 oz.	195	4.1
(Planters)	1 oz.	206	3.5

PENNE RIGATI, dry (See
**PASTA, DRY OR FRESH,
REFRIGERATED**)

Food	Measure	Cals.	Carbs.
PEPPER, BANANA (Vlasic)			
hot rings	1 oz.	4	1.0
PEPPER, BLACK (French's):			
Regular	1 tsp. (2.3 grams)	9	1.5
Seasoned	1 tsp.	8	1.0
PEPPER, CHERRY (Vlasic)			
mild	1 oz.	8	2.0
PEPPER, CHILI:			
Raw, green (USDA) without seeds	4 oz.	42	10.3
Canned:			
(Goya)	1 piece	5	1.0
(La Victoria):			
Marinated	1 T.	4	1.0
Nacho	1 T.	2	1.0
(Old El Paso) green, chopped or whole	1 oz.	7	1.4
(Ortega):			
Green, diced, strips or whole	1 oz.	10	2.6
Jalapeño, diced or whole	1 oz.	9	1.7
(Vlasic) Jalapeño	1 oz.	8	2.0
PEPPER, STUFFED:			
Home recipe (USDA) with beef & crumbs	2¾" × 2½" pepper with 1⅛ cups stuffing	314	31.1
Frozen:			
(Celentano) red, with beef, in sauce	12½-oz. pkg.	290	21.0
(Stouffer's) green, with beef in tomato sauce	7¾-oz. serving	180	19.0
PEPPER, SWEET:			
Raw (USDA):			
Green:			
Whole	1 lb. (weighed untrimmed)	82	17.9
Without stem & seeds	1 med. pepper (2.6 oz.)	13	2.9
Chopped	½ cup (2.6 oz.)	16	3.6
Slices	½ cup (1.4 oz.)	9	2.0

Food	Measure	Cals.	Carbs.
Red:			
Whole	1 lb. (weighed untrimmed)	112	25.8
Without stem & seeds	1 med. pepper (2.2 oz.)	19	2.4
Boiled, green, without salt, drained	1 med. pepper (2.6 oz.)	13	2.8
Frozen:			
(Bel-Air) green, diced	1 oz.	6	1.0
(Frosty Acres):			
Green	1-oz. serving	6	1.0
Red & green	2-oz. serving	15	2.0
(Larsen) green	1 oz.	6	1.0
(Southland):			
Green, diced	2-oz. serving	10	2.0
Red & green, cut	2-oz. serving	15	2.0
PEPPER & ONION, frozen (Southland)	2-oz. serving	15	2.0
PEPPER STEAK, frozen:			
(Armour):			
Classic Lite, beef	11¼-oz. meal	220	29.0
Dining Lite, oriental	9-oz. meal	260	33.0
(Budget Gourmet) with rice	10-oz. meal	300	39.0
(Healthy Choice) beef:			
Dinner	11-oz. dinner	290	35.0
Entree	9½-oz. entree	250	36.0
(La Choy) *Fresh & Lite*, with rice & vegetables	10-oz. meal	280	33.1
(Le Menu)	11½-oz. meal	370	36.0
(Stouffer's)	10½-oz. pkg.	330	36.0
*PEPPER STEAK MIX (Chun King) stir fry	6-oz. serving	249	8.6
PEPPERONI:			
(Eckrich)	1-oz. serving	135	1.0
(Hormel):			
Regular, chub, *Rosa* or *Rosa Grande*	1 oz.	140	0.0
Canned bits	1 T.	35	0.0
Leoni Brand	1 oz.	130	0.0
Packaged, sliced	1 slice	40	0.0

Food	Measure	Cals.	Carbs.
PERCH, OCEAN:			
Raw Atlantic, (USDA):			
Whole	1 lb. (weighed whole)	124	0.0
Meat only	4 oz.	108	0.0
Pacific, raw, whole	1 lb. (weighed whole)	116	0.0
Frozen:			
(Captain's Choice)	3-oz. fillet	103	0.0
(Frionor) *Norway Gourmet*	4-oz. piece	120	0.0
(Gorton's) *Fishmarket Fresh*	4 oz.	140	2.0
(Van de Kamp's):			
Regular batter, dipped, french fried	2-oz. piece	135	10.0
Light & crispy	2-oz. piece	170	10.0
Today's Catch	4 oz.	110	0.0
PERKINS RESTAURANT:			
Broccoli, raw	4-oz. serving	31	5.9
Carrots, raw	4-oz. serving	49	11.5
Cauliflower, raw	4-oz. serving	27	5.6
Chicken dinner, lemon pepper, with rice pilaf, broccoli & salad	1 serving	620	59.6
Fruit cup	4½-oz. serving	48	11.9
Margarine	1 T.	60	0.0
Muffin:			
Regular:			
Plain	1 muffin	586	81.0
Apple	1 muffin	543	76.0
Banana nut	1 muffin	586	75.0
Blueberry	1 muffin	506	71.0
Bran	1 muffin	478	83.0
Carrot	1 muffin	560	88.0
Chocolate chocolate chip	1 muffin	546	73.0
Corn	1 muffin	683	121.0
Cranberry nut	1 muffin	558	71.0
Oat bran	1 muffin	513	87.0
Dietetic, plain, 98% fat free	1 muffin	495	111.0
Mushroom, raw	4-oz. serving	29	5.3
Omelet:			
Country Club:			
Plain	1 serving	932	5.8
With hash browns	1 serving	1033	22.5
Deli ham & cheese:			
Plain	1 serving	962	8.2
With hash browns	1 serving	1063	24.9

Food	Measure	Cals.	Carbs.
Denver, with fruit cup	1 serving	235	22.3
Everything:			
Plain	1 serving	697	8.6
With hash browns	1 serving	798	25.3
Granny's country:			
Plain	1 serving	941	6.9
With hash browns	1 serving	1245	56.9
Ham & cheese:			
Plain	1 serving	644	2.6
With hash browns	1 serving	745	19.3
Mushroom & cheese:			
Plain	1 serving	687	4.9
With hash browns	1 serving	788	33.5
Seafood, with fruit cup	1 serving	271	27.5
Pancakes:			
Buttermilk	1 pancake	147	23.2
Harvest Grain:			
Regular with 1½ oz. low-calorie syrup	5 pancakes	473	93.0
Short stack	1 pancake	89	18.6
Pie:			
Apple, regular	1 slice	521	72.0
Cherry, regular	1 slice	571	84.0
Coconut cream	1 slice	437	56.0
French silk	1 slice	551	59.0
Lemon meringue	1 slice	395	63.0
Peanut butter brownie	1 slice	455	44.0
Pecan	1 slice	669	106.0
Potatoes, hash browns	3-oz. serving	101	16.7
Salad:			
Chef, mini	1 serving	214	6.8
Dinner, Lite & Healthy	1 serving	103	14.7
Syrup, low calorie	1½-oz. serving	26	6.6
Toast, with .5-oz. margarine & ¾-oz. grape jelly	1 slice	219	27.7
Vegetable sandwich, pita, stir fry:			
Plain	1 serving	308	41.1
With coleslaw	1 serving	441	53.9
With coleslaw & pasta salaad	1 serving	626	62.9
With pasta salad	1 serving	493	50.1
PERNOD (Julius Wile)	1 fl. oz.	79	1.1
PERSIMMON (USDA):			
Japanese or Kaki, fresh:			
With seeds	4.4-oz. piece	79	20.1
Seedless	4.4-oz. piece	81	20.7

Food	Measure	Cals.	Carbs.
Native, fresh, flesh only	4-oz. serving	144	38.0
PETIT SIRAH WINE			
(Louis M. Martini):			
Regular, 12½% alcohol	3 fl. oz.	61	.2
White, 12.3% alcohol	3 fl. oz.	54	Tr.
PHEASANT, raw (USDA) meat only	4-oz. serving	184	0.0
PICKLE:			
Cucumber, fresh or bread & butter			
(USDA)	3 slices (.7 oz.)	15	3.8
(Fannings)	1.2-oz. serving	17	3.9
(Featherweight) low sodium	1-oz. pickle	12	3.0
(Vlasic):			
Chips	1-oz. serving	30	7.0
Chunks	1-oz. serving	25	6.0
Stix	1-oz. serving	18	5.0
Dill:			
(USDA)	4.8-oz. pickle	15	3.0
(Claussen) halves	2 oz.	7	1.3
(Featherweight) low sodium, whole kosher	1-oz. serving	4	1.0
(Smucker's):			
Candied sticks	4" piece (.8 oz.)	45	11.0
Hamburger, sliced	1 slice (.13 oz.)	Tr.	0.0
Polish, whole	3½" pickle (1.8 oz.)	8	1.0
Spears	3½" spear (1.4 oz.)	6	1.0
(Vlasic):			
No garlic	1-oz. serving	4	1.0
Original	1-oz. serving	2	1.0
Hamburger (Vlasic) chips	1-oz. serving	2	1.0
Hot & spicy (Vlasic) garden mix	1-oz. serving	4	1.0
Kosher dill:			
(Featherweight) low sodium	1-oz. serving	4	1.0
(Smucker's):			
Baby	2¾"-long pickle	4	.5
Slices	1 slice (.1 oz.)	Tr.	0.0
Whole	3½"-long pickle (.5 oz.)	8	1.0
(Vlasic):			
Deli	1-oz. serving	4	1.0

Food	Measure	Cals.	Carbs.
Spear, regular or half-the-salt	1-oz. serving	4	1.0
Sour (USDA) cucumber	1 oz.	3	.6
Sweet:			
(Nalley's) *Nubbins*	1-oz. serving	28	7.9
(Smucker's):			
Candied mix	1 piece (.3 oz.)	14	3.3
Gherkins	2" long pickle (9 grams)	15	3.5
Slices	1 slice (.2 oz.)	11	2.3
Whole	2½" long pickle	18	4.0
(Vlasic) butter chips, half-the-salt	1-oz. serving	30	7.0
Sweet & sour (Claussen) slices	1 slice	3	.8
PICKLING SPICE			
(Tone's)	1 tsp.	10	1.0
PIE:			
Regular, non-frozen:			
Apple:			
Home recipe (USDA), 2-crust	⅙ of 9" pie	404	60.2
(Dolly Madison)	4½-oz. pie	490	59.0
(Entenmann's) homestyle	2.1-oz. serving	140	21.0
(Hostess) regular or French	1 piece	430	60.0
(Tastykake):			
Regular	1 piece	290	45.0
French	1 piece	360	61.0
Banana, home recipe (USDA), cream or custard, 1-crust	⅙ of 9" pie	336	46.7
Blackberry, home recipe (USDA) 2 crust	⅙ of 9" pie	384	54.4
Blueberry:			
Home recipe (USDA), 2-crust	⅙ of 9" pie	382	55.1
(Dolly Madison)	4½-oz. pie	430	56.0
(Hostess)	1 piece	420	59.0
(Tastykake)	1 piece	320	54.0
Boston cream (USDA), home recipe, 1-crust	1/12 of 8" pie	208	34.4
Butterscotch (USDA), home recipe, 1-crust	⅙ of 9" pie	406	58.2

Food	Measure	Cals.	Carbs.
Cherry:			
Home recipe (USDA), 2-crust	⅙ of 9" pie	412	60.7
(Dolly Madison):			
Regular	4½-oz. pie	470	53.0
N' cream	4½-oz. pie	440	63.0
(Hostess)	1 piece	460	65.0
Chocolate (Dolly Madison):			
Regular	4½-oz. pie	560	74.0
Pudding	4½-oz. pie	500	53.0
Chocolate chiffon (USDA) home recipe, made with vegetable shortening, 1-crust	⅙ of 9" pie	459	61.2
Chocolate meringue (USDA), home recipe, made with vegetable shortening, 1-crust	⅙ of 9" pie	353	46.9
Coconut custard:			
Home recipe (USDA) 1-crust	⅙ of 9" pie	357	37.8
(Entenmann's)	1.8-oz. serving	140	16.0
Lemon (Dolly Madison)	4½-oz. pie	460	60.0
Lemon meringue (USDA) 1-crust	⅙ of 9" pie	357	52.8
Mince, home recipe, (USDA) 2-crust	⅙ of 9" pie	428	65.1
Peach (Dolly Madison)	4½-oz. pie	460	54.0
Pecan, home recipe (USDA) 1-crust, made with lard or vegetable shortening	⅙ of 9" pie	577	70.8
Pineapple, home recipe (USDA) 1-crust, made with lard or vegetable shortening	⅙ of 9" pie	344	48.8
Pineapple custard, home recipe (USDA) made with lard or vegetable shortening	⅙ of 9" pie (5.4 oz.)	400	60.2
Pumpkin, home recipe (USDA) 2-crust, made with lard or vegetable shortening	⅙ of 9" pie (5.4 oz.)	321	37.2
Raisin, home recipe (USDA) 2-crust, made with lard or vegetable shortening	⅙ of 9" pie (5.6 oz.)	427	67.9

Food	Measure	Cals.	Carbs.
Rhubarb, home recipe (USDA) 2-crust, made with lard or vegetable shortening	⅙ of 9" pie (5.6 oz.)	400	60.4
Strawberry, home recipe (USDA) made with lard or vegetable shortening—1-crust	⅙ of 9" pie (5.6 oz.)	313	48.8
Vanilla (Dolly Madison) pudding	4½-oz. pie	500	52.0
Frozen:			
Apple:			
(Banquet) family size	⅙ of 20-oz. pie	250	37.0
(Mrs. Smith's):			
Regular:			
Plain	⅛ of 8" pie (3¼ oz.)	220	31.0
Plain	⅛ of 10" pie (5¾ oz.)	390	55.0
Dutch	⅛ of 8" pie (3¼ oz.)	250	37.0
Dutch	⅛ of 10" pie (5¾ oz.)	430	64.0
Natural Juice:			
Plain	⅛ of 9" pie (4.6 oz.)	370	45.0
Dutch	⅛ of 9" pie (5.11 oz.)	380	56.0
Pie In Minutes	⅛ of 25-oz. pie	210	29.0
(Pet-Ritz)	⅙ of 26-oz. pie	330	53.0
(Sara Lee):			
Free & Light, streusel	⅛ of pie	170	36.0
Homestyle:			
Regular	⅒ of a 9" pie	280	42.0
Regular, high	⅒ of a 10" pie	400	46.0
Dutch	⅒ of a 9" pie	300	45.0
(Weight Watchers)	3½-oz. serving	200	39.0
Banana cream:			
(Banquet)	⅙ of 14-oz. pie	180	21.0
(Pet-Ritz)	⅙ of 14-oz. pie	170	22.0
Blackberry (Banquet)	⅙ of 20-oz. pie	270	40.0
Blueberry:			
(Banquet)	⅙ of 20-oz. pie	270	40.0
(Mrs. Smith's):			
Regular	⅛ of 8" pie (3¼ oz.)	210	30.0

Food	Measure	Cals.	Carbs.
Natural Juice	⅛ of 9" pie (4.6 oz.)	350	49.0
Pie In Minutes	⅛ of 26-oz. pie	220	32.0
(Pet-Ritz)	⅙ of 26-oz. pie	370	50.0
Boston cream (Weight Watchers)	3-oz. pie	160	34.0
Cherry:			
(Banquet) family size	⅙ of 24-oz. pie	250	36.0
(Mrs. Smith's)			
Regular:			
Small	⅛ of 26-oz. pie	220	31.0
Large	⅛ of 46-oz. pie	390	55.0
Natural Juice	⅛ of 36.8-oz. pie	350	49.0
Pie In Minutes	⅛ of 25-oz. pie	220	32.0
(Pet-Ritz)	⅙ of 26-oz. pie	300	48.0
(Sara Lee):			
Free & Light	⅒ of a 9" pie	160	34.0
Homestyle	⅒ of a 9" pie	270	37.0
Chocolate cream:			
(Banquet)	⅙ of 14-oz. pie	185	24.0
(Pet-Ritz)	⅙ of 14-oz. pie	190	27.0
Chocolate mocha (Weight Watchers) *Sweet Celebrations*	2¾-oz. serving	160	23.0
Coconut cream:			
(Banquet)	⅙ of 14-oz. pie	187	22.0
(Pet-Ritz)	⅙ of 14-oz. pie	190	27.0
Coconut custard (Mrs. Smith's):			
8" pie	⅛ of 25-oz. pie	180	22.0
10" pie	⅛ of 44-oz. pie	280	36.0
Custard, egg (Pet-Ritz)	⅙ of 24-oz. pie	200	28.0
Lemon cream:			
(Banquet)	⅙ of 14-oz. pie	173	23.0
(Pet-Ritz)	⅙ of 14-oz. pie	190	26.0
Lemon meringue (Mrs. Smith's)	⅛ of 8" pie (3 oz.)	210	38.0
Mincement:			
(Banquet) Family size	⅙ of 20-oz. pie	260	38.0
(Mrs. Smith's):			
Small	⅛ of 26-oz. pie	220	30.0
Large	⅛ of 46-oz. pie	430	64.0
(Pet-Ritz)	⅙ of 26-oz. pie	280	48.0
(Sara Lee) homestyle	⅒ of a 9" pie	300	43.0
Mud, Mississippi (Pepperidge Farm)	2¼-oz. serving	310	23.0
Neapolitan (Pet-Ritz)	⅙ of 14-oz. pie	180	17.0

Food	Measure	Cals.	Carbs.
Peach:			
(Banquet) Family size	⅙ of 20-oz. pie	245	35.0
(Mrs. Smith's):			
Regular:			
Small	⅛ of 26-oz. pie	200	28.0
Large	⅛ of 46-oz. pie	360	49.0
Natural juice	⅛ of 36.8-oz. pie	330	46.0
Pie In Minutes	⅛ of 25-oz. pie	210	29.0
(Pet-Ritz)	⅙ of 26-oz. pie	320	51.0
(Sara Lee) homestyle	⅒ of a 9" pie	280	41.0
Pecan (Mrs. Smith's):			
Regular	⅛ of 24-oz. pie	330	51.0
Pie In Minutes	⅛ of 24-oz. pie	330	51.0
Pumpkin:			
(Banquet)	⅙ of 20-oz. pie	200	29.0
(Mrs. Smith's) *Pie In Minutes*	⅛ of 25-oz. pie	190	30.0
(Sara Lee) homestyle	⅒ of a 9" pie	240	34.0
Pumpkin custard:			
(Mrs. Smith's):			
Small	⅛ of 26-oz. pie	180	28.0
Large	⅛ of 46-oz. pie	300	48.0
(Pet-Ritz)	⅙ of 26-oz. pie	250	39.0
Raspberry (Mrs. Smith's) red	⅛ of 26-oz. pie	220	32.0
Strawberry cream:			
(Banquet)	⅙ of 14-oz. pie	170	22.0
(Pet-Ritz)	⅙ of 14-oz. pie	170	20.0
Strawberry rhubarb (Mrs. Smith's)	⅛ of 26-oz. pie	230	33.0
PIECRUST:			
Home recipe (USDA), 9" pie, baked, made with vegetable shortening	1 crust	900	78.8
Frozen:			
(Empire Kosher)	7 oz.	1001	105.0
(Mrs. Smith's):			
8" shell	⅛ of 10-oz. shell	80	8.0
9" shell:			
Regular	⅛ of 12-oz. shell	90	10.0
Shallow	⅛ of 10-oz. shell	80	8.0
9⅝" shell	⅛ of 15-oz. shell	120	12.0
(Oronoque):			
Regular	⅙ of 7.4-oz. shell	170	14.0
Deep dish	⅙ of 8.5-oz. shell	200	16.0
(Pet-Ritz):			
Regular	⅙ of 5-oz. shell	110	11.0

Food	Measure	Cals.	Carbs.
Deep dish:			
Regular	⅙ of 6-oz. shell	130	12.0
Vegetable shortening	⅙ of 6-oz. shell	140	12.0
Graham cracker	⅙ of 5-oz. shell	110	8.0
Refrigerated (Pillsbury)	⅛ of 2-crust shell	240	24.0
*PIECRUST MIX:			
(Betty Crocker):			
Regular	1/16 of pkg.	120	10.0
Stick	⅛ of stick	120	10.0
(Flako)	⅙ of 9" pie shell	245	25.2
(Pillsbury) mix			
or stick	⅙ of 2-crust pie	270	25.0
PIE FILLING (See also **PUDDING OR PIE FILLING**):			
Regular:			
Apple:			
(Thank You Brand)	3½ oz.	91	23.0
(White House)	½ cup (4.8 oz.)	163	39.0
Apple rings or slices (See **APPLE,** canned)			
Apricot (Comstock)	⅙ of 21-oz. can	110	24.0
Banana cream (Comstock)	⅙ of 21-oz. can	110	22.0
Blueberry (White House)	½ cup	159	38.0
Cherry:			
(Thank You Brand):			
Regular	3½ oz.	99	24.8
Sweet	3½ oz.	115	29.0
(White House)	½ cup (4.8 oz.)	190	45.0
Chocolate (Comstock)	⅙ of 21-oz. can	140	27.0
Coconut cream (Comstock)	⅙ of 21-oz. can	120	24.0
Coconut custard (USDA) home recipe, made with egg yolk & milk	5 oz. (inc. crust)	288	41.3
Lemon (Comstock)	⅙ of 21-oz. can	160	33.0
Mincemeat (Comstock)	⅙ of 21-oz. can	170	36.0
Peach (White House)	½ cup	158	39.0
Pineapple (Comstock)	⅙ of 21-oz. can	110	25.0
Pumpkin (See also **PUMPKIN,** canned):			
(Libby's)	1 cup	210	58.0
(Comstock)	⅙ of 27-oz. can	170	38.0
Raisin (Comstock)	⅙ of 21-oz. can	140	30.0
Strawberry (Comstock)	⅙ of 21-oz. can	130	28.0

Food	Measure	Cals.	Carbs.
Dietetic (Thank You Brand):			
Apple	3¼ oz.	60	.3
Cherry	3⅓ oz.	83	20.8
*PIE MIX:			
Banana cream (Jell-O)	⅛ of pie	240	27.0
Boston cream:			
(Betty Crocker) Classic	⅛ of pie	270	50.0
(Jell-O) no bake, mousse	⅛ of pie	260	25.0
Chocolate mint (Royal) no bake	⅛ of pie	260	25.0
Coconut cream (Jell-O) no bake	⅛ of pie	260	27.0
Lemon meringue (Royal) no bake	⅛ of pie	310	50.0
Pumpkin:			
(Jell-O) no bake	⅛ of pie	250	31.0
(Libby's)	⅙ of pie	390	53.0
PIEROGIES, frozen (Empire Kosher):			
Cheese	1½-oz. serving	81	14.2
Onion	1½-oz. serving	62	13.0
PIGEON (See **SQUAB**)			
PIGEONPEA (USDA):			
Raw, immature seeds in pods	1 lb.	207	37.7
Dry seeds	1 lb.	1551	288.9
PIGNOLI (See **PINE NUT**)			
PIGS FEET, pickled (USDA)	4-oz. serving	226	0.0
PIGS KNUCKLES, canned (Penrose) pickled	6 oz.	290	1.0
PIKE:			
Blue:			
Whole	1 lb. (weighed whole)	180	0.0
Meat only	4 oz.	102	0.0
Northern:			
Whole	1 lb. (weighed whole)	104	0.0
Meat only	4 oz.	100	0.0
Walleye:			

Food	Measure	Cals.	Carbs.
Whole	1 lb. (weighed whole)	140	0.0
Meat only	4 oz.	105	0.0
PIMIENTO, canned:			
(Dromedary) drained	1-oz. serving	10	2.0
(Sunshine) diced or sliced, solids & liq.	1 T.	4	.9
*PIÑA COLADA COCKTAIL:			
Canned (Mr. Boston)			
12½% alcohol	3 fl. oz.	249	34.2
*Mix (Bar-Tender's)	5 fl. oz.	254	24.0
PIÑA COLADA COCKTAIL MIX:			
Dry (Holland House)	.56-oz. pkg.	82	12.0
*Frozen (Bacardi)	4 fl. oz.	110	14.0
Liquid:			
*(Bar-Tender's)	5 fl. oz.	254	24.0
(Holland House)	1 fl. oz.	33	8.0
PINEAPPLE:			
Fresh (USDA):			
Whole	1 lb. (weighed untrimmed)	123	32.3
Diced	½ cup (2.8 oz.)	41	10.7
Sliced	⅜" × 3½" slice (3 oz.)	44	11.5
Canned, regular pack, solids & liq.:			
(USDA):			
Juice pack	4 oz.	66	17.1
Light syrup	5 oz.	76	17.5
Heavy syrup:			
Crushed	½ cup (5.6 oz.)	97	25.4
Slices	1 large slice & 2 T. syrup (4.3 oz.)	90	23.7
Tidbits	½ cup (4.6 oz.)	95	25.0
(Del Monte):			
Juice pack:			
Chunks, slices or tidbits	½ cup (4 oz.)	70	18.0
Spears	2 spears (3.1 oz.)	50	14.0
Syrup pack	½ cup (4 oz.)	90	23.0

Food	Measure	Cals.	Carbs.
(Dole) Juice pack, chunk, crushed or sliced	½ cup (4 oz.)	70	18.0
(Town House) juice pack	½ cup	70	18.0
Canned, unsweetened or dietetic, solids & liq.:			
(Diet Delight) juice pack	½ cup (4.4 oz.)	70	18.0
(Libby's) Lite	½ cup (4.4 oz.)	60	16.0
(S&W) *Nutradiet*, blue label	1 slice	30	7.5

PINEAPPLE, CANDIED

(USDA)	1-oz. serving	90	22.7

PINEAPPLE & MANDARIN ORANGE, canned (Dole) in light syrup, solids & liq.

	½ cup (4.4-oz.)	75	19.0

PINEAPPLE JUICE:

Canned:			
(Ardmore Farms)	6 fl. oz.	102	25.2
(Dole) unsweetened	6 fl. oz.	100	25.0
(Minute Maid):			
Regular	8.45-fl.-oz. container	139	34.1
On the Go	10-fl.-oz. bottle	165	40.4
(Mott's)	9½-fl.-oz. can	169	42.0
(Town House)	6 fl.-oz.	100	25.0
(Tree Top)	6 fl.-oz.	100	24.0
Chilled (Minute Maid)	6 fl.-oz.	99	24.2
*Frozen:			
(Dole) unsweetened	6 fl.-oz.	90	22.0
(Minute Maid)	6 fl.-oz.	99	24.2

PINEAPPLE & GRAPEFRUIT JUICE DRINK, canned:

(Del Monte) regular or pink	6 fl. oz.	90	24.0
(Dole) pink	6 fl. oz.	101	25.4
(Texsun)	6 fl. oz.	91	22.0

*PINEAPPLE-ORANGE JUICE:

Canned:			
(Ardmore Farms)	6 fl.-oz.	102	25.2
(Dole)	6 fl.-oz.	100	23.0
(Johanna Farms) *Tree Ripe*	8.45 fl.-oz. container	132	32.4
*Frozen:			
(Dole)	6 fl.-oz.	90	22.0

Food	Measure	Cals.	Carbs.
(Minute Maid)	6 fl.-oz.	98	23.9
*PINEAPPLE-ORANGE-BANANA JUICE, frozen (Dole)	6 fl.-oz.	90	23.0
*PINEAPPLE-ORANGE-GUAVA JUICE, frozen (Dole)	6 fl.-oz.	100	22.0
*PINEAPPLE-PASSION-BANANA JUICE, frozen (Dole)	6 fl.-oz.	100	21.0
PINEAPPLE PRESERVE OR JAM, sweetened (Smucker's)	1 T. (.7 oz.)	54	12.0
PINE NUT (USDA):			
Pignoli, shelled	4 oz.	626	13.2
Pinon, whole	4 oz. (weighed in shell)	418	13.5
Pinon, shelled	4 oz.	720	23.2
PINOT CHARDONNAY WINE			
(Paul Masson) 12% alcohol	3 fl. oz.	71	2.4
PISTACHIO NUT:			
Raw (USDA):			
In shell	4 oz. (weighed in shell)	337	10.8
Shelled	½ cup (2.2 oz.)	368	11.8
Shelled	1 T. (8 grams)	46	1.5
Roasted:			
(Fisher) salted:			
In shell	1 oz.	84	2.7
Shelled	1 oz.	174	5.4
(Flavor House) dry roasted	1 oz.	168	5.4
(Planters) dry roasted	1 oz.	170	6.0
PITANGA, fresh (USDA)			
Whole	1 lb. (weighed whole)	187	45.9
Flesh only	4 oz.	58	14.2

Food	Measure	Cals.	Carbs.
PIZZA HUT:			
Hand-tossed:			
Beef	1 slice of medium pizza	261	28.0
Cheese	1 slice of medium pizza	253	27.0
Meat Lovers	1 slice of medium pizza	321	28.0
Pepperoni	1 slice of medium pizza	283	28.0
Pepperoni Lovers	1 slice of medium pizza	335	28.0
Pork	1 slice of medium pizza	270	28.0
Sausage, Italian	1 slice of medium pizza	313	27.0
Super Supreme	1 slice of medium pizza	276	28.0
Supreme	1 slice of medium pizza	289	28.0
Veggie Lovers	1 slice of medium pizza	222	28.0
Bigfoot:			
Cheese	1 slice	186	24.0
Pepperoni	1 slice	195	24.0
Pepperoni, Italian sausage & mushroom	1 slice	214	25.0
Pan:			
Beef	1 slice of medium pizza	288	28.0
Cheese	1 slice of medium pizza	260	28.0
Meat Lovers	1 slice of medium pizza	340	28.0
Pepperoni	1 slice of medium pizza	265	26.0
Pepperoni Lovers	1 slice of medium pizza	362	27.0
Pork	1 slice of medium pizza	294	27.0
Sausage, Italian	1 slice of medium pizza	399	26.0
Super Supreme	1 slice of medium pizza	323	27.0
Supreme	1 slice of medium pizza	311	28.0

Food	*Measure*	*Cals.*	*Carbs.*
Personal Pan:			
Pepperoni	1 pizza	675	76.0
Supreme	1 pizza	647	76.0
PIZZA NUGGETS, frozen			
(Hormel) *Quick Meal*	1 piece (.6 oz.)	42	5.0
PIZZA PIE (See also ***SHAKEY'S, LITTLE CAESAR, PIZZA HUT***, etc.):			
Regular, non-frozen:			
Home recipe (USDA) with cheese topping	⅛ of 14" pie	177	21.2
(*Domino's*):			
Cheese:			
Plain:			
Small	⅛ of 12" pizza	157	24.3
Large	1/12 of 16" pizza	239	28.4
Double:			
Small	⅛ of 12" pizza	240	24.7
Large	1/12 of 16" pizza	350	29.1
Double, with pepperoni:			
Small	⅛ of 12" pizza	227	24.8
Large	1/12 of 16" pizza	389	29.1
Mushroom & sausage:			
Small	⅛ of 12" pizza	183	24.6
Large	1/12 of 16" pizza	266	28.9
Pepperoni:			
Plain:			
Small	⅛ of 12" pizza	192	24.3
Large	1/12 of 16" pizza	278	28.5
With sausage:			
Small	⅛ of 12" pizza	215	48.9
Large	1/12 of 16" pizza	303	57.3
Sausage:			
Small	⅛ of 12" pizza	180	24.4
Large	1/12 of 16" pizza	264	28.6
(Godfather's):			
Cheese:			
Original:			
Mini	¼ of pizza (2.8 oz.)	140	20.0
Small	⅙ of pizza (3.6 oz.)	240	32.0
Medium	⅛ of pizza (4 oz.)	242	35.0
Large:			

Food	Measure	Cals.	Carbs.
Regular	1/10 of pizza (4.4 oz.)	270	37.0
Hot slice	1/8 of pizza (5½ oz.)	370	48.0
Stuffed:			
Small	1/6 of pizza (4.4 oz.)	310	38.0
Medium	1/8 of pizza (4.8 oz.)	350	42.0
Large	1/10 of pizza (5.2 oz.)	381	44.0
Thin crust:			
Small	1/6 of pizza (2.6 oz.)	180	21.0
Medium	1/8 of pizza (3 oz.)	310	26.0
Large	1/10 of pizza (3.4 oz.)	228	28.0
Combo:			
Original:			
Mini	1/4 of pizza (3.8 oz.)	165	20.0
Small	1/6 of pizza (5.6 oz.)	300	35.0
Medium	1/8 of pizza (6.2 oz.)	320	37.0
Large:			
Regular	1/10 of pizza (6.8 oz.)	332	38.0
Hot Slice	1/8 of pizza (8.5 oz.)	550	52.0
Stuffed:			
Small	1/6 of pizza (6.3 oz.)	430	41.0
Medium	1/8 of pizza (7 oz.)	480	45.0
Large	1/10 of pizza (7.6 oz.)	521	47.0
Thin crust:			
Small	1/6 of pizza (4.3 oz.)	270	23.0
Medium	1/8 of pizza (4.9 oz.)	310	29.0
Large	1/10 of pizza (5.4 oz.)	336	31.0
Frozen:			
Bacon (Totino's)	½ of 10-oz. pizza	370	35.0

Food	Measure	Cals.	Carbs.
Bagel (Empire Kosher)	2-oz. serving	140	17.0
Canadian style bacon:			
(Jeno's) Crisp 'N Tasty	½ of 7.7-oz. pizza	250	27.0
(Stouffer's) french bread	½ of 11⅝-oz. pkg.	360	41.0
(Totino's)	½ of 10.2-oz. pizza	310	35.0
Cheese:			
(Banquet) Zap, french bread	4½-oz. serving	310	41.0
(Celentano):			
Nine-slice	2.7-oz. piece	150	22.0
Thick crust	⅓ of 13-oz. pizza	290	35.0
(Empire Kosher):			
Regular	⅓ of 10-oz. pie	195	27.0
Family size	⅕ of 15-oz. pie	215	30.0
3-pack	⅑ of 27-oz. pie	215	30.0
(Jeno's):			
Crisp 'N Tasty	½ of 7.4-oz. pizza	270	28.0
4-pack	¼ of 8.9-oz. pkg.	160	17.0
(Kid Cuisine)	6½-oz. serving	240	41.0
(Pappalo's) french bread	5.7-oz. piece	360	40.0
(Pepperidge Farm) croissant crust	1 pizza	430	41.0
(Pillsbury) microwave:			
Regular	½ of 7.1-oz. pizza	240	28.0
French bread	5.7-oz. piece	370	41.0
(Stouffer's) french bread:			
Regular:			
Plain	½ of 10⅜-oz. pkg.	340	41.0
Double cheese	½ of 11⅜-oz. pkg.	410	43.0
Lean Cuisine:			
Plain	5⅛-oz. serving	310	40.0
Extra Cheese	5½-oz. serving	350	39.0
(Totino's):			
Microwave	3.9-oz. pizza	250	34.0
My Classic, deluxe	⅙ of 18.6-oz. pizza	210	23.0
Pan, three cheese	⅙ of pizza (3.9 oz.)	290	33.0
Party	½ of 9.8-oz. pizza	340	34.0

Food	Measure	Cals.	Carbs.
Slices	2½-oz. slice	170	20.0
(Weight Watchers):			
Regular	5¾-oz. serving	310	39.0
French bread	5.1-oz. serving	310	31.0
Combination:			
(Jeno's):			
Crisp 'N Tasty	½ of 7.8-oz. pizza	300	27.0
4-pack	¼ of 9.6-oz. pkg.	180	17.0
(Pappalo's):			
French bread	6½-oz. serving	430	41.0
Pan	⅙ of 26.5-oz. pizza	340	34.0
Thin crust	⅙ of 22-oz. pizza	260	29.0
(Pillsbury) microwave	½ of 9-oz. pizza	310	29.0
(Totino's):			
My Classic, deluxe	1⅙ of 22½-oz. pizza	270	23.0
Party	½ of 10½-oz. pizza	380	35.0
Slices	2.7-oz. piece	200	20.0
(Weight Watchers) deluxe	6¾-oz. serving	300	37.0
Deluxe:			
(Banquet) Zap	4.8-oz. serving	330	39.0
(Pepperidge Farm) crois- sant crust	1 pizza	440	43.0
(Stouffer's) french bread:			
Regular	6.2-oz. serving	430	41.0
Lean Cuisine	6⅛-oz. serving	350	40.0
(Weight Watchers) french bread	6.12-oz. serving	310	31.0
English muffin (Empire Kosher)	2-oz. serving	140	17.0
Golden topping (Fox Deluxe)	½ of 6.8-oz. pizza	240	25.0
Hamburger:			
(Fox Deluxe)	½ of 7.6-oz. pizza	260	26.0
(Jeno's):			
Crisp 'N Tasty	½ of 8.1-oz. pizza	290	28.0
4-pack	¼ of 10-oz. pkg.	180	17.0
(Pappalo's):			
Pan	⅙ of 26.3-oz. pizza	310	34.0
Thin crust	⅙ of 22.2-oz. pizza	240	28.0

Food	Measure	Cals.	Carbs.
(Stouffer's) french bread	½ of 12¼-oz. pkg.	410	40.0
(Totino's) party	½ of 10.6-oz. pizza	370	35.0
Mexican style (Totino's)	½ of 10.2-oz. pizza	380	35.0
Pepperoni:			
(Banquet) Zap, french bread	4½-oz. serving	350	36.0
(Fox Deluxe)	½ of 7-oz. pizza	250	26.0
(Jeno's):			
Crisp 'N Tasty	½ of 7.6-oz. pizza	280	27.0
4-pack	¼ of 9.2-oz. pkg.	170	17.0
(Pappalo's):			
French bread	6-oz. serving	410	41.0
Pan	⅙ of 25.2-oz. pizza	330	34.0
Thin crust	⅙ of 22-oz. pizza	270	28.0
(Pepperidge Farm) croissant crust	1 pizza	420	43.0
(Pillsbury) microwave:			
Regular	½ of 8½-oz. pizza	300	29.0
French bread	6-oz. serving	430	46.0
(Stouffer's) french bread:			
Regular	½ of 11¼-oz pkg.	410	41.0
Lean Cuisine	5½-oz. serving	340	40.0
(Totino's):			
Microwave, small	4-oz. pizza	280	34.0
My Classic	⅙ of 21.1-oz. pizza	260	23.0
Pan	⅙ of 25.2-oz. pizza	330	34.0
Party	½ of 10.2-oz. pizza	370	35.0
Slices	2.6-oz. slice	190	20.0
(Weight Watchers):			
Regular	5.87-oz. serving	320	38.0
French bread	5¼-oz. serving	310	28.0
Sausage:			
(Fox Deluxe)	½ of 7.2-oz. pizza	260	26.0
(Jeno's):			
Crisp 'N Tasty	½ of 7.8-oz. pizza	300	28.0

Food	Measure	Cals.	Carbs.
4-pack	¼ of 9.6-oz. pkg.	180	17.0
(Pappalo's):			
French bread	6.3-oz. piece	410	41.0
Pan	⅙ of 26.3-oz.		
	pizza	360	34.0
Thin crust	⅙ of 22-oz. pizza	250	28.0
(Pillsbury) microwave:			
Regular	½ of 8¾-oz.		
	pizza	280	29.0
French bread	6.3-oz. piece	410	48.0
(Stouffer's) french bread:			
Regular	½ of 12-oz. pkg.	420	41.0
Lean Cuisine	6-oz. serving	350	40.0
(Totino's):			
Microwave, small	4.2-oz. pizza	320	33.0
Pan	⅙ of 26.3-oz.		
	pizza	320	34.0
Party	½ of 10.6-oz.		
	pizza	390	35.0
Slices	2.7-oz. slice	200	20.0
(Weight Watchers)	6¼-oz. serving	310	37.0
Sausage & pepperoni			
(Stouffer's) french bread	½ of 12½-oz.		
	pkg.	450	40.0
Vegetable (Stouffer's)	½ of 12¾-oz.		
french bread	pkg.	420	41.0
*Mix (Ragu) *Pizza Quick*	¼ of pie	300	37.0
PIZZA PIE CRUST:			
*Mix, *Gold Medal*	⅙ of mix	110	22.0
Fresh (Boboli):			
6" size	1 crust	300	49.0
12" size	1 crust	1200	196.0
Refrigerated (Pillsbury)	⅛ of crust	90	16.0
PIZZA POPS (Totino's):			
Pepperoni	1 piece	320	30.0
Sausage	1 piece	310	30.0
Sausage & pepperoni	1 piece	320	28.0
Supreme	1 piece	305	30.0
PIZZA ROLL, frozen (Jeno's):			
Cheese	½ of 6-oz. pkg.	240	23.0
Hamburger	½ of 6-oz. pkg.	240	21.0
Pepperoni & cheese:			
Regular	½ of 6-oz. pkg.	230	22.0

Food	Measure	Cals.	Carbs.
Microwave	⅓ of 9-oz. pkg.	240	23.0
Sausage & pepperoni:			
Regular	½ of 6-oz. pkg.	230	22.0
Microwave	⅓ of 9-oz. pkg.	250	24.0
PIZZA SAUCE:			
(Contadina):			
Regular or with cheese	½ cup (4.2 oz.)	80	10.0
With pepperoni	½ cup (4.2 oz.)	90	10.0
With tomato chunks	½ cup (4.2 oz.)	50	10.0
(Ragu):			
Regular	15½-oz. jar	250	30.0
Pizza Quick:			
Chunky	14-oz. jar	332	44.2
Mushroom, sausage or			
traditional	14-oz. jar	329	32.9
Pepperoni	14-oz. jar	412	32.9
PIZZA SEASONING SPICE			
(French's)	1 tsp. (.1 oz.)	5	1.0
PLANTAIN, raw (USDA):			
Whole	1 lb. (weighed with skin)	389	101.9
Flesh only	4 oz.	135	35.4
PLUM:			
Fresh (USDA):			
Damson:			
Whole	1 lb. (weighed with pits)	272	73.5
Flesh only	4 oz.	75	20.2
Japanese & hybrid:			
Whole	1 lb. (weighed with pits)	205	52.5
	2.1-oz. plum (2" dia.)	27	6.9
Diced	½ cup (2.9 oz.)	39	10.1
Halves	½ cup (3.1 oz.)	42	10.8
Slices	½ cup (3 oz.)	40	10.3
Prune type:			
Whole	1 lb. (weighed with pits)	320	84.0
Halves	½ cup (2.8 oz.)	60	52.8
Canned, purple, regular pack solids & liq.:			

Food	Measure	Cals.	Carbs.
(USDA):			
Extra heavy syrup	4 oz.	116	30.3
Heavy syrup, with pits	½ cup (4.5 oz.)	106	27.6
Heavy syrup, without pits	½ cup (4.2 oz.)	100	25.9
Light syrup	4 oz.	71	18.8
(Stokely-Van Camp)	½ cup	120	30.0
(Thank You Brand):			
Heavy syrup	½ cup (4.8 oz.)	109	27.2
Light syrup	½ cup (4.7 oz.)	80	20.0
Canned, unsweetened or low calorie, solids & liq.:			
(Diet Delight) purple:			
Juice pack	½ cup (4.4 oz.)	70	19.0
Water pack	½ cup (4.4 oz.)	50	13.0
(S&W) *Nutradiet*, purple, juice pack	½ cup	80	20.0
(Thank You Brand)	½ cup (4.8 oz.)	49	12.2
PLUM JELLY:			
Sweetened (Bama)	1 T. (.7 oz.)	45	12.0
Dietetic or low calorie (Featherweight)	1 T.	16	4.0
PLUM PRESERVE OR JAM, sweetened (Smucker's)	1 T. (.7 oz.)	53	13.5
PLUM PUDDING (Richardson & Robbins)	2" wedge (3.6 oz.)	270	61.0
POLENTA (San Gennaro):			
Regular	½" slice	35	7.5
Basil & garlic	½" slice	36	7.5
Sun-dried tomato	½" slice	37	8.0
POLISH-STYLE SAUSAGE (See **SAUSAGE**)			
POMEGRANATE, raw (USDA):			
Whole	1 lb. (weighed whole)	160	41.7
Pulp only	4 oz.	71	18.6
PONDEROSA **RESTAURANT:**			
A-1 Sauce	1 tsp.	4	1.0
Beef, chopped, patty only (see also Bun):			
Regular	3½ oz.	209	0.0

Food	Measure	Cals.	Carbs.
Big	4.8 oz.	295	0.0
Double Deluxe	5.9 oz.	362	0.0
Junior *(Square Shooter)*	1.6 oz.	98	0.0
Steakhouse Deluxe	2.96 oz.	181	0.0
Beverages:			
Coca-Cola	8 fl. oz.	96	24.0
Coffee	6 fl. oz.	2	.5
Dr Pepper	8 fl. oz.	96	24.8
Lemon	8 fl. oz.	110	28.5
Milk:			
Regular	8 fl. oz.	159	12.0
Chocolate	8 fl. oz.	208	25.9
Orange drink	8 fl. oz.	110	30.0
Root beer	8 fl. oz.	104	25.6
Sprite	8 fl. oz.	95	24.0
Bun:			
Regular	2.4-oz. bun	190	35.0
Hot dog	1 bun	108	18.9
Junior	1.4-oz. bun	118	21.0
Steakhouse deluxe	2.4-oz. bun	190	35.0
Chicken strips:			
Adult portion	2⅜ oz.	282	15.8
Children's portion	1.4 oz.	141	7.9
Cocktail sauce	1½ oz.	57	.2
Filet mignon	3.8 oz. (edible portion)	152	.2
Filet of sole, fish only (See also Bun)	3-oz. piece	125	4.4
Fish, baked	4.9-oz. serving	268	11.6
Gelatin dessert	½ cup	97	23.5
Gravy, au jus	1 oz.	3	Tr.
Ham & cheese:			
Bun (See Bun)			
Cheese, Swiss	2 slices (.8 oz.)	76	.5
Ham	2½ oz.	184	1.4
Hot dog, child's, meat only (See also Bun)	1.6-oz. hot dog	140	2.0
Margarine:			
Pat	1 pat	36	Tr.
On potato, as served	½ oz.	100	.1
Mustard sauce, sweet & sour	1 oz.	50	9.5
New York strip steak	6.1 oz. (edible portion)	362	0.0
Onion, chopped	1 T. (.4 oz.)	4	.9
Pickle, dill	3 slices (.7 oz.)	2	.2
Potato:			
Baked	7.2-oz. potato	145	32.8

Food	Measure	Cals.	Carbs.
French fries	3-oz. serving	230	30.2
Prime ribs:	4.2 oz. (edible		
Regular	portion)	286	0.0
Imperial	8.4 oz. (edible		
	portion)	572	0.0
King	6 oz. (edible		
	portion)	409	0.0
Pudding:			
Butterscotch	4½ oz.	200	27.4
Chocolate	4½ oz.	213	27.1
Vanilla	4½ oz.	195	27.5
Ribeye	3.2 oz. (edible		
	portion)	197	0.0
Ribeye & shrimp:			
Ribeye	3.2 oz.	197	0.0
Shrimp	2.2 oz.	139	0.0
Roll, kaiser	2.2-oz. roll	184	33.0
Salad bar:			
Bean sprouts	1 oz.	13	1.5
Beets	1 oz.	5	.9
Broccoli	1 oz.	9	1.7
Cabbage, red	1 oz.	9	2.0
Carrots	1 oz.	12	2.8
Cauliflower	1 oz.	8	1.5
Celery	1 oz.	4	1.1
Chickpeas (Garbanzos)	1 oz.	102	17.3
Cucumber	1 oz.	4	.7
Mushrooms	1 oz.	8	1.2
Onion, white	1 oz.	11	2.6
Pepper, green	1 oz.	6	1.4
Radish	1 oz.	5	1.0
Tomato	1 oz.	6	1.3
Salad dressing:			
Blue cheese	1 oz.	129	2.1
Italian, creamy	1 oz.	138	2.8
Low calorie	1 oz.	14	.8
Oil & vinegar	1 oz.	124	.9
Sweet'n Tart	1 oz.	129	9.2
1000 Island	1 oz.	117	6.7
Shrimp dinner	7 pieces (3½ oz.)	220	9.8
Sirloin:			
Regular	3.3 oz. (edible		
	portion)	197	0.0
Super	6½ oz. (edible		
	portion)	383	0.0
Tips	4 oz. (edible		
	portion)	192	0.0

Food	Measure	Cals.	Carbs.
Steak sauce	1 oz.	23	4.0
Tartar sauce	1.5 oz.	285	4.5
T-bone	4.3 oz. (edible portion)	240	0.0
Tomato (See also Salad Bar):			
Slices	2 slices (.9 oz.)	5	1.2
Whole, small	3.5 oz.	22	4.7
Topping, whipped	¼ oz.	19	1.2
Worcestershire sauce	1 tsp.	4	.9
POPCORN:			
*Plain, popped fresh:			
(General Mills) *Top Secret*	1 cup	33	3.7
(Jiffy Pop)	½ of 5-oz. pkg.	244	29.8
(Jolly Time):			
Regular, no added butter or salt:			
White	1 cup	19	4.0
Yellow	1 cup	22	4.7
Microwave:			
Natural	1 cup	53	5.0
Butter flavor	1 cup	53	5.3
Cheese flavor	1 cup	60	5.7
(Orville Redenbacher's)			
Original:			
Plain	1 cup (.2 oz.)	22	4.5
With oil & salt	1 cup (.3 oz.)	40	5.3
Caramel crunch	1 cup	140	19.0
Hot air corn	1 cup	25	4.5
Microwave:			
Regular, butter flavored	1 cup	27	2.5
Regular, natural	1 cup	27	2.7
Flavored:			
Caramel	1 cup	96	11.6
Cheese	1 cup	50	4.0
Sour cream & onions	1 cup	50	4.3
(Pillsbury) microwave:			
Regular	1 cup	70	6.5
Butter flavor, regular or frozen	1 cup	70	6.7
Salt free, frozen	1 cup	57	7.7
Butter flavor	1 cup	65	6.0
Dry popped	1 oz.	100	20.0
Oil popped	1 oz.	220	20.0
Packaged:			
Plain:			
Cape Cod	1 oz.	160	12.0

Food	Measure	Cals.	Carbs.
(Eagle)	1 oz.	160	12.0
(Wise) butter flavored	1 oz.	140	16.0
Caramel-coated:			
(Bachman)	1-oz. serving	110	25.0
(Old Dutch)	1 oz.	109	DNA
(Old London) without			
peanuts	1⅜-oz. serving	195	43.6
Cheese flavored (Snyder's)	1-oz. serving	180	14.0
Cracker Jack	1-oz. serving	120	22.0
POPCORN BAR (Pop Secret)			
caramel or chocolate	1 piece	80	15.0
POPCORN CAKES (Orville			
Redenbacher):			
Apple cinnamon, mini	1.1-oz. serving	100	26.0
Butter:			
Regular	1 piece	38	8.7
Mini	1.1-oz. serving	100	23.0
Caramel	1 piece	40	11.5
Cheddar, white:			
Regular	1 piece	37	8.7
Mini	1.1-oz. serving	100	23.0
POPCORN POPPING OIL			
(Orville Redenbacher's)			
gourmet, buttery flavor	1 T.	120	0.0
***POPEYE'S* RESTAURANT:**			
Biscuit	2.3-oz. piece	250	26.1
Chicken, mild or spicy:			
Breast	3.7-oz. serving	270	9.2
Leg	1.7-oz. serving	120	4.4
Thigh	3.1 oz. serving	300	9.3
Chicken nuggets	4.2-oz. serving	410	17.9
Coleslaw	4-oz. serving	149	13.6
Corn on the cob	5.2-oz. serving	90	21.4
French fries	3-oz. serving	240	30.8
Onion rings	3.1-oz. serving	310	31.1
Pie, apple	3.1-oz. serving	290	36.6
Red beans & rice	5.9-oz. serving	270	29.7
POPOVER:			
Home recipe (USDA)	1 average		
	popover (2 oz.)	128	14.7
*Mix (Flako)	1 popover	170	25.0

Food	Measure	Cals.	Carbs.
POPPY SEED (French's)	1 tsp.	13	.8
POPSICLE, twin	3-fl.-oz. pop	70	17.0
PORGY, raw (USDA):			
Whole	1 lb. (weighed whole)	208	0.0
Meat only	4 oz.	127	0.0
PORK, medium-fat:			
Fat, separable, cooked	1 oz.	219	0.0
Fresh (USDA):			
Boston butt:			
Raw:	1 lb. (weighed with bone & skin)	1220	0.0
Roasted, lean & fat	4 oz.	400	0.0
Roasted, lean only	4 oz.	277	0.0
Chop:			
Broiled, lean & fat	1 chop (4 oz., weighed with bone)	295	0.0
Broiled, lean & fat	1 chop (3 oz., weighed without bone)	332	0.0
Broiled, lean only	1 chop (3 oz., weighed without bone)	230	0.0
Ham:			
Raw	1 lb. (weighed with bone & skin)	1188	0.0
Roasted, lean & fat	4 oz.	424	0.0
Roasted, lean only	4 oz.	246	0.0
Loin:			
Raw	1 lb. (weighed with bone)	1065	0.0
Roasted, lean & fat	4 oz.	411	0.0
Roasted, lean only	4 oz.	288	0.0
Picnic:			
Raw	1 lb. (weighed with bone & skin)	1083	0.0
Simmered, lean & fat	4 oz.	424	0.0
Simmered, lean only	4 oz.	240	0.0

Food	Measure	Cals.	Carbs.
Spareribs:			
Raw, with bone	1 lb. (weighed with bone)	976	0.0
Braised, lean & fat	4 oz.	499	0.0
Cured, light commercial cure:			
Bacon (See **BACON**)			
Boston butt (USDA):			
Raw	1 lb. (weighed with bone & skin)	1227	0.0
Roasted, lean & fat	4 oz.	374	0.0
Roasted, lean only	4 oz.	276	0.0
PORK, CANNED, chopped luncheon meat (USDA):			
Regular	1 oz.	83	.4
Chopped	1 cup (4.8 oz.)	400	1.8
Diced	1 cup	415	1.8
PORK DINNER OR ENTREE:			
*Canned:			
(Hunt's) *Minute Gourmet*	6.6-oz. serving	500	46.0
(La Choy) sweet & sour	¾ cup	250	48.0
Frozen (Swanson) loin of	10¾-oz. dinner	280	27.0
PORK, PACKAGED (Eckrich)	1-oz. serving	45	1.0
PORK, SALT (See **SALT PORK**)			
PORK SANDWICH, frozen (Hormel) *Quick Meal*, barbecue	4.3-oz. serving	350	40.0
PORK, SWEET & SOUR, frozen:			
(Chun King)	13-oz. entree	400	78.0
(La Choy)	12-oz. entree	360	64.0
PORK & BEANS (See **BEAN, BAKED**)			
PORK RINDS (Old Dutch)	1-oz. serving	154	1.0
PORT WINE:			
(Gallo) 16% alcohol	3 fl. oz.	94	7.8

Food	Measure	Cals.	Carbs.
(Louis M. Martini) 19½% alcohol	3 fl. oz.	165	2.0
*POSTUM, instant, regular or coffee flavored	6 fl. oz.	11	2.6
POTATO (See also SWEET POTATO):			
Cooked (USDA)			
Au gratin, with cheese	½ cup (4.3 oz.)	177	16.6
Baked, peeled	2½" dia. potato (3.5 oz.)	92	20.9
Boiled, peeled before boiling, no salt	4.3-oz. potato	79	17.7
French-fried in deep fat, no salt	10 pieces (2 oz.)	156	20.5
Hash-browned, home recipe, after holding overnight	½ cup (3.4 oz.)	223	28.4
Mashed, milk & butter added	½ cup (3.5 oz.)	92	12.1
Canned, solids & liq.:			
(Allen's) Butterfield	½ cup	45	10.0
(Hunt's)	4 oz.	55	12.0
(Larsen) *Freshlike*	½ cup	60	13.0
(Town House)	½ cup	55	12.0
Frozen:			
(Bel-Air):			
With cheese	5-oz. serving	220	31.0
French fries:			
Regular	3-oz. serving	120	40.0
Crinkle cut	3-oz. serving	120	20.0
Hash brown	4-oz. serving	80	19.0
Shoestring	3-oz. serving	140	20.0
Sour cream & chives	5-oz. serving	230	31.0
(Birds Eye):			
Cottage fries	2.8-oz. serving	119	17.3
Crinkle cuts:			
Regular	3-oz. serving	115	18.4
Deep Gold	3-oz. serving	138	25.5
French fries:			
Regular	3-oz. serving	113	16.8
Deep Gold	3-oz. serving	161	24.4
Hash browns:			
Regular	4-oz. serving	74	16.5
Shredded	¼ of 12-oz. pkg.	61	13.1
Steak fries	3-oz. serving	109	17.9
Tasti Fries	2½-oz. serving	136	16.5

Food	Measure	Cals.	Carbs.
Tasti Puffs	¼ of 10-oz. pkg.	192	19.4
Tiny Taters	⅕ of 16.oz. pkg.	204	22.0
Whole, peeled	3.2-oz. serving	59	12.8
(Empire Kosher) french fries	3-oz. serving	110	18.0
(Green Giant) One Serving:			
Au gratin	5½-oz. serving	200	20.0
& broccoli in cheese sauce	5½-oz. serving	130	14.0
(Larsen) diced	4-oz. serving	80	19.0
(McKenzie) whole, white, boiled	3-oz. serving	70	15.0
(Ore-Ida):			
Cheddar Browns	3-oz. serving	80	14.0
Cottage fries	3-oz. serving	120	19.0
Country Style Dinner Fries or *Home Style Potato Wedges*	3-oz. serving	110	19.0
Crispers!	3-oz. serving	230	25.0
Crispy Crowns	3-oz. serving	170	20.0
Golden Crinkles or *Golden Fries*	3-oz. serving	120	20.0
Golden Patties	2½-oz. serving	140	15.0
Golden Twirls	3-oz. serving	160	21.0
Hash browns:			
Microwave	2-oz. serving	120	13.0
Shredded or Southern style	3-oz. serving	70	15.0
Toaster	1¾-oz. serving	100	12.0
Lite Crinkle Cuts	3-oz. serving	90	16.0
Pixie Crinkles	3-oz. serving	140	21.0
Potatoes O'Brien	3-oz. serving	60	14.0
Shoestring	3-oz. serving	150	22.0
Tater Tots:			
Plain:			
Regular	3-oz. serving	150	20.0
Microwave	4-oz. serving	200	29.0
With onions	3-oz. serving	150	20.0
Whole, small, peeled	3-oz. serving	70	16.0
(Stouffer's):			
Au gratin	⅓ of 11½-oz. pkg.	110	10.0
Scalloped	⅓ of 11½-oz. pkg.	90	11.0

POTATO, STUFFED, BAKED,
  frozen (Green Giant):

Food	Measure	Cals.	Carbs.
With cheese flavored topping	½ of 10-oz. pkg.	200	33.0
With sour cream & chives	½ of 10-oz. pkg.	230	31.0

Food	Measure	Cals.	Carbs.
POTATO CHIPS:			
(Cape Cod) any style	1 oz.	150	16.0
(Cottage Fries) unsalted	1 oz.	160	14.0
Delta Gold	1 oz.	160	14.0
(Energy Food Factory) *Potato Pops:*			
Au gratin	1 oz.	120	24.0
Fat free	1 oz.	100	26.0
Herb & garlic, regular or salt & vinegar	1 oz.	100	22.0
Mesquite	1 oz.	100	24.0
(Frito-Lay):			
All flavors except sour cream & onion	1 oz.	150	15.0
Sour cream & onion	1 oz.	160	15.0
Ruffles:			
Regular:			
All flavors	1 oz.	150	15.0
Light	1 oz.	130	19.0
Cottage fries:			
BBQ	1 oz.	150	14.0
Sour cream & chives or unsalted	1 oz.	160	14.0
(Laura Scudder's):			
Barbecue	1 oz.	150	15.0
Sour cream & onion	1 oz.	150	14.0
(New York Deli)	1 oz.	160	14.0
(Old Dutch) *O'Grady's:*	1 oz.	150	16.0
All flavors except BBQ	1 oz.	150	16.0
BBQ	1 oz.	140	16.0
(Snyder's)	1 oz.	150	15.0
(Tom's):			
Regular, BBQ, rippled or sour cream & onion	1 oz.	160	14.0
Hot or vinegar and salt	1 oz.	160	15.0
(Weight Watchers) *Great Snackers,* barbecue, cheddar cheese or sour cream & onion	1 oz.	140	20.0
(Wise):			
Regular:			
Barbecue, garlic & onion	1 oz.	150	14.0
Lightly salted, natural or salt & vinegar	1 oz.	160	14.0

Food	Measure	Cals.	Carbs.
Cottage Fries:			
BBQ	1 oz.	150	14.0
No salt added or sour cream & chives	1 oz.	160	14.0
Ridgies	1 oz.	160	14.0
*POTATO MIX:			
Au gratin:			
(Betty Crocker)	½ cup	150	21.0
(French's) tangy	½ cup	130	20.0
(Lipton) & sauce	¼ of pkg.	108	22.4
(Town House)	½ cup	150	21.0
Beef & mushroom (Lipton)	½ cup	95	20.4
Casserole (French's) cheddar cheese & bacon	½ cup	130	18.0
Cheddar bacon (Lipton) & sauce	½ cup	106	20.5
Cheddar broccoli (Lipton)	½ cup	104	20.5
Chicken flavored mushroom (Lipton) & sauce	½ cup	90	19.2
Hash browns (Betty Crocker) with onion	½ cup	160	24.0
Italian (Lipton)	½ cup	107	20.8
Julienne (Betty Crocker)	½ cup	130	18.0
Mashed:			
(Betty Crocker) *Buds*	½ cup	130	17.0
(French's):			
Big Tate	½ cup	140	16.0
Idaho	½ cup	120	16.0
(Pillsbury) *Hungry Jack*, flakes	½ cup	140	17.0
(Town House)	½ cup	120	16.0
Nacho (Lipton) & sauce	½ cup	103	20.9
Scalloped:			
(Betty Crocker) plain	½ cup	140	19.0
(French's):			
Creamy Italian	½ cup	120	19.0
Crispy top or real cheese	½ cup	140	19.0
(Lipton) & sauce	½ cup	102	19.5
Sour cream & chive:			
(Betty Crocker)	½ cup	160	21.0
(French's)	½ cup	150	19.0
(Lipton)	¼ pkg.	113	21.0
*POTATO PANCAKE MIX			
(French's)	3" pancake	30	5.3

Food	Measure	Cals.	Carbs.
POTATO SALAD, home recipe (USDA):			
With cooked salad dressing seasonings	4 oz.	112	18.5
With mayonnaise & French dressing, hard-cooked eggs, seasonings	4 oz.	164	15.2
POTATO TOPPERS (Libby's)	1 T.	30	4.0
POT ROAST, frozen:			
(Armour) *Dinner Classics*	10-oz. meal	310	26.0
(Budget Gourmet) *Light and Healthy*	10-oz. meal	230	19.0
(Healthy Choice) Yankee	11-oz. meal	260	36.0
(Stouffer's) homestyle, with browned potatoes	8⅞-oz. meal	280	24.0
(Swanson) Yankee:			
Regular	11½-oz. meal	270	35.0
Hungry Man	16-oz. meal	420	49.0
POUND CAKE (See **CAKE,** Pound)			
PRESERVE OR JAM (See individual flavors)			
PRETZELS:			
(Eagle) *A & Eagle*	1 oz.	110	22.0
(Estee) unsalted	1 piece (1.3 grams)	7	1.6
(Nabisco) *Mister Salty:*			
Regular:			
Dutch	1 piece	55	11.0
Logs	1 piece	12	2.3
Mini	1 piece	7	1.3
Mini mix or nuggets	1 piece	5	1.0
Rings	1 piece	5	.9
Rods	1 piece	55	10.5
Sticks	1 piece	1	.2
Twists	1 piece	22	4.2
Juniors	1 piece	4	.7
(Old Dutch)	1-oz. serving	120	23.0
(Rokeach) Dutch style:			
Regular	1 oz.	110	24.0

Food	Measure	Cals.	Carbs.
Unsalted	1 oz.	110	20.0
Rold Gold	1 oz.	110	22.0
(Seyfert's) rods, butter	1 oz.	110	21.0
(Snyder's)			
Hard	1 oz.	102	22.7
Sticks or thins	1 oz.	110	22.0
(Tom's) twists	1 oz.	100	22.0
(Wise) nuggets	1 oz.	110	21.0
PRICKLY PEAR, fresh (USDA):			
Whole	1 lb. (weighed with rind & seeds)	84	21.8
Flesh only	4 oz.	48	12.4
PRODUCT 19, cereal (Kellogg's)	1 cup (1 oz.)	100	24.0
PRUNE:			
Canned:			
(Featherweight) stewed, water pack	½ cup	130	35.0
(Sunsweet) stewed	½ cup (4.6 oz.)	120	32.0
Dried:			
(Sunsweet):			
Whole	2 oz.	120	31.0
Pitted	2 oz.	140	36.0
PRUNE JUICE:			
(Algood) *Lady Betty*	6 fl. oz.	130	30.0
(Ardmore Farms)	6 fl. oz.	148	36.6
(Knudsen & Sons)	6 fl. oz.	127	31.5
(Mott's) regular	6 fl. oz.	130	32.0
(S&W) unsweetened	6 fl. oz.	120	31.0
(Town House)	6 fl. oz.	120	31.0
PRUNE WHIP (USDA) home recipe	1 cup (4.8 oz.)	211	49.8
PUDDING OR PIE FILLING (See also **CUSTARD**) Home recipe (USDA): Bread (See **BREAD PUDDING**)			

Food	Measure	Cals.	Carbs.
Rice, made with raisins	½ cup (4.7 oz.)	1983	35.2
Tapioca:			
Apple	½ cup (4.4 oz.)	146	36.8
Cream	½ cup (2.9 oz.)	110	14.0
Canned, regular pack:			
Banana:			
(Del Monte) *Pudding Cup*	5-oz. container	180	30.0
(Hunt's) *Snack Pack*	4-oz. container	158	25.0
(Thank You Brand)	½ cup	150	33.8
(Town House)	5-oz. container	160	28.0
Butterscotch:			
(Del Monte) *Pudding Cup*	5-oz. container	180	31.0
(Hunt's) *Snack Pack*	4¼-oz. container	170	26.0
(Swiss Miss)	4-oz. container	160	23.0
(Town House)	5-oz. container	160	28.0
Chocolate:			
(Del Monte) *Pudding Cup*	5-oz. container	190	31.0
(Hunt's) *Snack Pack:*			
Regular	4¼-oz. container	160	28.0
Fudge	4¼-oz. container	170	24.0
German	4¼-oz. container	190	30.0
Marshmallow	4¼-oz. container	170	26.0
(Swiss Miss):			
Regular	4-oz. container	180	27.0
Fudge:			
Regular	4-oz. container	170	26.0
Fruit on bottom:			
Black cherries	4-oz. container	170	30.0
Strawberries	4-oz. container	170	29.0
(Town House)	5-oz. container	160	28.0
Lemon (Thank You Brand)	½ cup	174	37.7
Rice (Hunt's) *Snack Pack*	4¼-oz. container	190	23.0
Tapioca:			
(Hunt's) *Snack Pack*	4¼-oz. container	160	28.0
(Swiss Miss)	4-oz. container	150	26.0
(Thank You Brand)	½ cup	144	24.7
(Town House)	5-oz. container	160	26.0
Vanilla:			
(Hunt's) *Snack Pack*	4¼-oz. container	170	28.0
(Swiss Miss)	4-oz. container	160	26.0
(Thank You Brand)	½ cup	150	26.0
(Town House)	5-oz. container	160	25.0
Canned, dietetic pack (Estee)	½ cup	70	13.0
Chilled (Swiss Miss):			

Food	Measure	Cals.	Carbs.
Butterscotch, chocolate malt			
or vanilla	4-oz. container	150	24.0
Chocolate or double rich	4-oz. container	160	24.0
Chocolate malt	4-oz. container	150	22.0
Chocolate sundae	4-oz. container	170	26.0
Rice	4-oz. container	150	24.0
Tapioca	4-oz. container	130	22.0
Vanilla sundae	4-oz. container	170	25.0
Frozen (Rich's):			
Butterscotch	4½-oz. container	198	27.2
Chocolate	4½-oz. container	212	27.0
Vanilla	4½-oz. container	194	27.4
*Mix, sweetened, regular &			
instant:			
Banana:			
(Jell-O) cream:			
Regular	½ cup	161	26.7
Instant	½ cup	174	30.0
(Jell-Well) cream	½ cup	180	31.0
(Royal) regular	½ cup	160	27.0
Butter pecan (Jell-O)			
instant	½ cup	175	29.1
Butterscotch:			
(Jell-O):			
Regular	½ cup	172	29.7
Instant	½ cup	175	30.0
(Jell-Well)	½ cup	180	31.0
(Royal) regular	½ cup	160	27.0
Chocolate:			
(Jell-O):			
Plain:			
Regular	½ cup	174	28.8
Instant	⅓ cup	181	30.6
Fudge:			
Regular	½ cup	169	27.8
Instant	½ cup	182	30.9
Milk:			
Regular	½ cup	171	28.2
Instant	½ cup	184	34.0
(Jell-Well)	½ cup	180	31.0
(Royal)	½ cup	190	35.0
Coconut:			
(Jell-O) cream:			
Regular	½ cup	176	24.4
Instant	½ cup	182	26.1

Food	Measure	Cals.	Carbs.
(Royal) instant	½ cup	170	30.0
*Flan (Knorr):			
Without sauce	½ cup	130	19.0
With sauce	½ cup	190	34.0
Lemon:			
(Jell-O):			
Regular	½ cup	181	38.8
Instant	½ cup	179	31.1
(Jell-Well)	½ cup	180	31.0
Lime (Royal) Key Lime, regular	½ cup	160	30.0
Pineapple (Jell-O) cream, instant	½ cup	176	30.4
Pistachio (Jell-O) instant	½ cup	174	28.4
Raspberry (Salada) *Danish Dessert*	½ cup	130	32.0
Rice (Jell-O) *Americana*	½ cup	176	29.9
Strawberry (Salada) *Danish Dessert*	½ cup	130	32.0
Tapioca (Jell-O) *Americana:*			
Chocolate	½ cup	173	27.8
Vanilla	½ cup	162	27.4
Vanilla:			
(Jell-O):			
Plain, instant	½ cup	179	31.0
French, regular	½ cup	172	29.7
(Royal)	½ cup	180	29.0
*Mix, dietetic:			
Butterscotch:			
(D-Zerta)	½ cup	68	12.0
(Weight Watchers)	½ cup	90	16.0
Chocolate:			
(D-Zerta)	½ cup (4.6 oz.)	68	11.5
(Estee)	½ cup	70	13.0
(Louis Sherry)	½ cup (4.2 oz.)	50	9.0
(Weight Watchers)	½ cup	90	18.0
Vanilla:			
(D-Zerta)	½ cup	70	13.0
(Estee) instant	½ cup	70	13.0
(Royal)	½ cup	100	16.0
(Weight Watchers)	½ cup	90	17.0

Food	Measure	Cals.	Carbs.
PUDDING POPS (See *JELL-O PUDDING POPS*)			
PUDDING ROLL-UPS, *Fruit Corners* (General Mills):			
Butterscotch	.5-oz. piece	60	11.0
Chocolate fudge or milk chocolate	.5-oz. piece	60	10.0
PUDDING SUNDAE (Swiss Miss):			
Caramel or mint	4-oz. container	170	25.0
Chocolate	4-oz. container	190	29.0
Peanut butter	4-oz. container	200	23.0
Vanilla	4-oz. container	180	28.0
PUFF PASTRY (See **PASTRY SHEET, PUFF**)			
PUFFED RICE:			
(Malt-O-Meal)	1 cup (.5 oz.)	54	12.2
(Quaker)	1 cup	55	12.7
PUFFED WHEAT:			
(Malt-O-Meal)	1 cup (.5 oz.)	53	10.4
(Quaker)	1 cup (.5 oz.)	54	10.8
PUMPKIN:			
Fresh (USDA):			
Whole	1 lb. (weighed with rind & seeds	83	20.6
Flesh only	4 oz.	29	7.4
Canned:			
(Libby's) solid pack	½ of 16-oz. can	40	10.0
(Stokely-Van Camp)	½ cup (4.3 oz.)	45	9.5
PUMPKIN BUTTER (Smucker's) *Autumn Harvest*	1 T.	36	9.0
PUMPKIN SEED, dry (USDA):			
Whole	4 oz. (weighed in hull)	464	12.6
Hulled	4 oz.	627	17.0

Food	Measure	Cals.	Carbs.
PUNCH DRINK (Minute Maid):			
Canned:			
Regular	8.45-fl. oz. container	131	32.7
On the Go	10-fl. oz. bottle	155	38.7
Tropical	8.45-fl. oz. container	130	32.0
Chilled, citrus	6 fl. oz.	93	23.1
*Frozen, citrus	6 fl. oz.	93	23.1
PURE & LIGHT, fruit juice, canned (Dole):			
Country raspberry or orchard peach	6 fl. oz.	90	24.0
Mandarin tangerine	6 fl. oz.	100	24.0
Mountain cherry	6 fl. oz.	90	20.0

Q

Food	Measure	Cals.	Carbs.
QUAIL, raw (USDA) meat & skin	4 oz.	195	0.0
QUIK (Nestlé):			
Chocolate	1 tsp. (.4 oz.)	45	9.5
Strawberry	1 tsp. (.4 oz.)	45	11.0
Sugar free	1 tsp. (.2 oz.)	18	3.0
QUINCE JELLY, sweetened (Smucker's)	1 T.	54	12.0

Food	Measure	Cals.	Carbs.

R

RABBIT (USDA)
  Domesticated:
    Raw, ready-to-cook

	1 lb. (weighed with bones)	581	0.0

    Stewed, flesh only — 4 oz. — 245 — 0.0
  Wild, ready-to-cook

	1 lb. (weighed with bones)	490	0.0

RACCOON, roasted, meat only — 4 oz. — 289 — 0.0

RADISH (USDA):
  Common, raw:
    Without tops

	½ lb. (weighed untrimmed)	34	7.4

    Trimmed, whole — 4 small radishes (1.4 oz.) — 7 — 1.4
    Trimmed sliced — ½ cup (2 oz.) — 10 — 2.1
  Oriental, raw, without tops — ½ lb. (weighed unpared) — 34 — 7.4
  Oriental, raw, trimmed & pared — 4 oz. — 22 — 4.8

RAISIN:
  Dried:
    (USDA):
      Whole, pressed down — ½ cup (2.9 oz.) — 237 — 63.5
      Chopped — ½ cup (2.9 oz.) — 234 — 62.7
      Ground — ½ cup (4.7 oz.) — 387 — 103.7
    (Dole) regular or golden — ¼ cup (1½-oz.) — 125 — 33.0
    (Sun-Maid) seedless, natural Thompson — 1 oz. — 96 — 23.0
    (Town House) — ¼ cup — 130 — 33.0
  Cooked (USDA) added sugar, solids & liq. — ½ cup (4.3 oz.) — 260 — 68.8

RAISIN BRAN (See **BRAN BREAKFAST CEREAL**)

Food	Measure	Cals.	Carbs.
RAISIN SQUARES, cereal (Kellogg's)	½ cup (1 oz.)	90	22.0
RASPBERRY:			
Black (USDA):			
Fresh:			
Whole	1 lb. (weighed with caps & stems)	160	34.6
Without caps & stems	½ cup (2.4 oz.)	49	10.5
Canned, water pack unsweetened, solids & liq.	4 oz.	58	12.1
Red (USDA):			
Fresh:			
Whole	1 lb. (weighed with caps & stems)	126	29.9
Without caps & stems	½ cup (2.5 oz.)	41	9.8
Canned, water pack, unsweetened or low calorie, solids & liq.	4 oz.	40	10.0
Frozen (Birds Eye) quick thaw:			
Regular	5-oz. serving	155	37.0
In lite syrup	5-oz. serving	110	25.7
RASPBERRY DRINK, mix (Funny Face)	8 fl. oz.	88	22.0
RASPBERRY JUICE, canned:			
(Santa Cruz Natural) red	8 fl. oz.	120	28.0
(Smucker's) red	8 fl. oz.	120	30.0
RASPBERRY JUICE FLOAT, canned (Knudsen & Sons)	8 fl. oz.	130	31.0
RASPBERRY NECTAR, canned (Knudsen & Sons)	8 fl. oz.	120	30.0
RASPBERRY-PEACH JUICE, canned (Knudsen & Sons)	8 fl. oz.	115	28.0
RASPBERRY PRESERVE OR JAM:			
Sweetened (Smucker's)	1 T. (.7 oz.)	53	13.5
Dietetic:			
(Estee; Louis Sherry)	1 T. (.6 oz.)	6	0.0
(Featherweight) red	1 T.	16	4.0

Food	Measure	Cals.	Carbs.
(S&W) *Nutradiet*, red label	1 T.	12	3.0
RAVIOLI:			
Fresh, refrigerated:			
(Contadina) beef or cheese	3 oz.	270	30.0
(Di Giorno) cooked:			
With Italian herb cheese	1 cup	280	35.0
With Italian sausage	1 cup	270	34.0
Canned, regular pack:			
(Chef Boyardee):			
Beef:			
Regular	7½-oz. serving	190	31.0
Supreme, Microwave			
Main meal	10½-oz. serving	290	52.0
Cheese:			
Regular, in meat sauce	7½-oz. serving	200	37.0
Microwave Main Meal,			
supreme	10½-oz. serving	290	52.0
(Franco-American)			
beef, *RavioliOs*	7½-oz. serving	250	35.0
(Hormel) *Micro Cup*, beef	7½-oz. serving	270	34.0
(Libby's) Diner, beef in			
sauce	7½-oz. serving	240	35.0
(Pathmark) no frills, regular			
or bite size	7½-oz. can	180	28.0
Canned, dietetic (Estee)			
beef	7½-oz. can	230	25.0
Frozen:			
(Budget Gourmet) *Light and*			
Healthy, cheese	9½-oz. meal	290	34.0
(Buitoni):			
Regular, square:			
Cheese	4.8-oz. serving	331	45.2
Meat	4.8-oz. serving	318	44.9
Ravioletti:			
Cheese	2.6-oz. serving	221	36.9
Meat	2.6-oz. serving	233	37.1
(Celentano) cheese:			
Regular	½ of 13-oz. box	380	50.0
Mini	½ of 8-oz. box	250	39.0
(Healthy Choice) cheese,			
baked	9-oz. meal	250	44.0
(Kid Cuisine)	8¾-oz. meal	250	52.0
(Weight Watchers) baked	9-oz. meal	240	27.0
RAZZLEBERRY JUICE,			
canned (Knudsen & Sons)	8 fl. oz.	90	21.0

Food	Measure	Cals.	Carbs.
RED & GRAY SNAPPER, raw (USDA):			
Whole	1 lb. (weighed whole)	219	0.0
Meat only	4 oz.	105	0.0
RED LOBSTER **RESTAURANT**			
Calamari, breaded & fried:			
Lunch, portion	5-oz. raw	360	30.0
Dinner portion	10-oz. raw	720	60.0
Catfish:			
Breast	4 oz.	120	0.0
Lunch portion	5-oz. raw	170	0.0
Dinner portion	10-oz. raw	340	0.0
Chicken breast, skinless	4-oz. serving	140	0.0
Clam, cherrystone:			
Lunch portion	5-oz. raw.	130	11.0
Dinner portion	10-oz. raw	260	22.0
Cod, Atlantic, fillet:			
Lunch portion	5-oz. raw	100	0.0
Dinner portion	10-oz. raw	200	0.0
Crab legs:			
King	1-lb. serving	150	33.0
Snow	1-lb. serving	170	32.0
Flounder:			
Lunch portion	5-oz. raw	100	1.0
Dinner portion	10-oz. raw	200	2.0
Grouper:			
Lunch portion	5-oz. raw	110	0.0
Dinner portion	10-oz. raw	220	0.0
Haddock:			
Lunch portion	5-oz. raw	110	2.0
Dinner portion	10-oz. raw	220	4.0
Halibut:			
Lunch portion	5-oz. raw	110	1.0
Dinner portion	10-oz. raw	220	2.0
Hamburger, no bun	5.3-oz. serving	320	0.0
Langostino:			
Lunch portion	5-oz. raw	120	2.0
Dinner portion	10-oz. raw	240	4.0
Lobster:			
Maine	1½ lb.	240	5.0
Rock	1 tail	230	2.0
Mackerel:			
Lunch portion	5 oz. raw	190	20.0
Dinner portion	10 oz. raw	380	40.0

Food	Measure	Cals.	Carbs.
Monkfish:			
Lunch portion	5 oz. raw	110	24.0
Dinner portion	10-oz. raw	220	48.0
Mussel	3 oz.	70	3.0
Oyster, raw, on half shell	6 oysters	110	11.0
Red snapper:			
Lunch portion	5-oz raw	110	0.0
Dinner portion	10-oz. raw	220	0.0
Salmon:			
Norwegian:			
Lunch portion	5-oz. raw	230	3.0
Dinner portion	10-oz. raw	460	6.0
Sockeye:			
Lunch portion	5-oz. raw	160	3.0
Dinner portion	10-oz. raw	320	6.0
Scallop:			
Calico:			
Lunch portion	5-oz. raw	180	8.0
Dinner portion	10-oz. raw	360	16.0
Deep sea:			
Lunch portion	5-oz. raw	130	2.0
Dinner portion	10-oz. raw	260	4.0
Shark:			
Blacktip:			
Lunch portion	5-oz. raw	150	0.0
Dinner portion	10-oz. raw	300	0.0
Mako:			
Lunch portion	5-oz. raw	140	0.0
Dinner portion	10-oz. raw	280	0.0
Shrimp	8–12 pieces	120	0.0
Steak, strip	7-oz. serving	690	0.0
Swordfish:			
Lunch portion	5-oz. raw	100	0.0
Dinner portion	10-oz. raw	200	0.0
Trout:			
Lunch portion	5-oz. raw	170	0.0
Dinner portion	10-oz. raw	340	0.0
RELISH:			
Dill (Vlasic)	1 oz.	2	1.0
Hamburger:			
(Heinz)	1 T.	30	8.0
(Vlasic)	1 oz.	40	9.0
Hot dog:			
(Heinz)	1 oz.	35	8.0
(Vlasic)	1 oz.	40	8.0
India (Heinz)	1 oz.	35	9.0

Food	Measure	Cals.	Carbs.
Sour (USDA)	1 T. (.5 oz.)	3	.4
Sweet:			
(Heinz)	1 oz.	25	6.6
(Vlasic)	1 oz.	30	8.0
RHINE WINE:			
(Great Western) 12% alcohol	3 fl. oz.	73	2.9
(Taylor) 12½% alcohol	3 fl. oz.	75	.3
RHUBARB (USDA)			
Cooked, sweetened, solids & liq.	½ cup (4.2 oz.)	169	43.2
Fresh:			
Partly trimmed	1 lb. (weighed with part leaves, fends & trimmings)	54	12.6
Trimmed	4 oz.	18	4.2
Diced	½ cup (2.2 oz.)	10	2.3
*RICE:			
Basmate (Fantastic Foods):			
With butter	½ cup	115	22.0
Without butter	½ cup	102	22.0
Brown (Uncle Ben's)			
parboiled, with added butter & salt	⅔ cup	152	26.4
White:			
(USDA) instant or pre-cooked	⅔ cup (3.3 oz.)	101	22.5
(Minute Rice) instant, no added butter	⅔ cup (4.3 oz.)	120	27.4
(River)	½ cup	100	22.0
(Success) long grain	½ cup	110	23.0
*(Uncle Ben's):			
Cooked without butter or salt	⅔ cup	129	28.9
Cooked with butter and salt	⅔ cup	148	28.9
White & wild (Carolina)	½ cup	90	20.0
RICE, FRIED (See also RICE MIX):			
*Canned (La Choy)	⅓ of 11-oz. can	190	40.0
Frozen:			
(Birds Eye)	3.7-oz. serving	104	22.8
(Chun King):			
Chicken	8 oz.	254	40.0
Pork	8 oz.	263	43.0
(La Choy) & meat	8-oz. serving	280	52.0

Food	Measure	Cals.	Carbs.
RICE & VEGETABLE, frozen:			
(Birds Eye):			
For One:			
& broccoli, au gratin	5-oz. pkg.	229	25.0
with green beans &			
almonds	5½-oz. pkg.	200	23.6
Mexican, with corn	5½-oz. pkg.	158	29.9
Pilaf	5½-oz. pkg.	215	27.6
International:			
Country style	⅓ of 10-oz. pkg.	87	19.0
French style	⅓ of 10-oz. pkg.	106	23.0
Spanish style	⅓ of 10-oz. pkg.	111	24.0
(Green Giant):			
One Serving Vegetable:			
& broccoli in cheese sauce	4½-oz. pkg.	180	25.0
with peas & mushrooms			
with sauce	5½-oz. pkg.	130	27.0
Rice Originals:			
& broccoli in cheese sauce	4 oz.	120	18.0
Medley	4 oz.	100	19.0
& wild rice	4 oz.	130	24.0
*RICE & VEGETABLE MIX:			
(Knorr) risotto:			
With mushroom or onions	½ cup	130	24.0
With peas & corn	½ cup	130	23.0
(Lipton) & sauce:			
Asparagus with			
hollandaise sauce	½ cup	123	24.9
& broccoli, with			
cheddar cheese sauce	½ cup	131	26.1
RICE BRAN (USDA)	1 oz.	78	14.4
RICE CAKE:			
(Hain):			
Regular, any type	1 piece	40	8.0
Mini:			
Plain, apple cinnamon			
or teriyaki	½-oz. serving	50	12.0
Barbecue or			
nacho cheese	½-oz. serving	70	10.0
Cheese	½-oz. serving	60	10.0
Honeynut	½-oz. serving	60	12.0
Ranch	½-oz. serving	40	4.0
Heart Lovers (TKI			
Foods)	.3-oz. piece	35	6.0

Food	Measure	Cals.	Carbs.
(Pritikin)	1 piece	35	6.0
(Quaker):			
Apple cinnamon:			
Regular	1 piece	40	9.0
Mini	1 piece	10	2.4
Caramel corn, mini	1 piece	10	2.4
Cinnamon crunch, fat free	1 piece	50	11.0
Corn	1 piece	35	7.4
Multi-grain	.32-oz-piece	34	6.9
Plain	.32-oz. piece	35	7.1
Ranch	1 piece	35	6.5
Wheat	1 piece	34	6.7
*RICE MIX:			
Alfredo (Uncle Ben's) *Country Inn Recipes*	½ cup	140	23.0
Asparagus:			
(Lipton) & sauce, with hollandaise sauce:			
Made with butter	½ cup	170	25.0
Made with margarine	½ cup	150	25.0
(Uncle Ben's) au gratin, *Country Inn Recipes*	½ cup	130	22.0
Beef:			
(Lipton) & sauce, prepared with butter	½ cup	150	26.0
(Minute Rice) prepared with butter:			
Family size	½ cup	160	25.0
Single size	½ cup	150	25.0
(Rice-A-Roni)	½ cup	140	24.0
(Success Rice)	½ cup	100	19.0
Beef broccoli (Rice-A-Roni)	½ cup	140	24.0
Beef with mushrooms (Rice-A-Roni)	½ cup	150	26.0
Broccoli:			
(Rice-A-Roni) *Savory Classics*	½ cup	180	21.0
(Uncle Ben's) *Country Inn Recipes:*			
Amondine	½ cup	130	23.0
Au gratin	½ cup	130	22.0
Broccoli & cheddar cheese (Minute Rice) made with butter	½ cup	160	26.0
Brown & wild:			
(Success Rice)	½ cup	120	23.0

Food	Measure	Cals.	Carbs.
(Uncle Ben's)	½ cup	130	27.0
Brown & Wild with mushrooms (Uncle Ben's)	½ cup	130	27.0
Cajun (Lipton) & sauce, made with butter	½ cup	150	26.0
Cauliflower, au gratin:			
(Rice-A-Roni) *Savory Classics*	½ cup	170	23.0
(Uncle Ben's) *Country Inn Classics*	½ cup	130	23.0
Cheddar cheese (Rice-A-Roni):			
White, with herbs	½ cup	65	26.0
Zesty, *Savory Classics*	½ cup	180	25.0
Chicken:			
(Lipton) & sauce, made with butter	½ cup	150	25.0
(Minute Rice):			
Family size	½ cup	160	27.0
Single size	½ cup	150	27.0
(Rice-A-Roni)	½ cup	110	18.0
Chicken with broccoli (Rice-A-Roni)	½ cup	150	25.0
Chicken with creamy mushroom (Uncle Ben's) *Country Inn Recipes*	½ cup	140	25.0
Chicken with mushrooms:			
(Rice-A-Roni)	½ cup	180	26.0
(Uncle Ben's) *Mushroom Royale, Country Inn Recipes*	½ cup	120	25.0
Drumstick (Minute Rice made with butter	½ cup	150	25.0
Florentine (Uncle Ben's)	½ cup	140	24.0
Fried:			
(Minute Rice) made with oil, without butter or salt	½ cup	160	25.0
(Rice-A-Roni):			
Plain	½ cup	110	21.0
With almonds, ½ less salt	½ cup	130	26.0
Green bean amondine:			
(Rice-A-Roni) *Savory Classics*	½ cup	210	22.0
(Uncle Ben's) casserole, *Country Inn Recipes*	½ cup	120	23.0
Herb, au gratin:			
(Success Rice)	½ cup	100	20.0

Food	Measure	Cals.	Carbs.
(Uncle Ben's) *Country Inn Recipe*	½ cup	140	25.0
Herb butter:			
(Lipton) & sauce, made with butter	½ cup	150	24.0
(Rice-A-Roni)	½ cup	130	22.0
Long grain & wild:			
(Lipton) & sauce, made with butter	½ cup	150	26.0
(Minute Rice):			
Without salt or butter	½ cup	120	20.2
With salted butter	½ cup	150	25.0
(Rice-A-Roni) original	½ cup	130	23.0
(Uncle Ben's):			
Regular:			
Without salt or butter	½ cup	100	22.0
With salt & butter	½ cup	120	22.0
Fast cooking; made with salt and butter	½ cup	130	21.0
Long grain & wild with chicken & almonds (Rice-A-Roni)	½ cup	140	24.0
Mushrooms (Lipton) & sauce, made with butter	½ cup	150	26.0
Mushrooms with oriental-style sauce (Ultra Slim Fast)	½ cup	120	29.0
Pilaf:			
(Lipton) & sauce:			
Made with 2 T. butter	½ cup	170	25.0
Made with 1 tsp. margarine	½ cup	140	25.0
(Rice-A-Roni)	½ cup	150	25.0
(Success Rice)	½ cup	120	24.0
Rib roast (Minute rice) made with salted butter	½ cup	150	25.0
Risotto (Rice-A-Roni)	½ cup	200	32.0
Spanish:			
(Lipton) & sauce, made with 1 T. butter	½ cup	140	26.0
(Rice-A-Roni)	½ cup	150	25.0
*(Carolina) *Bake-It-Easy*	¼ of pkg.	110	23.0
*(Lipton) & sauce	½ cup	120	25.7
*(Minute Rice)	½ cup (5.2 oz.)	150	25.6
Rice-A-Roni	⅓ of 7½-oz. pkg.	110	22.0
*Tomato (Knorr)	½ cup	130	23.0

Food	Measure	Cals.	Carbs.
RICE PUDDING (See **PUDDING OR PIE FILLING**)			
RICE SEASONING MIX:			
Fried:			
*(Durkee)	1 cup	213	46.5
(Kikkoman)	1-oz. pkg.	91	15.6
Spice Your Rice (French's):			
Beef flavor & onion, cheese & chives or chicken flavor & parmesan	½ cup	160	27.0
Buttery herb	½ cup	170	27.0
Chicken flavor & herb	½ cup	160	26.0
RICE WINE (HEW/FAO):			
Chinese, 20.7% alcohol	1 fl. oz.	38	1.1
Japanese, 10.6% alcohol	1 fl. oz.	72	13.1
RIGATONI:			
Dry and fresh, refrigerated (See **PASTA, DRY OR FRESH, REFRIGERATED**)			
Frozen:			
(Budget Gourmet) *Light and Healthy,* in cream sauce with broccoli & chicken	10.8-oz. meal	290	44.0
(Healthy Choice):			
Regular, with meat sauce	9½-oz. meal	260	34.0
Extra Portion, with chicken & vegetables	12½-oz. meal	360	50.0
(Stouffer's):			
Regular, homestyle, with meat sauce	12-oz. meal	400	49.0
Lean Cuisine, baked, with meat sauce & cheese	9¾-oz. meal	250	27.0
ROCK & RYE (Mr. Boston) 27% alcohol	1 fl. oz.	75	6.8
ROCKY ROAD, cereal (General Mills)	⅔ cup (1 oz.)	120	23.0

Food	Measure	Cals.	Carbs.
ROE (USDA):			
Raw:			
Carp, cod haddock, herring, pike or shad	4 oz.	147	1.7
Salmon, sturgeon or turbot	4 oz.	235	1.6
Baked or broiled, cod & shad	4 oz.	143	2.2
Canned, cod, haddock or herring, solids & liq.	4 oz.	134	.3
ROLL OR BUN:			
Commercial type, non-frozen:			
Apple (Dolly Madison)	2-oz. piece	180	33.0
Banquet (Mrs. Wright's)	1-oz. roll	90	17.0
Biscuit (Mrs. Wright's)	1-oz. piece	90	15.0
Blunt (Mrs. Wright's)	2-oz. piece	150	28.0
Brown & serve:			
(Interstate Brands) *Merita*	1-oz. roll	70	14.0
(Mrs. Wright's):			
Buttermilk, cloverleaf, gem or twin	1 piece	90	13.0
Half & half	1 piece	100	15.0
Sesame	1 piece	80	15.0
Sesame seed	1 piece	90	15.0
(Pepperidge Farm):			
Club	1 piece	100	19.0
French	1 piece	240	48.0
Hearth	1 piece	50	10.0
(Roman Meal)	1-oz. piece	72	12.6
Cherry (Dolly Madison)	2-oz. piece	180	33.0
Cinnamon (Dolly Madison)	1¾-oz. piece	180	28.0
Country (Pepperidge Farm)	1 piece	50	9.0
Crescent (Pepperidge Farm) butter	1-oz. piece	110	13.0
Croissant:			
(Pepperidge Farm)	1 piece	170	22.0
(Awrey's):			
Butter	3-oz. roll	300	32.0
Margarine	2½-oz. roll	250	26.0
Wheat	2½-oz. roll	240	24.0
(Pepperidge Farm)	1 piece	170	22.0
Danish:			
(Awrey's) filled:			
Apple:			
Miniature	1.7-oz. piece	160	21.0

Food	Measure	Cals.	Carbs.
Round	2¾-oz. piece	270	34.0
Square	3-oz. piece	220	34.0
Cheese:			
Miniature	1.7-oz. piece	170	21.0
Round	2¾-oz. piece	280	34.0
Square	2½-oz. piece	210	25.0
Cinnamon-raisin, square	3-oz. piece	290	41.0
Pineapple, miniature	1.7-oz. piece	157	21.0
Strawberry:			
Miniature	1.7-oz. piece	160	21.0
Round	2¾-oz. piece	270	34.0
(Dolly Madison) *Danish Twirls:*			
Apple	2-oz. piece	240	28.0
Cheese, cream	3½-oz. piece	380	43.0
Cherry	2-oz. piece	230	28.0
Cinnamon-raisin	2-oz. piece	250	28.0
Deli krisp (Mrs. Wright's)	1.3-oz. roll	120	20.0
Dinner:			
(Awrey's):			
Regular	1 piece	60	11.0
Black Forest	1 piece	50	10.0
Cracked wheat	1 piece	50	10.0
Crusty	1 piece	70	12.0
Dinner party	1 piece	51	9.4
Sesame seed	1 piece	60	11.0
Butternut	1-oz. roll	90	15.0
Eddy's	1-oz. roll	75	14.0
Holsum	1-oz. roll	90	15.0
(Mrs. Wright's) split top	1.1-oz. roll	80	14.0
(Roman Meal)	1-oz. roll	75	12.7
Egg, *Weber's*	1-oz. bun	70	12.0
Farmstyle (Mrs. Wright's)	1-oz. piece	90	15.0
Finger (Pepperidge Farm) poppy seed	1 piece	50	8.0
Frankfurter:			
(Awrey's) oat bran	1 roll	110	20.0
(Mrs. Wright's):			
Regular	1 piece	110	19.0
Sesame	1 piece	120	21.0
Wheat, crushed	1.5-oz. piece	110	22.0
(Pepperidge Farm):			
Regular	1 piece	140	24.0
Dijon	1 piece	160	23.0
(Roman Meal) original	1.5-oz. roll	104	19.3

Food	Measure	Cals.	Carbs.
French (Arnold) *Francisco:*			
Regular	2-oz. roll	160	31.0
Sourdough	1.1-oz. piece	90	16.0
Golden Twist			
(Pepperidge Farm)	1-oz. piece	110	14.0
Hamburger:			
(Mrs. Wright's):			
Regular	2.3-oz. piece	190	35.0
Giant, plain	2½-oz. piece	200	37.0
Lite	1 piece	80	15.0
Multi-meal or onion	1 piece	130	24.0
Sesame	1.7-oz. piece	140	25.0
Sesame	2.3-oz. piece	200	34.0
Wheat, crushed:			
Regular	1.6-oz. piece	120	24.0
Giant	2.3-oz. piece	170	34.0
(Pepperidge Farm)	1.5-oz. piece	130	22.0
(Roman Meal)	1.6-oz. piece	122	20.6
Hard (USDA)	1.8-oz. piece	156	29.8
Hoagie (Pepperidge Farm)	1 piece	210	34.0
Honey (Dolly Madison)	3½-oz. piece	420	47.0
Lemon (Dolly Madison)	2-oz. piece	180	31.0
Old fashioned (Pepperidge Farm)	.6-oz. piece	50	7.0
Parkerhouse (Pepperidge Farm)	.6-oz. piece	50	9.0
Party (Pepperidge Farm)	.4-oz. piece	30	5.0
Potato:			
(Mrs. Wright's)	1 piece	100	18.0
(Pepperidge Farm):			
Hearty, classic	1 piece	90	14.0
Sandwich bun	1 piece	160	28.0
Pull-apart (Mrs. Wright's)	2-oz. piece	170	23.0
Raspberry (Dolly Madison)	2-oz. piece	190	31.0
Soft (Pepperidge Farm)	1¼-oz. piece	100	18.0
Steak, *Butternut*	1-oz. roll	80	14.0
Sub (Mrs. Wright's):			
Regular	5-oz. piece	310	70.0
Jr.	3-oz. piece	220	45.0
Tea (Mrs. Wright's)	1 piece	70	4.0
Frozen:			
(Pepperidge Farm):			
Crescent, *Deli Classic*	1 piece	110	13.0
Danish, cinnamon	1 piece	280	34.0
Hoagie, *Deli classic*	1 piece	210	34.0

Food	Measure	Cals.	Carbs.
(Sara Lee):			
Croissant, butter	1 piece	170	19.0
Danish:			
Apple:			
Free & Light	⅛ of pkg.	130	30.0
Individual	1.3-oz. piece	120	15.0
Twist	⅛ of pkg.	190	22.0
Cheese	1.3-oz. piece	130	13.0
Cinnamon-raisin	1.3-oz. piece	150	17.0
*ROLL OR BUN DOUGH:			
Frozen (Rich's) home style	1 roll	75	14.0
Refrigerated (Pillsbury):			
Butterflake	1 piece	140	20.0
Caramel danish, with nuts	1 piece	160	19.0
Cinnamon:			
Regular	1 piece	210	29.0
With icing:			
Regular	1 piece	110	17.0
& raisin	1 piece	140	19.5
Crescent	1 piece	100	11.0
*ROLL MIX, HOT (Pillsbury)	1 piece	100	17.0
ROMAN MEAL CEREAL, HOT:			
Regular:			
Cream of rye	⅓ cup (1.3 oz.)	112	27.3
Multi bran with cinnamon apples	⅓ cup (1.2 oz.)	112	23.8
Oat bran	¼ cup (1 oz.)	93	17.4
Oats, wheat, dates, raisins & almonds	⅓ cup (1.3 oz.)	136	25.6
Original:			
Plain	⅓ cup (1 oz.)	82	20.3
With oats	⅓ cup (1.2 oz.)	106	23.3
Instant, oats, wheat, honey, coconut & almond	⅓ cup (1.3 oz.)	154	23.9
ROSEMARY LEAVES			
(French's)	1 tsp.	5	.8
ROSÉ WINE:			
Corbett Canyon (Glenmore)	3 fl. oz.	63	<1.0
(Great Western) 12% alcohol	3 fl. oz.	80	2.4

Food	Measure	Cals.	Carbs.
(Paul Masson):			
Regular, 11.8% alcohol	3 fl. oz.	76	4.2
Light, 7.1% alcohol	3 fl. oz.	49	3.9
ROY ROGERS:			
Biscuit	1 biscuit	231	26.2
Breakfast crescent sandwich:			
Regular	4.5-oz. sandwich	408	28.0
With bacon	4.7-oz. sandwich	446	28.0
With ham	5.8-oz. sandwich	456	29.0
With sausage	5.7-oz. sandwich	564	28.0
Cheeseburger:			
Regular	1 serving	525	37.0
Bacon	1 serving	552	31.0
Express:			
Plain	1 serving	613	30.0
With bacon	1 serving	641	33.0
Small	1 serving	275	24.0
Chicken:			
Breast	1 piece (5.1 oz.)	412	16.9
Breast & wing	6.9-oz. piece	604	25.4
Leg	1 piece (1.9 oz.)	140	5.5
Thigh	1 piece (3.5 oz.)	296	11.7
Thigh & leg	5.3-oz. piece	436	17.2
Wing	1 piece (1.8 oz.)	192	8.5
Chicken nugget	1 piece	48	3.5
Coleslaw	3½-oz. serving	110	11.0
Danish, swirl:			
Apple	1 piece	328	62.0
Cheese	1 piece	383	54.0
Drinks:			
Coffee, black	6 fl. oz.	Tr.	Tr.
Cola:			
Regular	12 fl. oz.	145	37.0
Diet	12 fl. oz.	1	0.0
Hot chocolate	6 fl. oz.	123	22.0
Milk	8 fl.oz.	150	11.4
Orange juice:			
Regular	7 fl. oz.	99	22.8
Large	10 fl. oz.	136	31.2
Shake:			
Chocolate	1 shake	358	61.3
Strawberry	1 shake	306	45.0
Vanilla	1 shake	315	49.4

Food	Measure	Cals.	Carbs.
Tea, iced, plain	8 fl.oz.	0	0.0
Egg & biscuit platter:			
Regular	1 meal	559	44.0
With bacon	1 meal	607	44.0
With ham	1 meal	607	44.0
With sausage	1 meal	713	44.0
Hamburger:			
Regular	1 serving	472	37.0
Express	1 serving	561	42.0
Roy Rogers Bar	1 serving	573	38.0
Small	1 serving	222	23.0
Pancake platter, with syrup & butter			
Plain	1 order	386	63.0
With bacon	1 order	436	63.0
With ham	1 order	434	64.0
With sausage	1 order	542	63.0
Potato:			
Baked, plain	1 serving	211	48.0
French fried:			
Regular	4 oz.	320	39.0
Small	3 oz.	238	29.0
Large	5½ oz.	440	54.0
Potato salad	3½-oz. order	107	10.9
Roast beef sandwich:			
Plain:			
Regular	1 sandwich	350	37.0
Large	1 sandwich	373	35.0
With cheese:			
Regular	1 sandwich	403	29.0
Large	1 sandwich	427	30.3
Roy's Roasters:			
Skin on:			
Breast/wing	1 serving	500	3.0
Thigh/leg quarter	1 serving	490	2.0
Skin off:			
Breast/wing	1 serving	190	2.0
Thigh/leg quarter	1 serving	190	1.0
Salad bar:			
Bacon bits	1 T.	33	2.2
Beets, sliced	¼ cup	18	2.0
Broccoli	½ cup	12	3.5
Carrot, shredded	¼ cup	12	9.7
Cheese, cheddar	¼ cup	112	.8
Croutons	1 T.	35	7.0

Food	Measure	Cals.	Carbs.
Cucumber	1 slice	Tr.	.2
Egg, chopped	1 T.	27	.3
Lettuce	1 cup	10	4.0
Macaroni salad	1 T.	30	3.1
Mushrooms	¼ cup	5	.7
Noodle, Chinese	¼ cup	55	6.5
Pea, green	¼ cup	7	1.2
Pepper, green	1 T.	2	.5
Potato salad	1 T.	25	2.8
Sunflower seeds	1 T.	78	2.5
Tomato	1 slice	7	1.6
Salad dressing:			
Regular:			
Bacon & tomato	1 T.	68	3.0
Bleu cheese	1 T.	75	1.0
Ranch	1 T.	77	2.0
1000 Island	1 T.	80	2.0
Low calorie, Italian	1 T.	35	1.0
Sundae:			
Caramel	1 sundae	293	51.5
Hot fudge	1 sundae	337	53.3
Strawberry	1 sundae	216	33.1

RUM (See **DISTILLED LIQUOR**)

RUTABAGA:
Raw (USDA):

Without tops	1 lb. (weighed with skin)	177	42.4
Diced	½ cup (2.5 oz.)	32	7.7
Boiled (USDA) drained, diced	½ cup (3 oz.)	30	7.1
Canned (Sunshine) solids & liq.	½ cup (4.2 oz.)	32	6.9

RYE, whole grain (USDA)	1 oz.	95	20.8

RYE FLOUR (See **FLOUR**)

RYE WHISKEY (See **DISTILLED LIQUOR**)

Food	Measure	Cals.	Carbs.

S

SABLEFISH, raw (USDA):

Whole	1 lb. (weighed whole)	362	0.0
Meat only	4 oz.	215	0.0

SAFFLOWER SEED (USDA) in hull

hull	1 oz.	89	1.8

SAKE WINE (HEW/FAO)

19.8% alcohol	1 fl. oz.	39	1.4

*SALAD BAR PASTA (Buitoni):

Country buttermilk or homestyle	⅙ of pkg.	250	22.0
Italian:			
Creamy	⅙ of pkg.	290	20.0
Zesty	⅙ of pkg.	140	21.0

SALAD, MIXED, fresh (Dole):

Regular:			
Classic or french	3½-oz. serving	25	4.0
Italian	3½-oz. serving	25	3.0
Salad-in-a-Minute:			
Caesar	3½-oz. serving	170	9.0
Oriental	3½-oz. serving	110	12.0
Spinach	3½-oz. serving	180	19.0

SALAD DRESSING:

Regular:			
Bacon & tomato (Henri's)	1 T.	70	4.0
Bleu or blue cheese:			
(USDA)	1 T. (.5 oz.)	76	1.1
(Henri's)	1 T.	60	3.0
(Nu Made)	1 T.	60	1.0
(Wish-Bone) chunky	1 T.	73	.8
Boiled (USDA) home recipe	1 T. (.6 oz.)	26	2.4

Food	Measure	Cals.	Carbs.
Buttermilk:			
(Hain)	1 T.	70	0.0
(Nu Made)	1 T.	50	1.0
Caesar:			
(Hain) creamy	1 T.	60	1.0
(Wish-Bone)	1 T.	78	.9
Cheddar bacon (Wish-Bone)	1 T. (.5 oz.)	70	1.0
Cucumber, creamy:			
(Nu Made)	1 T.	70	1.0
(Wish-Bone)	1 T. (.5 oz.)	80	1.0
Cucumber dill (Hain)	1 T.	80	0.0
Dijon vinaigrette:			
(Hain)	1 T.	50	0.0
(Wish-Bone)	1 T.	60	1.0
French:			
Home recipe (USDA)	1 T.	101	.6
(Hain) creamy	1 T.	60	1.0
(Henri's):			
Hearty	1 T.	70	4.0
Original	1 T.	60	3.0
Sweet 'n saucy	1 T.	70	5.0
(Nu Made) savory	1 T.	60	2.0
(Wish-Bone):			
Deluxe	1 T.	57	2.3
Red	1 T.	64	3.9
French mustard (Hain)	1 T.	50	1.0
Green tomato vinaigrette			
(Hain)	1 T.	60	1.0
Garlic & sour cream (Hain)	1 T.	70	0.0
Green goddess (Nu Made)	1 T.	60	1.0
Honey & sesame (Hain)	1 T.	60	2.0
Italian:			
(Hain):			
Canola oil	1 T.	50	1.0
& cheese vinaigrette	1 T.	55	0.0
Creamy or traditional	1 T.	80	0.0
(Henri's):			
Authentic	1 T.	80	1.0
Creamy garlic	1 T.	50	3.0
(Wish-Bone):			
Creamy	1 T.	56	1.7
Herbal	1 T.	70	1.2
Robusto	1 T.	70	1.3
Mayonnaise (See **MAYONNAISE**)			
Mayonnaise-type:			
(Luzianne) Blue Plate	1 T.	70	3.0

Food	Measure	Cals.	Carbs.
Miracle Whip (Kraft)	1 T.	70	2.0
Ranch (Henri's) *Chef's Recipe*	1 T.	70	2.0
Red wine vinegar & oil (Wish-Bone)	1 T.	50	4.3
Roquefort (USDA)	1 T. (.5 oz.)	76	1.1
Russian:			
(USDA)	1 T.	74	1.6
(Henri's)	1 T.	60	4.0
(Wish-Bone)	1 T.	45	5.9
Swiss cheese vinaigrette (Hain)	1 T.	60	0.0
Tangy citrus (Hain)	1 T.	50	1.0
Tas-Tee (Henri's)	1 T.	60	4.0
1000 Island:			
(USDA)	1 T.	80	2.5
(Hain)	1 T.	50	0.0
(Henri's)	1 T.	50	2.0
(Nu Made)	1 T.	60	3.0
(Wish-Bone)	1 T.	61	3.2
Dietetic or low calorie:			
Bleu or blue cheese:			
(Estee)	1 T. (.5 oz.)	8	1.0
(Henri's)	1 T.	35	5.0
Herb Magic (Luzianne Blue Plate) creamy	1 T.	8	2.0
(Hidden Valley Ranch) low fat	1 T.	10	3.0
(S&W) *Nutradiet*	1 T.	25	2.0
(Walden Farms) chunky	1 T.	27	1.7
(Wish-Bone) chunky	1 T.	40	1.0
Caesar:			
(Hain) low salt	1 T.	60	1.0
(Weight Watchers)	¾-oz. pouch	6	1.0
Catalina (Kraft)	1 T.	16	3.0
Chef's Recipe (Henri's) ranch	1 T.	40	6.0
Creamy (S&W) *Nutradiet*:			
Regular	1 T.	10	1.0
No oil	1 T.	2	0.0
Cucumber:			
(Kraft) creamy	1 T.	30	1.0
(Luzianne Blue Plate) *Herb Magic,* creamy	1 T. (.6 oz.)	8	2.0
Cucumber & onion (Henri's) creamy	1 T.	35	6.0
Dijon (Estee)	1 T.	8	1.0

Food	Measure	Cals.	Carbs.
French:			
(Estee)	1 T. (.5 oz.)	4	1.0
(Henri's):			
Hearty	1 T.	30	5.0
Original	1 T.	40	6.0
(Pritikin)	1 T.	10	2.0
(S&W) *Nutradiet*	1 T.	18	3.0
(Walden Farms)	1 T.	33	2.6
(Wish-Bone):	1 T.	31	2.1
Regular	1 T.	30	1.9
Red	1 T.	17	3.2
Sweet & spicy	1 T.	18	3.2
Garlic (Estee)	1 T. (.5 oz.)	2	0.0
Herb basket, *Herb Magic*			
(Luzianne Blue Plate)	1 T.	6	2.0
Italian:			
(Estee) creamy	1 T. (.5 oz.)	4	0.0
(Estee) spicy	1 T.	4	1.0
(Hain) creamy	1 T.	80	1.0
(Henri's) authentic	1 T.	20	2.0
Herb Magic (Luzianne			
Blue Plate)	1 T.	4	1.0
(Kraft) zesty	1 T.	6	1.0
(Pritikin):			
Regular	1 T.	6	2.0
Creamy	1 T.	16	3.0
(Walden Farms):			
Regular or low sodium	1 T.	9	1.5
No sugar added	1 T.	6	Tr.
(Weight Watchers) regular	1 T.	50	2.0
(Wish-Bone)	1 T	7	.9
Ranch:			
Herb Magic (Luzianne			
Blue Plate)	1 T.	6	1.0
(Pritikin)	1 T.	18	4.0
(Weight Watchers)	¾-oz. pkg.	35	8.0
(Wish-Bone)	1 T.	46	2.3
Red wine vinegar			
(Estee)	1 T.	2	0.0
Russian:			
(Pritikin)	1 T.	12	3.0
(Weight Watchers)	1 T. (.5 oz.)	50	2.0
(Wish-Bone)	1 T. (.5 oz.)	22	3.9
Tas-Tee (Henri's)	1 T.	30	4.0
1000 Island:			
(Estee)	1 T.	8	2.0
(Henri's)	1 T.	30	4.0

Food	Measure	Cals.	Carbs.
Herb Magic (Luzianne Blue Plate)	1 T.	8	2.0
(Kraft)	1 T.	30	2.0
(Walden Farms)	1 T.	24	3.1
(Weight Watchers)	1 T.	50	2.0
(Wish-Bone)	1 T.	36	1.9
Vinaigrette (Pritikin)	1 T.	10	2.0
Whipped (Weight Watchers)	1 T. (.5 oz.)	45	2.0
*SALAD DRESSING MIX:			
Regular (Good Seasons):			
Blue cheese & herbs	1 T. (.6 oz.)	72	1.0
Buttermilk, farm style	1 T. (.6 oz.)	58	1.2
Classic dill	1 T.	70	.5
Garlic, cheese	1 T.	72	1.0
Garlic & herb	1 T.	71	1.0
Italian:			
Regular, cheese or zesty	1 T. (.6 oz.)	71	.6
Mild	1 T. (.6 oz.)	73	1.0
Ranch	1 T.	57	1.0
Dietetic:			
Blue cheese (Hain)	1 T.	14	1.0
Buttermilk (Hain)	1 T.	11	1.0
Caesar (Hain) no oil	1 T.	6	1.0
French (Hain) no oil	1 T.	12	3.0
Garlic & cheese (Hain)	1 T.	6	1.0
Herb (Hain)	1 T.	2	1.0
Italian:			
(Good Seasons):			
Regular	1 T.	8	1.8
Regular, fat free	1 T.	6	1.0
Creamy, fat free	1 T.	8	2.0
Lite	1 T.	27	.8
(Hain) no oil	1 T.	2	1.0
Ranch (Good Seasons)	1 T.	29	2.0
Russian (Weight Watchers)	1 T.	4	1.0
1000 Island:			
(Hain)	1 T.	12	3.0
(Weight Watchers)	1 T.	12	1.0
SALAD SUPREME			
(McCormick)	1 tsp. (.1 oz.)	11	.5
SALAD TOPPERS (Pepperidge Farm) any flavor	1 T.	35	4.0

Food	Measure	Cals.	Carbs.
SALAMI:			
(USDA):			
Dry	1 oz.	128	.3
Cooked	1 oz.	88	.4
(Eckrich):			
Beer or cooked	1 oz.	70	1.0
Cotto:			
Beef	.7-oz. slice	50	1.0
Meat	1-oz. slice	70	1.0
Hard	1 oz.	130	1.0
Hebrew National	1 oz.	80	1.0
(Hormel):			
Beef	1 slice	25	0.0
Cotto:			
Chub	1 oz.	100	0.0
Sliced	1 slice	52	5.
Genoa:			
Regular or *Gran Value*	1 oz.	110	0.0
Di Lusso	1 oz.	100	0.0
Hard:			
Packaged, sliced	1 slice	40	0.0
Whole:			
Regular	1 oz.	110	0.0
National Brand	1 oz.	120	0.0
Party slice	1 oz.	90	0.0
Piccolo, stick	1 oz.	120	0.0
(Ohse) cooked	1 oz.	65	1.0
(Oscar Mayer):			
Beer:			
Regular	.8-oz. slice	50	.4
Beef	.8-oz. slice	64	.4
Cotto:			
Regular	.8-oz. slice	53	.4
Beef	.5-oz. slice	29	.2
Beef	.8-oz. slice	46	.4
Genoa	.3-oz. slice	34	.1
Hard	.3-oz. slice	33	.1
(Smok-A-Roma):			
Beef or cotto	1-oz. slice	80	1.0
Turkey	1-oz. slice	45	1.0
SALISBURY STEAK:			
Canned (Top Shelf):			
Regular	10-oz. serving	320	22.0
Microwave bowl, with			
potatoes	1 serving	250	22.0
Frozen:			

Food	Measure	Cals.	Carbs.
(Armour):			
Classics Lite	11½-oz. meal	300	29.0
Dinner Classics:			
Regular	11¼-oz. meal	350	26.0
Parmigiana	11½-oz. meal	410	32.0
(Banquet):			
Regular	11-oz. dinner	500	26.0
Cookin' Bags, with gravy	5-oz. serving	190	8.0
Extra Helping, with			
mushroom gravy	18-oz. dinner	890	48.0
Family Entrees	8-oz. serving	300	12.0
Healthy Balance,			
charbroiled flavor	10½-oz. meal	270	34.0
Platter	10-oz. serving	460	20.0
(Budget Gourmet) sirloin	11½-oz. meal	410	28.0
(Healthy Choice):			
Regular	11½-oz. meal	300	41.0
Classics, with mushroom			
gravy	11-oz. meal	280	35.0
(Le Menu):			
Regular	11½-oz. meal	370	28.0
Lightstyle	10-oz. meal	280	31.0
(Morton)	10-oz. meal	300	23.0
(Stouffer's) *Lean Cuisine,*			
with gravy & potatoes	9½-oz. meal	240	22.0
(Swanson):			
Regular	10¾-oz. meal	400	43.0
Homestyle Recipe	10-oz. meal	320	22.0
Hungry Man	16½-oz. meal	680	37.0
SALMON:			
Atlantic (USDA):			
Raw:			
Whole	1 lb. (weighed		
	whole)	640	0.0
Meat only	4 oz.	246	0.0
Canned, solids & liq.,			
including bones	4 oz.	230	.9
Chinook or King (USDA)			
Raw:			
Steak	1 lb. (weighed		
	whole)	886	0.0
Meat only	4 oz.	252	0.0
Canned, solids & liq., in-			
cluding bones	4 oz.	238	0.0
Chum, canned (USDA), solids			
& liq., including bones	4 oz.	158	0.0

Food	Measure	Cals.	Carbs.
Coho, canned (USDA), solids & liq., including bones	4 oz.	174	0.0
Keta, canned (Peter Pan), solids & liq., including bones	½ cup (3.9 oz.)	140	0.0
Pink or Humpback (USDA):			
Raw:			
Steak	1 lb. (weighed whole)	475	0.0
Meat only	4 oz.	135	0.0
Canned, solids & liq.:			
(USDA) including bones	4 oz.	135	0.0
(Bumble Bee) including bones	½ cup (4 oz.)	155	0.0
(Del Monte)	7¾-oz. can	277	0.0
Sockeye or Red or Blueback, canned, solids & liq.:			
(USDA)	4 oz.	194	0.0
(Bumble Bee) including bones	½ cup (4 oz.)	155	0.0
(Del Monte)	½ of 7¾-oz. can	165	0.0
Unspecified kind of salmon (USDA) baked or broiled	4.2 oz. steak (approx. 4" × 3" × ½")	218	0.0
SALMON, SMOKED (USDA)	4 oz.	200	0.0
SALT:			
Regular:			
Butter-flavored (French's) imitation	1 tsp. (3.6 grams)	8	0.0
Garlic (Lawry's)	1 tsp. (4 grams)	5	1.0
Hickory smoke (French's)	1 tsp. (4 grams)	2	Tr.
Onion (Lawry's)	1 tsp.	4	.9
Seasoned (Lawry's)	1 tsp.	3	.6
Table:			
(USDA)	1 tsp.	0	0.0
(Morton) iodized	1 tsp. (7 grams)	0	0.0
Lite Salt (Morton) iodized	1 tsp. (6 grams)	0	0.0
Substitute:			
(Adolph's):			
Regular	1 tsp. (6 grams)	1	Tr.
Packet	8-gram packet	*1	Tr.
Seasoned	1 tsp.	6	1.1
(Estee) *Salt-It*	½ tsp.	0	0.0
(Morton):			

Food	Measure	Cals.	Carbs.
Regular	1 tsp. (6 grams)	Tr.	Tr.
Seasoned	1 tsp. (6 grams)	3	.5
SALT PORK, raw (USDA):			
With skin	1 lb. (weighed with skin)	3410	0.0
Without skin	1 oz.	222	0.0
SANDWICH DRESSING (Vlassic)			
Sandwich Zesters:			
Bell pepper salsa, garden onion or jalapeño salsa	1 T.	7	2.0
Italian tomato or mushroom & onion	1 T.	5	1.5
SANDWICH SPREAD:			
(USDA)	1 T. (.5 oz.)	57	2.4
(USDA)	½ cup (4.3 oz.)	466	19.5
(Hellmann's)	1 T. (.5 oz.)	55	2.4
(Nu Made)	1 T.	60	4.0
(Oscar Mayer)	1-oz. serving	67	3.6
SANGRIA (Taylor) 11.6% alcohol	3 fl. oz.	99	10.8
SARDINE:			
Raw (HEW/FAO):			
Whole	1 lb. (weighed whole)	321	0.0
Meat only	4 oz.	146	0.0
Canned:			
Atlantic:			
(USDA) in oil:			
Solids & liq.	3¾-oz. can	330	6
Drained solids, with skin & bones	3¾-oz. can	187	DNA
(Del Monte) in tomato sauce, solids & liq.	7½-oz. can	330	4.0
(Underwood):			
In mustard sauce	3¾-oz. can	220	2.0
In tomato sauce	3⅜-oz. can	220	2.0
Norwegian:			
(Granadaisa Brand) in tomato sauce	3¾-oz. can	195	0.0
(King David Brand) brisling, in olive oil	3¾-oz. can	293	0.0
(King Oscar Brand):			

Food	Measure	Cals.	Carbs.
In mustard sauce, solids & liq.	3¾-oz. can	240	2.0
In oil, drained	3-oz. can	260	1.0
In tomato sauce, solids & liq.	3¾-oz. can	240	2.0
(Queen Helga Brand) sild, in sild oil	3¾-oz. can	310	0.0
(Underwood) drained	3-oz. serving	230	1.0
Pacific (USDA) in brine or mustard, solids & liq.	4 oz.	222	1.9
SAUCE (See also **PASTA SAUCE** or **TOMATO SAUCE**)			
Regular:			
Alfredo:			
(Betty Crocker) *Recipe Sauces*	4 oz.	190	8.0
(Contadino):			
Fresh, refrigerated:			
Regular	6 oz.	540	10.0
Light	3.3 oz.	150	7.0
Canned	4 oz.	350	6.0
(Di Giorno)	4 oz.	400	4.0
A-1	1 T. (.6 oz.)	12	3.1
Barbecue:			
(USDA)	1 cup (8.8 oz.)	228	20.0
(Bull's Eye)	1 T. (.5 oz)	25	5.0
(Enrico's):			
Original	1 T.	18	3.0
Mesquite	1 T.	18	3.0
(French's) regular hot or smoky	1 T. (.6 oz.)	14	3.0
(Gold's)	1 T.	16	3.9
(Heinz):			
Regular	½ cup	160	27.0
Hickory smoked & hot	½ cup	160	31.0
Thick and Rich, original	1 oz.	35	8.0
(Hunt's) all natural:			
Original	1.2 oz.	40	9.4
Country style	1 T.	20	5.0
Hickory:			
Regular	1 T.	20	5.0
Bold	1 T.	19	4.2
Homestyle	1 T. (.5 oz.)	17	4.1
(Kraft):			
Plain or hot	½ cup	160	DNA

Food	Measure	Cals.	Carbs.
Onion bits	½ cup	200	DNA
(La Choy) oriental	1 T.	16	3.8
(Lawry's) dijon honey	¼ cup	203	27.0
(Watkins):			
Regular	1 T. (.2 oz.)	37	7.5
Bold	1 T.	37	7.5
Mesquite	1 T.	37	7.5
Smokehouse	1 T.	37	7.5
Cheese (Snow's) Welsh			
Rarebit	½ cup	170	10.0
Chicken:			
Chicken Sensations (Hunt's):			
Barbecue	2 T.	70	6.0
Italian garlic	2 T.	60	2.0
Lemon herb	2 T.	60	4.0
Chicken Tonight (Ragú):			
Cacciatore	4 oz.	70	12.0
Country French	4 oz.	140	6.0
Creamy:			
With mushrooms	4 oz.	110	5.0
Primavera	4 oz.	90	9.0
Herbed, with wine	4 oz.	100	13.0
Honey mustard, light	4 oz.	50	12.0
Chili (See **CHILI SAUCE**)			
Cocktail (See also Seafood cocktail):			
(Gold's)	1 oz.	31	7.5
(Pfeiffer)	1-oz. serving	50	6.0
Creole (Enrico's) Cajun, light	4 oz.	75	9.0
Grilling & broiling (Knorr):			
Chardonnay	⅛ of container	50	4.5
Spicy plum	⅛ of container	60	11.2
Tequila lime	⅛ of container	50	6.4
Tuscan herb	⅛ of container	55	4.6
Hollandaise (Knorr) microwave	¹⁄₁₂ of pkg. (1 oz.)	50	1.0
Hot dog, *Just Right*	2 oz.	60	6.0
Mandarin ginger (Knorr) microwave	⅛ of pkg.	55	5.3
Newberg (Snow's)	⅓ cup	120	10.0
Orange (La Choy)	1 T. (.6 oz.)	23	6.1
Parmesano (Knorr) microwave	⅛ of pkg.	50	3.3
Parmigiana (Betty Crocker) *Recipe Sauces*	3.9 oz.	50	9.0

Food	Measure	Cals.	Carbs.
Pepper steak (Betty Crocker)			
Recipe Sauces	3.8 oz.	45	8.0
Picante (Pace)	1 tsp.	2	.3
Plum (La Choy) tangy	1 oz.	44	10.8
Salsa Brava (La Victoria)	1 T.	6	1.0
Salsa Casera (La Victoria)	1 T.	4	1.0
Salsa Mexicana (Contadina)	4 fl. oz.		
	(4.4 oz.)	38	6.8
Salsa Ranchera (La Victoria)	1 T.	6	1.0
Salsa verde (Old El Paso)	1 T.	5	1.0
Seafood cocktail:			
(Del Monte)	1 T. (.6 oz.)	21	4.9
(Golden Dipt) regular or			
extra hot	1 T.	20	5.0
Soy:			
(USDA)	1 oz.	19	2.7
(Chun King)	1 tsp.	5	.7
(Gold's)	1 T.	10	1.0
(Kikkoman):			
Regular	1 T. (.6 oz.)	10	.9
Light, low sodium	1 T.	11	1.3
(La Choy)	1 T. (.5 oz.)	8	.9
Sparerib (Gold's)	1 oz.	60	14.0
Stir-fry (Kikkoman)	1 tsp.	6	2.3
Stroganoff (Betty Crocker)			
Recipe Sauces	3.8 oz.	60	6.0
Sweet & sour:			
(Chun King)	1.8-oz. serving	57	14.4
(Contadina)	4 fl. oz.		
	(4.4 oz.)	150	29.6
(Kikkoman)	1 T.	18	4.0
(La Choy)	1-oz. serving	30	7.0
Szechuan (La Choy)	1 oz.	48	12.0
Tabasco	¼ tsp.	Tr.	Tr.
Taco:			
(El Molino) red, mild	1 T.	5	1.0
(La Victoria):			
Green	1 T.	4	1.0
Red	1 T.	6	1.0
(Old El Paso), hot or mild	1 T.	5	1.2
(Ortega) hot or mild	1 oz.	13	3.1
Tartar:			
(USDA)	1 T. (.5 oz.)	74	.6
(Hellmann's)	1 T. (.5 oz.)	70	.1
Teriyaki (Kikkoman)	1 T. (.6 oz.)	15	2.7
Vera Cruz (Knorr)	¼ of pkg. (3.4		
microwave	oz.)	65	9.3

Food	Measure	Cals.	Carbs.
White (USDA) home recipe:			
Thin	¼ cup (2.2 oz.)	74	4.5
Medium	¼ cup (2.5 oz.)	103	5.6
Thick	¼ cup (2.2 oz.)	122	6.8
Worcestershire:			
(French's) regular or			
smoky	1 T. (.6 oz.)	10	2.0
(Gold's)	1 T.	42	3.3
(Lea & Perrins)	1 T. (.6 oz.)	12	3.0
Dietetic:			
Barbecue:			
(Estee)	1 T. (.6 oz.)	18	3.0
(Healthy Choice):			
Original or hot & spicy	1 T. (.6 oz.)	14	3.1
Hickory	1 T. (.6 oz.)	14	3.0
(Hunt's) light:			
Original	1.1 oz.	26	6.1
Hickory	1.1 oz.	27	6.2
Mexican (Pritikin)	1 oz.	12	2.0
Soy:			
(Kikkoman) lite	1 T.	9	.3
(La Choy)	1 T.	1	.8
Steak (Estee)	½ oz.	14	3.0
Tartar (USDA)	1 T. (.5 oz.)	31	.9
SAUCE MIX:			
*Au jus (Knorr)	2 fl. oz.	8	1.1
*Bearnaise (Knorr)	2 fl. oz.	170	5.0
*Carbonara (Knorr)	1 T.	35	2.5
*Demi-glace (Knorr)	2 fl. oz.	30	3.9
*Hollandaise (Knorr)	2 fl. oz.	170	5.0
*Hunter (Knorr)	2 fl. oz.	25	3.7
*Italian (Knorr) Napoli	4 fl. oz.	100	17.0
*Lyonnaise (Knorr)	2 fl. oz.	20	3.4
*Mushroom (Knorr)	2 fl. oz.	60	5.0
*Pepper (Knorr)	2 fl. oz.	20	3.0
*Sour cream:			
(Durkee)	⅔ cup	214	15.0
(French's)	2½ T.	60	5.0
*Stroganoff (French's)	⅓ cup	110	11.0
Sweet & sour:			
*(Durkee)	½ cup	115	22.5
*(French's)	½ cup	55	14.0
(Kikkoman)	1 T.	18	4.0
Teriyaki:			
*(French's)	1 T.	17	3.5
(Kikkoman)	1.5-oz. pkg.	125	22.3

Food	Measure	Cals.	Carbs.
*White (Durkee)	½ cup	119	20.5
SAUERKRAUT, canned:			
(USDA):			
Solids & liq.	½ cup (4.1 oz.)	21	4.7
Drained solids	½ cup (2.5 oz.)	15	3.1
(Claussen) drained	½ cup (2.7 oz.)	16	2.9
(Comstock) solids & liq.:			
Regular	½ cup (4.1 oz.)	30	4.0
Bavarian	½ cup (4.2 oz.)	35	7.0
(Frank's) solids & liq.:			
Regular	½ cup	28	4.0
Bavarian	½ cup	64	12.0
(Vlasic)	1 oz.	4	1.0
SAUERKRAUT JUICE, canned:			
(USDA) 2% salt	½ cup (4.3 oz.)	12	2.8
(S&W)	5 oz.	14	3.0
SAUSAGE:			
*Brown & serve:			
(USDA)	1 oz.	120	.8
(Eckrich) Lean Supreme	1 link	60	.5
(Hormel)	1 sausage	70	0.0
Country style (USDA) smoked	1 oz.	98	0.0
German (Smok-A-Roma)	4-oz. link	350	1.0
Italian style, hot or mild			
(Hillshire Farms)	3-oz. serving	263	*1.0
Knockwurst (*Hebrew National*)			
hot	1 oz.	79	.6
Links (Ohse) hot	1 oz.	80	4.0
Patty (Hormel) hot or mild	1 patty	150	0.0
Polish-style:			
(Eckrich) meat:			
Regular	1 oz.	95	1.0
Skinless	1-oz. link	90	1.0
With skin	1-oz. link	180	2.0
(Hillshire Farm):			
Regular:			
Bun size	2 oz.	180	2.0
Polska:			
Flavorseal:			
Regular	2 oz.	190	2.0
Lite	2 oz.	130	1.0
Links	2 oz.	190	2.0
Beef, Polska flavorseal	2 oz.	190	1.0
(Hormel):			

Food	Measure	Cals.	Carbs.
Regular	1 sausage	85	0.0
Kielbasa, skinless	½ a link	180	1.0
Kolbase	3 oz.	220	1.0
(Ohse):			
Regular	1 oz.	80	1.0
Hot	1 oz.	70	3.0
Pork:			
*(USDA)	1 oz.	135	Tr.
(Eckrich):			
Links	1-oz. link	110	.5
Patty	2-oz. patty	240	1.0
Roll, hot	2-oz. serving	240	1.0
*(Hormel):			
Little Sizzlers	1 link	51	0.0
Midget links	1 link	71	0.0
Smoked	1 oz.	96	.3
(Jimmy Dean)	2-oz. serving	227	Tr.
*(Oscar Mayer) *Little Friers*	1 link	79	.3
Roll (Eckrich) minced	1-oz. slice	80	1.0
Smoked:			
(Eckrich):			
Beef:			
Regular	2 oz.	190	1.0
Smok-Y-Links	.8-oz. link	70	1.0
Cheese	2 oz.	180	2.0
Ham, *Smok-Y-Links*	.8-oz. link	75	1.0
Lean Supreme	1 oz.	70	1.0
Maple flavored,			
Smok-Y-Links	.8-oz. link	75	1.0
Meat:			
Regular	2 oz.	190	1.0
Hot	2.7-oz. link	240	3.0
Skinless:			
Regular	2-oz. link	180	2.0
Smok-Y-Links	.8-oz. link	75	1.0
(Hormel) Smokies:			
Regular	1 link	80	.5
Cheese	1 link	84	.5
(Ohse)	1 oz.	80	1.0
(Oscar Mayer):			
Beef	1½-oz. link	126	.7
Cheese	1½-oz. link	127	.8
Little Smokies	1 link	28	.1
Meat	1.5-oz. link	126	.7
Thuringer (See **THURINGER**)			
Turkey (Louis Rich) links or			
tube	1-oz. serving	45	Tr.

Food	Measure	Cals.	Carbs.
Vienna, canned:			
(USDA)	1 link (5-oz. can)	38	Tr.
(Armour):			
In barbecue sauce	2½-oz. serving	190	4.0
In beef stock	2-oz. serving	180	1.0
Chicken, in beef stock	2-oz. serving	150	1.0
Smoked	2-oz. serving	180	1.0
(Hormel):			
Regular	1-oz. serving	69	2.0
Without broth	1 link	50	.2
Chicken	1-oz. serving	56	1.0
(Libby's):			
In barbecue sauce	2½-oz. serving	180	2.0
In beef broth:			
Regular	2-oz. serving	160	1.0
Chicken	2-oz. serving	130	3.0
SAUTERNE:			
(Great Western)	3 fl. oz.	79	4.5
(Taylor)	3 fl. oz.	81	4.8
SCALLION (See ONION, GREEN)			
SCALLOP:			
Raw (USDA) muscle only	4-oz. serving	92	3.7
Steamed (USDA)	4-oz. serving	127	DNA
Frozen:			
(Captain's Choice) fried	1 piece	33	1.5
(Mrs. Paul's) fried, light	3 oz.	160	18.0
SCHNAPPS:			
Apple (Mr. Boston) 27% alcohol	1 fl. oz.	78	8.0
Cinnamon (Mr. Boston) 27% alcohol	1 fl. oz.	76	8.0
Peppermint:			
(De Kuyper)	1 fl. oz.	79	7.5
(Mr. Boston) 50% alcohol	1 fl. oz.	115	8.0
Spearmint (Mr. Boston)	1 fl. oz.	78	7.8
Strawberry (Mr. Boston)	1 fl. oz.	68	6.2
SCOTCH WHISKY (See DISTILLED LIQUOR)			
SCREWDRIVER COCKTAIL			
(Mr. Boston) 12½% alcohol	3 fl. oz.	111	12.0

Food	Measure	Cals.	Carbs.
SCROD, frozen (Gorton's)	1 pkg.	320	17.0
SEA BASS, raw (USDA) meat only	4 oz.	109	0.0
SEASON-ALL **SEASONING** (McCormick)	1 tsp.	4	.6
SEAFOOD CREOLE, frozen (Swanson) *Homestyle Recipe*	9-oz. entree	240	40.0
SEAFOOD NEWBERG, frozen (Healthy Choice)	8-oz. meal	200	30.0
SEAWEED, dried (HHS/FAO):			
Agar	1 oz.	88	23.7
Lavar	1 oz.	67	12.6
SEGO **DIET FOOD,** canned:			
Regular:			
Very chocolate, very chocolate malt or very Dutch chocolate	10 fl. oz.	225	43.0
Very strawberry or very vanilla	10 fl. oz.	225	34.0
Lite:			
Chocolate, chocolate jamocha almond, chocolate malt or Dutch chocolate	10-fl.-oz. can	150	20.0
Double chocolate	10-fl.-oz. can	150	21.0
French vanilla, strawberry or vanilla	10-fl.-oz. can	150	17.0
SELTZER (See **MINERAL WATER**)			
SESAME NUT MIX, canned (Planters) roasted	1 oz.	160	8.0
SESAME SEEDS, dry (USDA):			
Whole	1 oz.	160	6.1
Hulled	1 oz.	165	5.0
7-ELEVEN:			
Burritos:			
Beef & bean:			
Plain	5-oz. serving	305	42.0

Food	Measure	Cals.	Carbs.
With green chili	10-oz. serving	615	84.0
With red chili	5-oz. serving	305	42.0
Red hot	5-oz. serving	310	42.0
Red hot, premium	5.2-oz. serving	359	41.0
Beef, bean & cheese	5.2-oz. serving	395	41.0
Beef & potato	5.2-oz. serving	394	48.0
Chicken & rice, premium	5-oz. serving	244	42.0
Chicken, breast of	4.8-oz. serving	405	48.0
Chimichanga, beef	5-oz. serving	360	42.0
Enchilada, beef & cheese	6½-oz. serving	369	27.6
Fajitas	5-oz. serving	310	40.4
Sandito:			
Ham & cheese	5-oz. serving	399	40.7
Pizza	5 oz. serving	345	38.0
Tacos, soft, twin	5.9-oz. serving	399	40.7
Deli-Shoppe microwave:			
Bacon cheeseburger	6-oz. serving	558	42.7
Bagel & cream cheese	4-oz. serving	338	37.2
Fish sandwich with cheese	5.2-oz. serving	433	20.4
Sausage, red hot	9.3-oz. serving	845	43.0
Turkey, wedge	3.4-oz. serving	193	20.3
SEVEN FRUIT JUICE DRINK, canned (Boku)	8 fl. oz.	120	29.0
7 GRAIN CEREAL (Loma Linda):			
Crunchy	1 oz.	110	21.0
No sugar	1 oz.	110	20.0
SHAD (USDA):			
Raw:			
Whole	1 lb. (weighed whole)	370	0.0
Meat only	4 oz.	193	0.0
Cooked, home recipe:			
Baked with butter or margarine & bacon slices	4 oz.	228	0.0
Creole	4 oz.	172	1.8
Canned, solids & liq.	4 oz.	172	0.0
SHAD, GIZZARD, raw (USDA):			
Whole	1 lb. (weighed whole)	229	0.0
Meat only	4 oz.	227	0.0

Food	Measure	Cals.	Carbs.
SHAD ROE (*See* **ROE**)			
SHAKE 'N BAKE:			
Chicken:			
Original recipe	5½-oz. pkg.	617	108.9
Barbecue	7-oz. pkg.	741	146.9
Country mild	4¾-oz. pkg.	610	79.5
Italian herb	5¾-oz. pkg.	613	111.0
Fish, original recipe	5¼-oz. pkg.	582	111.1
Pork or ribs:			
Original recipe	6-oz. pkg.	652	131.4
Barbecue	5¾-oz. pkg.	609	118.1
Extra crispy, *Oven Fry*	4.2-oz. pkg.	482	83.1
SHAKEY'S:			
Chicken, fried, & potatoes:			
3-piece	1 order	947	51.0
5-piece	1 order	1700	130.0
Ham & cheese sandwich	1 sandwich	550	56.0
Pizza:			
Cheese:			
Homestyle pan crust	⅒ of 12" pizza	303	31.0
Thick crust	⅒ of 12" pizza	170	21.6
Thin crust	⅒ of 12" pizza	133	13.2
Onion, green pepper, black olives & mushrooms:			
Homestyle pan crust	⅒ of 12" pizza	320	32.1
Thick crust	⅒ of 12" pizza	162	22.2
Thin crust	⅒ of 12" pizza	125	13.8
Pepperoni:			
Homestyle pan crust	⅒ of 12" pizza	343	31.1
Thick crust	⅒ of 12" pizza	185	21.8
Thin crust	⅒ of 12" pizza	148	13.2
Sausage & mushroom:			
Homestyle pan crust	⅒ of 12" pizza	343	31.4
Thick crust	⅒ of 12" pizza	178	21.8
Thin crust	⅒ of 12" pizza	141	13.3
Sausage & pepperoni:			
Homestyle pan crust	⅒ of 12" pizza	374	31.2
Thick crust	⅒ of 12" pizza	177	21.7
Thin crust	⅒ of 12" pizza	166	13.2
Special:			
Homestyle pan crust	⅒ of 12" pizza	384	31.6
Thick crust	⅒ of 12" pizza	208	22.3
Thin crust	⅒ of 12" pizza	171	13.5
Potatoes	15-piece order	950	120.0

Food	Measure	Cals.	Carbs.
Spaghetti with meat sauce & garlic bread	1 order	940	134.0
Super hot hero	1 sandwich	810	67.0
SHELLS, PASTA, STUFFED, frozen:			
(Buitoni) jumbo:			
Cheese stuffed	5½-oz. serving	288	25.1
Florentine	5½-oz. serving	264	23.1
(Celentano):			
Broccoli & cheese	13½-oz. pkg.	540	60.0
Cheese:			
Plain	½ of 12½-oz. pkg.	340	31.0
With sauce	½ of 16-oz. box	330	41.0
(Le Menu) healthy style, 3-cheese	10-oz. dinner	280	34.0
SHERBET OR SORBET:			
Fruit whip (Baskin-Robbins)	1 scoop	80	24.0
Lemon (Häagen-Dazs) Ice Cream Shop	4 fl. oz.	140	32.0
Lemonade (Edy's) pink	½ cup	130	27.0
Lime (Lucerne)	½ cup	120	26.0
Orange:			
(USDA)	½ cup	129	29.7
(Baskin-Robbins)	4 fl. oz.	158	33.4
(Borden)	½ cup	110	25.0
(Dole) Mandarin	½ cup	110	28.0
(Edy's) Swiss	½ cup	150	30.0
(Häagen-Dazs)	4 fl. oz.	113	30.0
(Lucerne)	½ cup	120	26.0
Peach (Dole)	½ cup	130	28.0
Pineapple:			
(Dole)	½ cup	120	28.0
(Lucerne)	½ cup	120	26.0
Raspberry:			
(Baskin-Robbins) red	4 fl. oz.	140	34.0
(Häagen-Dazs) Ice Cream Shop	4 fl. oz.	96	22.0
(Sealtest)	½ cup	130	30.0
Tropical (Edy's)	½ cup	130	27.0
SHERBET BAR:			
Regular (Fudgsicle) chocolate	1 bar	70	12.0
Dietetic:			

Food	Measure	Cals.	Carbs.
• (Creamsicle) with cream, all flavors, sugar free	1 bar	25	5.0
(Fudgsicle):			
Fat free, all flavors	1 bar	70	14.0
Sugar free, all flavors	1 bar	35	6.0
Sugar free, Fudge Nut Dip	1 bar	130	12.0

SHERBET OR SORBET & ICE CREAM:

(Häagen-Dazs):

Food	Measure	Cals.	Carbs.
Bar, orange & cream	2.6 fl.-oz. bar	130	18.0
Bulk:			
Blueberry & cream	4 fl. oz.	190	25.0
Key lime & cream	4 fl. oz.	200	29.0
Orange & cream	4 fl. oz.	190	27.0
Raspberry & cream	4 fl. oz.	180	23.0
(Lucerne) vanilla ice cream & orange sherbet	½ cup	130	21.0

SHERBET SHAKE, mix (Weight Watchers)

Food	Measure	Cals.	Carbs.
	1 envelope	70	11.0

SHONEY'S RESTAURANT:

Food	Measure	Cals.	Carbs.
Bacon	1 strip	36	Tr.
Biscuit	1 serving	170	21.6
Bread, Grecian	1 serving	80	13.2
Brownie, walnut, à la mode	1 serving	575	60.5
Cake:			
Carrot	1 serving	500	56.0
Hot fudge	1 serviing	522	81.9
Cheese sandwich, grilled:			
Plain	1 sandwich	454	29.0
With bacon	1 sandwich	440	27.9
Cheeseburger:			
Mushroom-Swiss burger	1 serving	161	26.8
Patty melt	1 serving	640	29.5
Chicken, charbroiled, *LightSide*	1 serving	239	1.0
Chicken sandwich:			
Charbroiled	1 sandwich	450	28.1
Fillet	1 sandwich	464	38.9
Chicken tenders, *America's Favorites*	1 serving	388	34.9
Croissant	1 serving	260	22.0
Egg, fried	1 egg	159	0.6
Fish:			
Baked, *LightSide*	1 serving	170	2.0
Fried, light	1 serving	297	21.5

Food	Measure	Cals.	Carbs.
Fish & chips entree, with fries	1 serving	639	50.4
Fish sandwich	1 sandwich	323	41.0
Fish N' Shrimp entree	1 serving	487	36.5
Gravy, country	3-oz. serving	114	5.7
Grits	3-oz. serving	57	6.2
Ham	1 slice	28	0.3
Ham sandwich:			
Baked	1 sandwich	500	26.8
Club, on whole wheat bread	1 sandwich	642	45.2
Hamburger:			
All American	1 burger	500	26.8
With bacon	1 burger	590	28.6
Old Fashioned	1 burger	470	25.6
Shoney Burger	1 burger	498	22.2
Hamburger patty, beef, light	1 serving	289	0.0
Italian feast entree	1 serving	500	43.8
Lasagna entree, *America's Favorites*	1 serving	297	44.9
Liver & onions entree, *America's Favorites*	1 serving	411	15.4
Mushrooms, sautéed	3-oz. serving	75	4.31
Onion, sautéed	2½-oz. serving	37	4.3
Onion rings	1 piece	52	5.0
Pancake	1 piece	91	19.9
Pie:			
Apple, à la mode	1 serving	490	67.0
Strawberry	1 serving	332	44.5
Potato:			
Baked	10-oz. serving	264	61.1
French-fried	3-oz. serving	189	28.9
French-fried	4-oz. serving	252	38.6
Hash browns	3-oz. serving	90	14.1
Home fries	3-oz. serving	115	18.7
Reuben sandwich	1 sandwich	595	31.5
Rice	3½-oz. serving	135	23.0
Salad bar:			
Ambrosia	¼ cup	75	11.5
Apple-grape surprise	¼ cup	19	4.9
Beet-onion	⅓ cup	25	3.0
Broccoli-cauliflower	¼ cup	53	2.7
Carrot-apple	¼ cup	99	4.2
Coleslaw	¼ cup	69	4.1
Cucumber, lite	¼ cup	12	2.7
Don's pasta salad	¼ cup	82	8.6
Fruit delight	¼ cup	54	10.1
Italian vegetable	¼ cup	11	2.5
Kidney bean	¼ cup	55	6.8

Food	Measure	Cals.	Carbs.
Macaroni salad	¼ cup	207	17.0
Oriental salad	¼ cup	79	13.4
Pea	¼ cup	73	2.5
Rotelli pasta salad	¼ cup	78	8.9
Snow peas	¼ cup	70	9.0
Spaghetti	¼ cup	81	8.7
Spring salad	¼ cup	38	2.4
Three-bean salad	¼ cup	96	11.9
Waldorf salad	¼ cup	80	8.5
Salad dressing:			
Regular:			
Blue cheese	2 T.	113	0.0
French	2 T.	124	2.0
Honey mustard	2 T.	165	2.4
Italian:			
Creamy	2 T.	135	1.0
Golden	2 T.	141	1.0
Ranch	2 T.	95	0.0
Thousand Island	2 T.	130	2.0
Dietetic:			
Biscayne	2 T.	62	1.0
Italian, nonfat	2 T.	10	2.4
Sauce, soufflé cup:			
Barbecue	1 serving	41	8.2
Cocktail	1 serving	36	8.7
Sweet & sour	1 serving	58	14.7
Tartar	1 serving	84	3.6
Sausage	1 patty	103	0.2
Seafood entree, platter	1 serving	566	45.7
Shrimp:			
Bite-size	1 serving	385	24.0
Charbroiled	1 serving	138	3.0
Shrimp entree:			
Boiled	1 serving	93	0.0
Sampler	1 serving	412	26.1
Shrimper's Feast:			
Regular	1 serving	383	29.9
Large	1 serving	575	44.9
Slim Jim sandwich	1 sandwich	484	40.4
Soup:			
Bean	6 oz.	63	9.8
Beef, with cabbage	6 oz.	85	9.4
Cheese, Florentine, with ham	6 oz.	110	11.8
Chicken, cream of	6 oz.	135	13.5
Chicken gumbo	6 oz.	60	7.0
Chicken noodle	6 oz.	62	9.2
Chicken rice	6 oz.	72	13.3

Food	Measure	Cals.	Carbs.
Onion	6 oz.	29	1.5
Potato	6 oz.	100	16.0
Tomato, Florentine	6 oz.	63	11.0
Vegetable	6 oz.	82	14.1
Spaghetti entree:			
America's Favorites	1 serving	496	63.4
LightSide	1 serving	248	32.0
Steak & chicken entree:			
Regular	8-oz. serving	435	0.0
Charbroiled:			
Regular	1 serving	239	1.3
Rib eye	1 serving	605	0.0
Sirloin	1 serving	357	0.0
Steak, entree, country fried,			
America's Favorites	1 serving	449	33.9
Steak sandwich:			
Country-fried	1 sandwich	588	67.0
Philly-style	1 sandwich	673	37.2
Steak N'Shrimp entree:			
Charbroiled	1 serving	361	1.0
Fried	1 serving	507	15.0
Steak, sirloin, charbroiled	6-oz. serving	357	0.0
Sundae:			
Hot fudge	1 serving	450	60.0
Strawberry	1 serving	380	47.7
Syrup, low calorie	2.2-oz. serving	98	24.4
Toast, buttered	1 slice	81	12.3
Turkey sandwich, club, on whole wheat bread	1 sandwich	635	44.1
SHREDDED WHEAT:			
(Nabisco):			
Regular	¾-oz. biscuit	90	19.0
& bran	1 oz.	110	23.0
Spoon Size	⅔ cup (1 oz.)	110	23.0
(Quaker)	1 biscuit (.6 oz.)	52	11.0
(Sunshine):			
Regular	1 biscuit	90	19.0
Bite size	⅔ cup (1 oz.)	110	22.0
Frosted:			
(Kellogg's) *Frosted Mini-Wheats,* regular & bite size	1 oz.	100	24.0
(Nabisco) *Frosted Wheat Squares*	1 oz.	100	24.0

Food	Measure	Cals.	Carbs.
SHRIMP:			
Raw (USDA):			
Whole	1 lb. (weighed in shell)	285	4.7
Meat only	4 oz.	103	1.7
Canned (Bumble Bee) solids & liq.	4½-oz. can	90	.9
Frozen:			
(Mrs. Paul's) fried	3-oz. serving	190	15.0
(Sau-Sea) cooked	5-oz. pkg.	90	0.0
SHRIMP & CHICKEN CANTONESE, frozen			
(Stouffer's) with noodles	10⅛-oz. meal	270	25.0
SHRIMP COCKTAIL, canned or frozen (Sau-Sea)	4 oz.	113	19.0
SHRIMP DINNER OR ENTREE:			
Canned (Ultra Slim Fast):			
Creole	12-oz. meal	240	45.0
Marinara	12-oz. meal	290	53.0
Frozen:			
(Armour) *Classics Lite:*			
Baby bay	9¾-oz. meal	220	31.0
Creole	11¼-oz. meal	260	53.0
(Budget Gourmet) with fettucini	9½-oz. meal	375	38.0
(Captain's Choice):			
Breaded:			
Gourmet	1 piece	18	.7
Jumbo	3 oz.	206	10.0
Cooked plain	3 oz.	84	0.0
(Gorton's):			
Crunchy, whole	5-oz. serving	380	35.0
Scampi	1 pkg.	470	33.0
(Healthy Choice):			
Creole	11¼-oz. meal	210	42.0
Marinara	10½-oz. meal	220	42.0
(La Choy) Fresh & Lite, with lobster sauce	10-oz. meal	240	36.4
(Stouffer's) *Right Course,* primavera	9⅝-oz. meal	240	32.0
(Weight Watchers) *Smart Ones,* marinara, with linguini	8-oz. meal	150	26.0

Food	Measure	Cals.	Carbs.
SHRIMP PASTE, canned			
(USDA)	1 oz.	51	.4
SIZZLER **RESTAURANT:**			
Avocado	½ avocado	153	6.0
Bacon bits	1 tsp.	27	2.0
Bean sprouts	¼ cup	8	2.0
Beans:			
Garbanzo	¼ cup	62	11.0
Kidney	¼ cup	52	10.0
Beef patty, ground:			
Regular	5.3-oz. serving	353	0.0
Large	8-oz. serving	530	0.0
Bread, focaccia	1 piece	54	4.51
Broccoli, raw	½ cup	12	2.0
Cantaloupe	½ cup	28	7.0
Carrots, raw	¼ cup	12	3.0
Cheese:			
Cheddar, imitation, shredded	1 oz.	85	4.5
Parmesan, grated	1 oz.	110	2.0
Swiss, sliced	1 oz.	100	1.0
Cheese toast	1 slice	273	16.0
Chicken:			
Breast, lemon herb	5-oz. serving	151	27.0
Patty, Malibu	1 patty	368	12.0
Wings:			
Regular	1 oz.	74	4.0
Cajun style, disjointed	3 oz.	301	1.8
Southern style:			
Disjointed	1 oz.	73	3.7
Whole	1 oz.	74	3.7
Chicken entree, with noodles	6-oz. serving	164	20.0
Chicken strips, breaded	1-oz. serving	68	DNA
Chili, with beans, grande	6-oz. serving	100	18.0
Corn nuggets	3-oz. serving	117	22.0
Crab:			
Imitation, shredded	3½-oz. serving	104	14.0
Snow, legs & claws	3½-oz. serving	91	0.0
Croissant, mini	1 piece	120	12.0
Egg:			
Cooked, diced	1-oz. serving	80	15.0
Cooked, salad topping	1-oz. serving	44	0.0
Fettuccini, whole egg	2-oz. serving	80	15.0
Fish nuggets	1-oz. serving	40	5.0
Halibut steak	6-oz. serving	180	0.0
Halibut steak	8-oz. serving	240	0.0

Food	Measure	Cals.	Carbs.
Hamburger, with lettuce & tomato	1 serving	626	36.0
Kiwifruit	2-oz. serving	35	8.0
Lasagna:			
Meat	8-oz. serving	327	23.0
Vegetable	8-oz. serving	245	29.0
Macaroni & cheese	6-oz. serving	214	22.0
Meatballs	1 piece	39	1.21
Onion, red, raw	1 T.	8	2.0
Pizza, Supreme round	5-inch pie (6½ oz.)	524	51.8
Potato:			
Baked	4-oz. serving	105	24.0
French fries	4-oz. serving	358	45.0
Skins	2-oz. serving	160	22.0
Salad:			
Beef teriyaki	2-oz. serving	49	45.0
Carrot & raisin	2-oz. serving	130	10.0
Chicken, Chinese	2-oz. serving	54	6.0
Fruit, Mediterranean Minted	2-oz. serving	29	7.0
Mexican Fiesta	2-oz. serving	54	10.0
Pasta:			
Italian	3½-oz. serving	90	18.3
Oriental	3½-oz. serving	114	22.6
Seafood Louis	2-oz. serving	64	9.0
Potato:			
German	3½-oz. serving	115	23.1
Old fashioned	3½-oz. serving	150	17.0
Red herb	3½-oz. serving	213	15.4
& egg	3½-oz. serving	140	166.0
Tuna	3½-oz. serving	353	7.3
Salad dressing:			
Regular:			
Blue cheese	1 oz.	111	1.0
Honey mustard	1 oz.	160	4.0
Hot bacon	1 T.	40	5.8
Parmesan Italian	1 oz.	100	2.0
Ranch	1 oz.	120	2.0
Thousand Island	1 oz.	143	3.0
Dietetic:			
Japanese rice vinegar, fat free	1 oz.	10	2.0
Ranch	1 oz.	90	4.0
Salmon	3½-oz. serving	125	0.0
Salmon	8-oz. serving	247	0.0
Sauce:			
Buttery dipping	1½ oz.	330	0.0

Food	Measure	Cals.	Carbs.
Cheese, nacho	2 oz.	120	3.0
Cocktail	1½ oz.	40	8.0
Hibachi	1½-oz.	57	11.0
Malibu	1½-oz.	283	0.0
Marinara	1 oz.	13	3.0
Tartar	1½ oz.	170	6.0
Scallop, breaded	4 oz. (approx. 30–40 pieces)	160	24.0
Shrimp:			
Broiled	5-oz. serving	150	0.0
Scampi	5-oz. serving	143	0.0
Tempura batter	3 oz. (approx. 21–25 pieces)	155	13.0
Soup:			
Broccoli cheese	4 oz.	139	10.0
Chicken noodle	4 oz.	31	4.0
Minestrone	4 oz.	36	7.0
Vegetable:			
Sirloin	4 oz.	60	6.0
Vegetarian	6 oz.	50	6.0
Spaghetti	2 oz.	80	16.0
Steak:			
Filet mignon	1 serving	179	0.0
Sirloin:			
Regular	6¼-oz. serving	447	0.0
Regular	9¼-oz. serving	655	0.0
Top sirloin	1 oz.	55	DNA
Strip, New York	1 serving	600	5.0
Tuna, yellowfin	1 serving	125	0.0
Yogurt, frozen, soft-serve, chocolate or vanilla	4 fl. oz.	136	24.0
SKATE, raw (USDA), meat only	4 oz.	111	0.0
SKIPPER'S **RESTAURANT:**			
Chicken meal, tenderloin strips:			
3 pieces, with small green salad, *Lite Catch*	1 serving	305	17.0
5 pieces, with fries	1 serving	793	69.0
Chicken sandwich, *Create A Catch*	1 serving	606	44.0
Chicken strips, *Create A Catch*	1 serving	82	4.0
Clam meal, strips with fries, in a basket	1 serving	1003	90.0
Cod meal, thick cut, with fries:			

Food	Measure	Cals.	Carbs.
3 pieces	1 serving	665	68.0
4 pieces	1 serving	759	74.0
5 pieces	1 serving	853	80.0
Coleslaw, *Create A Catch*	5-oz. serving	289	10.0
Combination meals:			
Chicken strips, fish & fries	1 serving	804	72.0
Chicken strips, shrimp & fries	1 serving	800	77.0
Clam strips, fish & fries	1 serving	868	81.0
Shrimp, fish & fries	1 serving	720	75.0
Oysters, fish & fries	1 serving	885	95.0
Fish fillet, *Create A Catch*	1 serving	175	11.0
Fish fillet meal:			
1 piece, with fries	1 serving	558	51.0
2 pieces, with small green salad, *Lite Catch*	1 serving	409	27.0
3 pieces, with fries	1 serving	908	82.0
Fish Sandwich, *Create A Catch:*			
Regular	1 serving	524	43.0
Double	1 serving	698	54.0
Oyster meal, with fries, in a basket	1 serving	1038	118.0
Potato:			
Baked	1 serving	145	21.0
French fries, *Create A Catch*	1 serving	383	50.0
Root beer float	1 serving	302	33.0
Salad:			
Green, small, *Lite Catch*	1 serving	59	6.0
Shrimp & seafood	1 serving	167	15.0
Side	1 serving	24	4.0
Salad dressing:			
Regular:			
Blue cheese	1 pouch	222	4.0
Italian	1 pouch	140	2.0
Ranch	1 pouch	188	2.0
Thousand Island	1 pouch	160	8.0
Dietetic, Italian	1 pouch	17	2.0
Salmon, baked	4.4-oz. serving	270	1.0
Sauce:			
Barbecue	1 T.	25	5.0
Tartar	1 T.	65	0.0
Seafood meal, with fries, *Skipper's Platter Basket*	1 serving	1038	97.0
Shrimp meal:			
In a basket, with fries:			
Original	1 serving	723	82.0
Jumbo	1 serving	707	79.0

Food	Measure	Cals.	Carbs.
Lite Catch, with seafood salad	1 serving	167	15.0
SLENDER (Carnation):			
Bar:			
Chocolate or chocolate chip	1 bar	135	13.0
Chocolate peanut butter or vanilla	1 bar	135	12.0
Dry	1 packet	110	21.0
Liquid	10-fl.-oz. can	220	34.0
SLOPPY JOE:			
Canned:			
(Hormel) *Short Orders*	7½-oz. can	340	15.0
(Libby's):			
Beef	⅓ cup (2.5 oz.)	110	7.0
Pork	⅓ cup	120	6.0
*(Hunt's) *Manwich*	1 sandwich	310	31.0
Frozen (Banquet) *Cookin' Bag*	5-oz. pkg.	210	12.0
SLOPPY JOE SAUCE, canned (Ragú) *Joe Sauce*	3½-oz.	50	11.0
SLOPPY JOE SEASONING MIX:			
*(Durkee)			
Regular	1¼ cup	128	32.0
Pizza flavor	1¼ cup	746	26.0
(French's)	1.5-oz. pkg.	128	32.0
*(Hunt's) *Manwich*	5.9-oz. serving	320	31.0
(McCormick)	1.3-oz. pkg.	103	23.4
SMELT, Atlantic, jack & bar (USDA):			
Raw:			
Whole	1 lb. (weighed whole)	244	0.0
Meat only	4 oz.	111	0.0
Canned, solids & liq.	4 oz.	227	0.0
S'MORES CRUNCH, cereal (General Mills)	¾ cup (1 oz.)	120	24.0
SMOKED SAUSAGE (See SAUSAGE)			

Food	Measure	Cals.	Carbs.
SNACKS (See **CRACKERS, PUFFS & CHIPS**; *NATURE SNACKS*; **POPCORN**; **POTATO CHIPS**; **PRETZELS**; etc.)			
SNAIL, raw (USDA):			
Unspecified kind	4 oz.	102	2.3
Giant African	4 oz.	83	5.0
SNAPPER (See **RED & GRAY SNAPPER**)			
SOAVE WINE (Antinori) 12% alcohol	3 fl. oz.	84	6.3
SOFT DRINK:			
Sweetened:			
Apple (Slice)	6 fl. oz.	98	24.0
Birch beer (Canada Dry)	6 fl. oz.	82	21.0
Bitter lemon:			
(Canada Dry)	6 fl. oz. (6.5 oz.)	75	19.5
(Schweppes)	6 fl. oz. (6.5 oz.)	82	20.0
Bubble Up	6 fl. oz.	73	18.5
Cactus Cooler (Canada Dry)	6 fl. oz. (6.5 oz.)	90	21.8
Cherry:			
(Canada Dry) wild	6 fl. oz. (6.5 oz.)	98	24.0
(Cragmont)	6 fl. oz.	91	23.0
(Shasta) black	6 fl. oz.	81	22.0
Cherry-lime (Spree) all natural	6 fl. oz.	79	21.5
Chocolate (Yoo-hoo)	6 fl. oz.	93	18.0
Citrus Mist (Shasta)	6 fl. oz.	85	23.0
Club	Any quantity	0	0.0
Cola:			
Coca-Cola:			
Regular, caffeine-free or cherry coke	6 fl. oz.	77	20.0
Classic	6 fl. oz.	72	19.0
(Cragmont) regular	6 fl. oz.	82	20.0
Pepsi-Cola, regular or *Pepsi Free*	6 fl. oz.	80	19.8

Food	Measure	Cals.	Carbs.
RC 100, caffeine-free	6 fl. oz.	86	21.4
(Royal Crown)	6 fl. oz.	86	21.4
(Shasta):			
Regular	6 fl. oz.	73	20.0
Cherry	6 fl. oz.	70	19.1
Shasta Free	6 fl. oz.	75	20.5
(Slice) cherry	6 fl. oz.	82	21.6
(Spree) all natural	6 fl. oz.	73	20.0
Collins mix (Canada Dry)	6 fl. oz.		
	(6.5 oz.)	60	15.0
Cream:			
(Canada Dry) vanilla	6 fl. oz. (6.6 oz.)	97	24.0
(Cragmont) regular or red	6 fl. oz.	84	21.0
(Shasta)	6 fl. oz.	77	21.0
Dr. Diablo (Shasta)	6 fl. oz.	70	19.0
Dr. Nehi (Royal Crown)	6 fl. oz.	82	20.4
Dr Pepper	6 fl. oz. (6.5 oz.)	75	19.4
Fruit punch:			
(Nehi)	6 fl. oz.	107	26.7
(Shasta)	6 fl. oz.	87	23.5
Ginger ale:			
(Canada Dry):			
Regular	6 fl. oz.	68	15.8
Golden	6 fl. oz.	75	18.0
(Cragmont)	6 fl. oz.	63	16.0
(Fanta)	6 fl. oz.	63	16.0
(Nehi)	6 fl. oz.	76	19.0
(Schweppes)	6 fl. oz.	65	16.0
(Shasta)	6 fl. oz.	60	16.5
(Spree) all natural	6 fl. oz.	60	16.5
Ginger beer (Schweppes)	6 fl. oz.	70	17.0
Grape:			
(Canada Dry) concord	6 fl. oz. (6.6 oz.)	97	24.0
(Cragmont)	6 fl. oz.	96	24.0
(Fanta)	6 fl. oz.	86	22.0
(Hi-C)	6 fl. oz.	74	19.5
(Nehi)	6 fl. oz.	97	24.4
(Schweppes)	6 fl. oz.	95	23.0
(Shasta)	6 fl. oz.	88	24.0
Grapefruit:			
(Schweppes)	6 fl. oz.	80	20.0
(Spree) all natural	6 fl. oz.	77	21.0
Half & half (Canada Dry)	6 fl. oz. (6.5 oz.)	82	19.5
Hi-Spot (Canada Dry)	6 fl. oz. (6.5 oz.)	75	18.7
Island Lime (Canada Dry)	6 fl. oz. (6.6 oz.)	97	24.8
Kick (Royal Crown)	6 fl. oz.	99	24.8
Lemon (Hi-C)	6 fl. oz.	71	17.1

Food	Measure	Cals.	Carbs.
Lemon-lime:			
(Cragmont):			
Regular	6 fl. oz.	74	19.0
Cherry	6 fl. oz	82	20.0
(Minute Maid)	6 fl. oz.	71	18.0
(Shasta)	6 fl. oz.	73	19.5
(Spree) all natural	6 fl. oz.	77	21.0
Lemon sour (Schweppes)	6 fl. oz.	79	19.0
Lemon-tangerine (Spree) all natural	6 fl. oz.	82	22.0
Mandarin-lime (Spree) all natural	6 fl. oz.	77	21.0
Mello Yello	6 fl. oz.	87	22.0
Mr. PiBB	6 fl. oz.	71	19.0
Mountain Dew	6 fl. oz.	89	22.2
Orange:			
(Canada Dry) *Sunripe*	6 fl. oz. (6.6 oz.)	97	24.7
(Cragmont)	6 fl. oz.	89	22.0
(Fanta)	6 fl. oz.	88	23.0
(Hi-C)	6 fl. oz.	74	19.5
(Minute Maid)	6 fl. oz.	87	22.0
(Nehi)	6 fl. oz.	104	26.0
(Orangina)	6 fl. oz.	67	15.6
(Schweppes) sparkling	6 fl. oz.	88	22.0
(Shasta)	6 fl. oz.	88	24.0
(Slice)	6 fl. oz.	97	25.2
Peach (Nehi)	6 fl. oz.	102	25.6
Punch (Hi-C)	6 fl. oz.	74	19.4
Quinine or tonic water:			
(Schweppes)	6 fl. oz.	64	16.0
(Shasta)	6 fl. oz.	60	16.5
Red berry (Shasta)	6 fl. oz.	79	22.5
Red pop (Shasta)	6 fl. oz.	79	22.5
Root beer:			
(Cragmont)	6 fl. oz.	84	21.0
(Fanta)	6 fl. oz.	78	20.0
(Nehi)	6 fl. oz.	97	24.4
(Ramblin')	6 fl. oz.	88	23.0
(Schweppes)	6 fl. oz.	76	19.0
(Shasta)	6 fl. oz.	77	21.0
(Spree) all natural	6 fl. oz.	77	21.0
Seltzer	Any quantity	0	0.0
7UP	6 fl. oz.	72	18.1
Slice	6 fl. oz.	76	19.8
Sprite	6 fl. oz.	71	18.0
Strawberry:			
(Cragmont)	6 fl. oz.	88	22.0

Food	Measure	Cals.	Carbs.
(Nehi)	6 fl. oz.	97	24.3
(Shasta)	6 fl. oz.	73	20.0
The Skipper (Cragmont)	6 fl. oz.	77	19.0
Tropical blend (Spree) all natural	6 fl. oz.	73	20.5
Upper 10 (Royal Crown)	6 fl. oz.	85	21.1
Dietetic:			
Apple (Slice)	6 fl. oz.	10	2.4
Birch beer (Shasta)	6 fl. oz.	2	.5
Blackberry (Schweppes) mid-calorie royal	6 fl. oz.	35	8.0
Cherry:			
(Cragmont) black	6 fl. oz.	0	0.0
Diet Rite	6 fl. oz.	2	.4
(Shasta) black	6 fl. oz.	Tr.	Tr.
Chocolate (Shasta)	6 fl. oz. (6.2 oz.)	0	0.0
Cola:			
Coca-Cola, regular, caffeine free or cherry	6 fl. oz.	Tr.	.1
(Cragmont) regular, lite or cherry	6 fl. oz.	0	0.0
Diet Rite (Royal Crown)	6 fl. oz.	Tr.	.2
Pepsi, diet, light or caffeine free	6 fl. oz.	Tr.	Tr.
RC	6 fl. oz.	Tr.	.2
(Shasta)	6 fl. oz.	0	0.0
(Slice) cherry	6 fl. oz.	10	2.4
Cream:			
(Cragmont)	6 fl. oz.	0	0.0
Diet Rite, caramel	6 fl. oz.	<1	.2
(Shasta)	6 fl. oz.	0	0.0
Fresca	6 fl. oz.	2	.1
Frolic (Shasta)	6 fl. oz.	0	0.0
Ginger ale:			
(Schweppes)	6 fl. oz.	2	<1.0
(Shasta)	6 fl. oz.	0	0.0
Grape (Shasta)	6 fl. oz.	0	0.0
Grapefruit, *Diet Rite*	6 fl. oz.	2	.4
Kiwi-passion fruit (Schweppes) mid-calorie royal	6 fl. oz.	35	8.0
Lemon-lime:			
(Cragmont) any type	6 fl. oz.	0	0.0
Diet Rite	6 fl. oz.	2	.6
(Minute Maid)	6 fl. oz.	10	2.0
(Shasta)	6 fl. oz.	0	0.0
Orange:			

Food	Measure	Cals.	Carbs.
(Fanta)	6 fl. oz.	<1	.1
(Minute Maid)	6 fl. oz.	4	.4
(No-Cal)	6 fl. oz.	1	0.0
(Shasta)	6 fl. oz.	0	0.0
(Slice)	6 fl. oz.	10	2.1
Peach, *Diet Rite,* golden	6 fl. oz.	1	.3
Peaches 'n Cream (Schweppes) mid-calorie royal	6 fl. oz.	35	8.0
Quinine or tonic (Canada Dry: No-Cal)	6 fl. oz.	3	Tr.
Raspberry, *Diet Rite*	6 fl. oz.	2	.5
Root beer:			
(Cragmont)	6 fl. oz.	0	0.0
(No-Cal)	6 fl. oz.	1	0.0
(Shasta)	6 fl. oz.	0	0.0
7UP	6 fl. oz.	2	0.0
Slice	6 fl. oz.	13	3.0
Sprite	6 fl. oz.	2	Tr.
Strawberry (Shasta)	6 fl. oz.	0	0.0
Strawberry-banana (Schweppes) mid-calorie royal	6 fl. oz.	35	8.0
Tangerine, *Diet Rite*	6 fl. oz.	2	.3
The Skipper (Cragmont)	6 fl. oz.	0	0.0
Tropical citrus (Schweppes) mid-calorie royal	6 fl. oz.	35	8.0
Upper 10 (RC)	6 fl. oz.	2	.6
SOLE, frozen:			
Raw, meat only (USDA)	4 oz.	90	0.0
Frozen:			
(Captain's Choice)	3-oz. fillet	99	0.0
(Frionor) *Norway Gourmet*	4-oz. fillet	60	0.0
(Gorton's):			
Fishmarket Fresh	4 oz.	90	1.0
Light Recipe, fillet, with lemon butter sauce	1 pkg.	250	8.0
(Healthy Choice):			
Au gratin	11-oz. meal	270	40.0
Lemon butter sauce	8¼-oz. meal	230	33.0
(Mrs. Paul's) fillet, light	1 piece	240	20.0
SOUFFLÉ:			
Cheese, home recipe (USDA)	1 cup (collapsed)	207	5.9
Corn, frozen (Stouffer's)	4-oz. serving	160	18.0
Spinach, frozen (Stouffer's)	4-oz. serving	140	8.0

Food	Measure	Cals.	Carbs.
SOUP:			
Canned, regular pack:			
*Asparagus (Campbell's),			
condensed, cream of	8-oz. serving	120	10.0
*Barley & bean (Rokeach)	8-oz. serving	90	15.0
Bean:			
(Campbell's):			
Chunky, with ham, old			
fashioned:			
Small	11-oz. can	290	38.0
Large	19¼-oz. can	500	66.0
*Condensed:			
Regular, with bacon	8-oz. serving	130	22.0
Homestyle	8-oz. serving	130	25.0
Home Cookin', & ham	9½-oz. can	180	26.0
Microwave, with			
bacon & ham	7½-oz. serving	230	38.0
(Grandma Brown's)	8-oz. serving	190	30.0
(Hormel) Hearty Soup	7½-oz. can	190	29.0
*(Town House) &			
bacon	8-oz. serving	140	20.0
Beef:			
(Campbell's):			
Chunky:			
Regular:			
Small	10¾-oz. can	200	24.0
Large	19-oz. can	340	42.0
Stroganoff style	10¾-oz. can	320	28.0
*Condensed:			
Regular	8-oz. serving	80	10.0
Broth	8-oz. serving	14	1.0
Consommé	8-oz. serving	25	2.0
Noodle:			
Regular	8-oz. serving	70	7.0
Homestyle	8-oz. serving	80	8.0
Home Cookin':			
Regular	10¾-oz. can	140	18.0
With vegetables &			
pasta	9½-oz. serving	120	16.0
(College Inn)	1 cup	18	1.0
(Hormel) vegetable,			
hearty	7½-oz. serving	90	15.0
(Lipton) *Hearty Ones*	11-oz. serving	229	40.0
(Progresso):			
Regular	½ of 19-oz. can	160	15.0
(Progresso) hearty	8 oz.	20	<2.0
Hearty	½ of 19-oz. can	160	15.0

Food	Measure	Cals.	Carbs.
Noodle	½ of 19-oz. can	170	17.0
Tomato, with rotini	½ of 19-oz. can	160	17.0
Vegetable	10½-oz. can	170	19.0
(Swanson)	7¼-oz. can	18	1.0
Beef barley (Progresso)	10½-oz. can	150	17.0
Borscht (See **BORSCHT**)			
*Broccoli (Campbell's)			
condensed, cream of	8-oz. serving	140	14.0
Celery:			
*(Campbell's) condensed,			
cream of	8-oz. serving	100	8.0
*(Rokeach):			
Prepared with milk	10-oz. serving	190	19.0
Prepared with water	10-oz. serving	90	12.0
*Cheese (Campbell's):			
Cheddar	8-oz. serving	110	10.0
Nacho	8-oz. serving	110	8.0
Chickarina (Progresso)	½ of 19-oz. can	130	13.0
Chicken:			
(Campbell's):			
Chunky:			
Mushroom, creamy	9.4-oz. serving	250	12.0
Noodle	10¾-oz. can	200	20.0
Nuggets	10¾-oz. can	190	24.0
Old fashioned:			
Small	10¾-oz. can	180	21.0
Large	19-oz. can	300	36.0
With rice	19-oz. can	280	32.0
Vegetable	19-oz. can	340	38.0
*Condensed:			
Alphabet	8-oz. serving	80	10.0
Broth:			
Plain	8-oz. serving	30	2.0
Noodles	8-oz. serving	45	8.0
Cream of	8-oz. serving	110	9.0
& dumplings	8-oz. serving	80	9.0
Gumbo	8-oz. serving	50	8.0
Mushroom, creamy	8-oz. serving	120	10.0
Noodle	8-oz. serving	60	8.0
NoodleOs	8-oz. serving	70	9.0
& rice	8-oz. serving	60	7.0
& stars	8-oz. serving	60	9.0
Vegetable	8-oz. serving	70	11.0
Home Cookin':			
Gumbo, with sausage	10¾-oz. can	140	15.0
With noodles	19-oz. can	220	20.0
Rice	10¾-oz. can	150	10.0

Food	Measure	Cals.	Carbs.
Microwave:			
Noodle	7¾-oz. serving	90	10.0
Rice	7¾-oz. serving	110	15.0
(College Inn) broth	1 cup (8.3 oz.)	35	0.0
(Hain):			
Broth	8¾-oz. can	70	0.0
Noodle	9½-oz. serving	120	12.0
Vegetable	9½-oz. serving	120	14.0
(Hormel) hearty:			
Noodle	7½-oz. serving	110	14.0
Rice	7½-oz. serving	110	17.0
(Lipton) *Hearty Ones,*			
homestyle	11-oz. serving	227	37.4
(Manischewitz):			
Clear	1 cup	46	DNA
Barley or rice	1 cup	83	DNA
Vegetable	1 cup	55	DNA
(Progresso):			
Barley	½ of 18½-oz.		
	can	100	13.0
Broth	8 oz.	16	0.0
Cream of	½ of 19-oz. can	190	13.0
Hearty	10½-oz. can	130	9.0
Homestyle	½ of 19-oz. can	110	11.0
Noodle	10½-oz. can	120	8.0
Rice	10½-oz. can	120	12.0
Vegetable	½ of 19-oz. can	140	16.0
(Swanson) broth:			
Regular	7¼-oz. can	30	2.0
Natural Goodness,			
clear	7¼-oz. can	20	1.0
Chili beef (Campbell's):			
Chunky:			
Small	11-oz. can	290	37.0
Large	19½-oz. can	520	66.0
*Condensed	8-oz. serving	140	20.0
Microwave	8-oz. serving	190	32.0
Chowder:			
Clam:			
Manhattan style:			
(Campbell's):			
Chunky:			
Small	10¾-oz. can	160	24.0
Large	19-oz. can	300	42.0
*Condensed	8-oz. serving	70	10.0
(Progresso)	½ of 19-oz. can	120	14.0
*(Snow's) condensed	7½-oz. serving	70	10.0

Food	Measure	Cals.	Carbs.
New England style:			
(Campbell's):			
Chunky:			
Small	10¾-oz. can	290	26.0
Large	19-oz. can	520	46.0
*Condensed:			
Made with milk	8-oz. serving	150	17.0
Made with water	8-oz. serving	80	12.0
Home Cookin'	9½-oz. serving	230	13.0
Microwave	7¾-oz. serving	200	15.0
*(Gorton's)	1 can	480	68.0
(Hain)	9¼-oz. serving	180	26.0
(Hormel) hearty	7½-oz. serving	130	16.0
(Progresso)	10½-oz. can	240	22.0
*(Snow's) condensed,			
made with milk	7½-oz. serving	140	13.0
*Corn (Snow's) New			
England, condensed,			
made with milk	7½-oz. serving	150	18.0
*Fish (Snow's) New			
England, condensed,			
made with milk	7½-oz. serving	130	11.0
*Seafood (Snow's) New			
England, condensed,			
made with milk	7½-oz. serving	130	11.0
*Corn (Campbell's) golden	8-oz. serving	110	18.0
Creole style (Campbell's)			
Chunky	19-oz. can	460	58.0
Escarole (Progresso) in	½ of 18½-oz.		
chicken broth	can	30	2.0
Ham'n butter bean			
(Campbell's) *Chunky*	10¾-oz. can	280	34.0
Italian vegetable pasta			
(Hain)	9½-oz. serving	160	25.0
Lentil:			
(Campbell's) *Home*			
Cookin'	10¾-oz. can	170	28.0
(Progresso):			
Regular	½ of 19-oz. can	140	25.0
With sausage	½ of 19-oz. can	180	20.0
Macaroni & bean			
(Progresso)	½ of 19-oz. can	150	25.0
Minestrone:			
(Campbell's):			
Chunky	19-oz. can	320	48.0
*Condensed	8-oz. serving	80	13.0
Home Cookin':			

Food	Measure	Cals.	Carbs.
Regular	10¾-oz. can	140	22.0
Chicken	½ of 19-oz. can	180	15.0
(Hain)	9½-oz. serving	160	27.0
(Hormel) hearty	7½-oz. serving	100	15.0
(Lipton) *Hearty Ones*	11-oz. serving	189	36.1
(Progresso):			
Beef	10½-oz. can	180	18.0
Chicken	½ of 19-oz. can	130	12.0
Hearty	½ of 18½-oz. can	110	16.0
Zesty	½ of 19-oz. can	150	19.0
*(Town House) condensed	8-oz. serving	80	12.0
Mushroom:			
*(Campbell's) condensed:			
Cream of	8-oz. serving	100	8.0
Golden	8-oz. serving	70	9.0
(Hain) creamy	9¼-oz. serving	110	16.0
(Progresso) cream of	½ of 18½-oz. can	160	14.0
*(Rokeach) cream of, prepared with water	10-oz. serving	150	3.0
*Noodle (Campbell's):			
Curly, & chicken	8-oz. serving	70	11.0
& ground beef	8-oz. serving	90	10.0
*Onion (Campbell's):			
Regular	8-oz. serving	60	9.0
Cream of:			
Made with water	8-oz. serving	100	12.0
Made with water & milk	8-oz. serving	140	15.0
*Oyster stew (Campbell's):			
Made with milk	8-oz. serving	140	10.0
Made with water	8-oz. serving	70	5.0
*Pea, green (Campbell's) condensed	8-oz. serving	150	25.0
Pea, split:			
(Campbell's):			
Chunky, with ham:			
Small	10¾-oz. can	230	33.0
Large	19-oz. can	420	60.0
*Condensed, with ham & bacon	8-oz. serving	160	24.0
Home Cookin', with ham	10¾-oz. can	230	38.0
(Grandma Brown's)	8-oz. serving	205	29.0
(Hain)	9½-oz. serving	170	28.0
(Progresso):			
Regular	½ of 19-oz. can	160	27.0

Food	Measure	Cals.	Carbs.
With ham	10½-oz. can	190	27.0
*Pepper pot (Campbell's)	8-oz. serving	90	9.0
*Potato (Campbell's):			
Cream of, made with water	8-oz. serving	80	12.0
Cream of, made with water & milk	8-oz. serving	120	15.0
*Scotch broth (Campbell's) condensed	8-oz. serving	80	9.0
Shav (Gold's)	8-oz. serving	25	4.0
Shrimp:			
*(Campbell's) condensed, cream of:			
Made with milk	8-oz. serving	160	13.0
Made with water	8-oz. serving	90	8.0
(Crosse & Blackwell)	6½-oz. serving	90	7.0
Sirloin burger (Campbell's) *Chunky:*			
Small	10¾-oz. can	220	23.0
Large	19-oz. can	400	40.0
Steak & potato (Campbell's) *Chunky:*			
Small	10¾-oz. can	200	24.0
Large	19-oz. can	360	42.0
Tomato:			
(Campbell's):			
Condensed:			
Regular:			
Made with milk	8-oz. serving	140	22.0
Made with water	8-oz. serving	90	17.0
Bisque	8-oz. serving	120	22.0
Homestyle, cream of:			
Made with milk	8-oz. serving	180	25.0
Made with water	8-oz. serving	110	20.0
& rice, old fashioned	8-oz. serving	110	22.0
Home Cookin', garden	10¾-oz. can	150	29.0
(Progresso)	8-oz. serving	90	18.0
*(Rokeach):			
Plain, made with water	10-oz. serving	90	20.0
& rice	10-oz. serving	160	25.0
Tortellini (Progresso):			
Regular	½ of 19-oz. can	80	12.0
Creamy	½ of 18½-oz. can	240	17.0
Tomato	½ of 18½-oz. can	130	16.0
Turkey (Campbell's):			
Chunky	18¾-oz. can	300	32.0

Food	Measure	Cals.	Carbs.
*Condensed:			
Noodle	8-oz. serving	70	9.0
Vegetable	8-oz. serving	70	8.0
Vegetable:			
(Campbell's):			
Chunky:			
Regular:			
Small	10¾-oz. can	160	28.0
Large	19-oz. can	300	50.0
Beef, old fashioned:			
Small	10¾-oz. can	190	20.0
Large	19-oz. can	320	34.0
Mediterranean	19-oz. can	320	48.0
*Condensed:			
Regular	8-oz. serving	90	14.0
Beef	8-oz. serving	70	10.0
Dinosaur	8-oz. serving	100	18.0
Homestyle	8-oz. serving	60	9.0
Old fashioned	8-oz. serving	60	9.0
Vegetarian	8-oz. serving	80	13.0
Home Cookin':			
Beef	10¾-oz. can	140	17.0
Country	10¾-oz. can	120	20.0
Microwave:			
Regular	7¾-oz. serving	100	17.0
Beef	7¾-oz. serving	100	14.0
(Hain):			
Broth	9½-oz. serving	45	10.0
Chicken	9½-oz. serving	120	14.0
Vegetarian	9½-oz. serving	150	22.0
(Hormel) hearty, country	7½-oz. serving	90	14.0
(Progresso)	½ of 19-oz. can	90	19.0
*(Rokeach) vegetarian	10-oz. serving	90	15.0
Vichyssoise (Crosse &			
Blackwell) cream of	6½-oz. serving	70	5.0
*Wonton (Campbell's)	8-oz. serving	40	5.0
Canned, dietetic pack:			
Bean:			
*(Campbell's) *Healthy*			
Request, & bacon	8-oz. serving	140	22.0
(Hain) 99% fat free	9½-oz. serving	120	29.0
(Health Valley) & carrots,			
fat free	7½-oz. serving	70	9.0
(Healthy Choice) & ham	7½-oz. serving	220	35.0
(Pritikin) navy	½ of 14¾-oz.		
	can	130	22.0
Beef:			

Food	Measure	Cals.	Carbs.
(Campbell's) Healthy Request, with vegetables	8-oz. serving	70	9.0
(Health Valley) broth	6.9-oz. serving	10	2.0
(Healthy Choice) vegetable, chunky	7½-oz. serving	110	14.0
(Pritikin) broth	½ of 13¾-oz. can	20	3.0
Chicken:			
(Campbell's):			
Regular:			
Broth, low sodium	10½-oz. can	30	2.0
Noodle, low sodium	10¾-oz. can	170	17.0
Healthy Request, hearty:			
Noodle	8-oz. serving	80	7.0
Rice	8-oz. serving	110	15.0
Vegetable	8-oz. serving	120	16.0
(Estee) & vegetable	7¼-oz. can	130	10.0
(Hain) no salt:			
Broth	9-oz. serving	45	2.0
Noodle	8-oz. serving	100	9.0
Vegetable	8-oz. serving	100	12.0
(Health Valley) fat free, broth	7½-oz. serving	20	1.0
(Healthy Choice):			
Noodle, old fashioned	7½-oz. serving	90	9.0
Rice	7½-oz. serving	140	18.0
(Pritikin):			
Broth defatted	½ of 13¾-oz. can	14	0.0
Gumbo or ribbon pasta	7¼-oz. serving	60	8.0
Vegetable	½ of 14½-oz. can	70	12.0
(Progresso) *Healthy Classics:*			
Noodle	8-oz. serving	80	10.0
Vegetables	8-oz. serving	80	11.0
Chowder:			
Clam			
(Campbell) New England, *Healthy Request,* hearty	8-oz. serving	100	14.0
(Pritikin):			
Manhattan	½ of 14¾-oz. can	100	17.0
New England	½ of 14¾-oz. can	118	20.0

Food	Measure	Cals.	Carbs.
Corn & vegetable (Health Valley) fat free	7½-oz. serving	70	13.0
Lentil:			
(Hain) 99% fat free, vegetarian			
Regular	9½-oz. serving	150	25.0
Salt free	9½-oz. serving	140	22.0
(Health Valley) & carrots, fat free	7½-oz. serving	70	10.0
(Pritikin)	½ of 14¾-oz. can	100	17.0
(Progresso) *Healthy Favorites*	8-oz. serving	120	18.0
Minestrone:			
(Campbell's) *Healthy Request*, hearty	8-oz. serving	90	13.0
(Estee)	7½-oz. can	165	19.0
(Hain) no salt	9½-oz. serving	160	28.0
(Health Valley)	7½-oz. serving	120	15.0
(Healthy Choice)	7½-oz. serving	160	30.0
(Pritikin)	½ of 14¾-oz. can	110	19.0
Mushroom:			
(Campbell's) cream of:			
Regular, low sodium	10½-oz. serving	210	18.0
Healthy Request	8-oz. serving	60	9.0
(Hain) 99% fat free	8-oz. serving	90	14.0
(Pritikin)	½ of 14¾-oz. can	60	11.0
(Weight Watchers) cream of	10½-oz. can	90	14.0
Pea, split:			
(Campbell's) low sodium	10¾-oz. can	230	37.0
(Hain) vegetarian, 99% fat free:			
Regular	9½-oz. serving	160	30.0
No salt	9½-oz. serving	150	25.0
(Pritikin)	½ of 15-oz. can	130	23.0
Tomato:			
(Campbell's):			
Low sodium, with tomato pieces	10½-oz. can	190	30.0
Condensed, Healthy Request	8-oz. serving	90	17.0
(Health Valley) vegetable, fat free	7½-oz. serving	50	8.0
(Healthy Choice) garden	7½-oz. serving	130	22.0

Food	Measure	Cals.	Carbs.
Turkey (Pritikin) vegetable, with ribbon pasta	½ of 14¾-oz. can	50	7.0
Vegetable:			
(Campbell's) *Healthy Request*:			
*Regular, condensed	8-oz. serving	90	14.0
Country	7½-oz. serving	120	23.0
Hearty	8-oz. serving	90	17.0
(Hain)			
Broth, vegetarian, 99% fat free:			
Regular	9½-oz. serving	40	8.0
No salt	9½-oz. serving	40	9.0
Vegetarian, no salt	9½-oz. serving	150	23.0
(Health Valley) fat free:			
Barley	7½-oz. serving	60	10.0
Beef	7½-oz. serving	130	20.0
5-bean	7½-oz. serving	100	15.0
(Pritikin)	½ of 14¾-oz. can	70	14.0
(Progresso) *Healthy Classics*	8-oz. serving	80	13.0
(Weight Watchers):			
with beef stock	10½-oz. can	90	13.0
Vegetarian, chunky	10½-oz. can	100	18.0
Wild rice (Hain) 99% fat free	9½-oz. can	80	16.0
Frozen:			
Asparagus (Kettle Ready) cream of	6 fl. oz.	62	5.1
*Barley & mushroom:	½ of 15-oz.		
(Empire Kosher)	polybag	69	12.0
(Tabatchnick)	8 oz.	92	16.0
Bean & barley (Tabatchnick)	8 oz.	63	22.0
Bean & ham (Kettle Ready):			
Black	6 fl. oz.	154	23.0
Savory	6 fl. oz.	113	20.2
Beef (Kettle Ready) vegetable	6 fl. oz.	85	10.7
Broccoli, cream of:			
(Kettle Ready):			
Regular	6 fl. oz.	94	6.4
Cheddar	6 fl. oz.	137	4.7
(Tabatchnick)	7½ oz.	90	10.0
Cauliflower (Kettle Ready) cream of	6 fl. oz.	93	5.5
Cheese (Kettle Ready) cheddar, cream of	6 fl. oz.	158	7.3

Food	Measure	Cals.	Carbs.
Chicken:			
(Empire Kosher):			
Corn	½ of 15-oz. polybag	71	7.0
Noodle	½ of 15-oz. polybag	267	13.0
(Kettle Ready):			
Cream of	6 fl. oz.	98	5.0
Gumbo	6 fl. oz.	93	12.1
Noodle	6 fl. oz.	94	12.0
Chili (Kettle Ready):			
Jalapeño	6 fl. oz.	173	14.7
Traditional	6 fl. oz.	161	13.8
Chowder:			
Clam:			
Boston (Kettle Ready)	6 fl. oz.	131	12.8
Manhattan:			
(Kettle Ready)	6 fl. oz.	69	7.9
(Tabatchnick)	7½ oz.	94	15.0
New England:			
(Kettle Ready)	6 fl. oz.	116	11.4
(Stouffer's)	8 oz.	180	16.0
(Tabatchnick)	7½-oz.	97	16.0
Corn & broccoli (Kettle Ready)	6 fl. oz.	101	12.8
Lentil (Tabatchnick)	8 oz.	173	27.0
Minestrone:			
(Kettle Ready)	6 fl. oz.	104	15.2
(Tabatchnick)	8 oz.	147	24.0
Mushroom (Kettle Ready) cream of	6 fl. oz.	85	6.2
Northern bean (Tabatchnick)	8 oz.	80	29.0
Onion (Kettle Ready) french	6 fl. oz.	42	4.9
Pea:			
(Empire Kosher)	7½ oz.	56	6.0
(Kettle Ready) split	6 fl. oz.	155	25.3
(Tabatchnick)	8 oz.	186	31.0
Potato (Tabatchnick)	8 oz.	95	19.0
Spinach, cream of:			
(Stouffer's)	8 oz.	210	12.0
(Tabatchnick)	7½ oz.	90	12.0
Tomato (Empire Kosher) with rice	7½ oz.	227	50.0
Tortellini (Kettle Ready)	6 fl. oz.	122	14.9
Turkey chili (Empire Kosher)	7½ oz.	200	DNA

Food	Measure	Cals.	Carbs.
Vegetable:			
(Empire Kosher)	7½ oz.	111	22.0
(Kettle Ready)	6 fl. oz.	85	12.3
(Tabatchnick)	8 oz.	97	18.0
Won ton (La Choy)	7½ oz.	50	6.0
*Mix, regular:			
Asparagus (Knorr)	8 fl. oz.	80	11.0
Barley (Knorr) country	10 fl. oz.	120	22.5
Bean (Hormel) *Micro-Cup,* with ham, hearty	1 pkg.	191	31.0
Bean, black (Knorr) Cup-A-Soup	1 serving	200	27.8
Bean, navy (Knorr) Cup-A-Soup	1 serving	140	26.9
Beef:			
(Campbell's) *Campbell's Cup,* microwave	1 container	130	23.0
Ramen:			
& noodle	8 fl. oz.	190	26.0
& vegetables, Cup-A-Ramen	8 fl. oz.	270	38.0
(Hormel) *Micro-Cup,* with vegetables, hearty	1 serving	71	12.0
(Lipton):			
Cup-A-Soup	6 fl. oz.	44	7.6
Hearty	6 fl. oz.	107	20.2
Broccoli, creamy (Lipton) Cup-A-Soup	6 fl. oz.	62	9.0
Broccoli, creamy, & cheese (Lipton) Cup-A-Soup	6 fl. oz.	70	10.0
Chicken:			
(Campbell's):			
Campbell's Cup:			
Creamy, with white meat	6 fl. oz.	90	12.0
Noodle, microwave	1.35-oz. container	140	22.0
Ramen:			
Noodle	8 fl. oz.	190	26.0
Noodle, with vegetables, Cup-A-Ramen	8 fl. oz.	270	38.0
Quality soup & recipe, noodle	8 fl. oz.	100	16.0
(Hormel) *Micro-Cup,* with vegetables & rice, hearty	1 serving	114	16.0
(Knorr):			

Food	Measure	Cals.	Carbs.
Noodle	8 fl. oz.	100	17.9
'n pasta	8 fl. oz.	90	16.2
(Lipton):			
Regular, noodle:			
Plain	8 fl. oz.	81	12.0
with white meat, diced	8 fl. oz.	81	12.1
Cup-A-Soup:			
Broth	6 fl. oz.	20	3.0
Cream of	6 fl. oz.	84	9.7
Creamy, with			
vegetables	6 fl. oz.	9	14.4
Hearty, country style	6 fl. oz.	69	11.1
Noodle:			
Regular	6 fl. oz.	48	6.6
Lots-A-Noodles:			
Hearty	7 fl. oz.	110	20.0
Hearty, creamy	7 fl. oz.	179	21.4
with meat	6 fl. oz.	45	6.5
With vegetables,	1 cup	75	12.0
hearty & rice	6 fl. oz.	45	7.5
Supreme, country			
style	6 fl. oz.	107	11.8
Vegetable	6 fl. oz.	45	7.8
Chili beef (Campbell's)			
microwave	7½ fl. oz.	190	32.0
Chowder, New England			
(Gorton's)	¼ of can	140	17.0
Herb (Knorr) fine	8 fl. oz.	130	15.0
Hot & Sour (Knorr) oriental	8 fl. oz.	80	9.0
Leek (Knorr)	8 fl. oz.	110	14.0
Lentil (Hain) savory	¾ cup	130	20.0
Minestrone:			
(Hain) savory	¾ cup	110	20.0
(Hormel) *Micro-Cup,*			
hearty	1 serving	104	15.0
(Knorr) hearty	10 fl.-oz.	130	22.7
(Manischewitz)	6 fl.-oz.	50	9.0
Mushroom:			
(Hain)	¾ cup	210	11.0
(Knorr)	8 fl. oz.	100	12.0
(Lipton):			
Regular:			
Beef	8 fl. oz.	38	6.7
Onion	8 fl. oz.	41	6.8
Cup-a-Noodles, cream of	6 fl. oz.	70	9.1
Noodle:			
(Campbell's):			

Food	Measure	Cals.	Carbs.
Campbell's Cup:			
Regular	1 cup	110	19.0
With chicken broth:			
Microwave	1.35-oz. container	130	23.0
2-minute soup	6 fl. oz.	90	15.0
With vegetables, hearty	1.7-oz. container	180	32.0
Quality Soup & Recipe:			
Regular	8 fl. oz.	110	19.0
Hearty	8 fl. oz.	90	15.0
Ramen:			
Oriental:			
Regular	8 fl. oz.	190	26.0
Cup-a-Ramen	8 fl. oz.	270	38.0
Pork flavor, regular	8 fl. oz.	200	26.0
(4C)	8 fl. oz.	50	7.0
(Lipton):			
Regular:			
Giggle Noodle	8 fl. oz.	77	11.4
Hearty, with vegetables	8 fl. oz	75	12.3
Ring-O-Noodle	8 fl. oz.	71	10.4
Cup-A-Soup, ring noodles	6 fl. oz.	47	7.6
Onion:			
(Campbell's) Quality Soup	8 fl. oz.	30	7.0
(Hain) Savory	¾ cup	50	6.0
(Knorr) french	8 fl. oz.	50	9.1
(Lipton):			
Regular:			
Plain	8 fl. oz.	20	4.3
Beefy	8 fl. oz.	24	4.1
Cup-a-Soup	6 fl. oz.	27	4.7
Oxtail (Knorr) hearty beef	8 fl. oz.	70	10.2
Pea, green (Lipton) *Cup-a-Soup*	6 fl. oz.	113	14.4
Pea, split (Manischewitz)	6 fl. oz.	45	8.0
Potato Leek (Hain)	¾ cup	260	20.0
Shrimp (Campbell's) *Cup-a-Ramen*, with vegetables	8 fl. oz.	280	40.0
Tomato:			
(Hain) savory	¾ cup	220	19.0
(Knorr) basil	8 fl. oz.	85	14.3
(Lipton) *Cup-A-Soup*	6 fl. oz.	103	21.2

Food	Measure	Cals.	Carbs.
Tortellini (Knorr) in broth	8 fl. oz.	60	10.9
Vegetable:			
(Campbell's) quality soup	8 fl. oz.	40	8.0
(Hain) savory	¾ cup	80	13.0
(Hormel) *Micro-Cup,* hearty	1 serving	89	13.0
(Knorr):			
Plain	8 fl. oz.	35	6.5
Spring, with herbs	8 fl. oz.	30	6.0
(Lipton):			
Regular:			
Plain	8 fl. oz.	39	6.9
Country	8 fl. oz.	80	15.7
Cup-a-Soup:			
Regular:			
Harvest	6 fl. oz.	91	18.8
Spring	6 fl. oz.	41	6.6
Lots-a-Noodles, garden	7 fl. oz.	123	23.1
(Manischewitz)	6 fl. oz.	50	9.0
*Mix, dietetic:			
Beef:			
(Campbell's) ramen:			
Noodle, low fat block	8 fl. oz.	160	32.0
With vegetables, Cup-A-Ramen, low fat	8 fl. oz.	220	44.0
(Estee)	6 fl. .oz.	20	3.0
(Ultra Slim Fast) with noodles	6 fl. oz.	45	7.0
Chicken:			
(Campbell's) ramen:			
Noodle, low fat block	8 fl. oz.	160	32.0
With vegetables, Cup-a-Ramen, low fat	8 fl. oz.	220	44.0
(Estee) noodle, instant	6 fl. oz.	25	4.0
(Featherweight) instant	1 tsp.	18	2.0
(Lipton) *Cup-a-Soup*, lite:			
Florentine	6 fl. oz.	42	7.6
Lemon	6 fl. oz.	48	9.1
(Ultra Slim Fast) with noodles	6 fl. oz.	45	6.0
(Weight Watchers) broth	1 packet	8	1.0
Chicken leek (Ultra Slim Fast) creamy	6 fl. oz.	50	7.0
Leek (Ultra Slim Fast) creamy	6 fl. oz.	80	15.0

Food	Measure	Cals.	Carbs.
Mushroom:			
(Estee) instant	6 fl. oz.	40	3.0
(Hain) savory soup & recipe mix, no salt added	6 fl. oz.	250	15.0
Noodle (Campbell's) ramen:			
Oriental noodle, low fat block	8 fl. oz.	150	31.0
Oriental, with vegetables, Cup-A-Ramen, low fat	8 fl. oz.	220	44.0
Pork flavor, low fat block	8 fl. oz.	150	31.0
Onion:			
(Estee)	6 fl. oz.	25	4.0
(4C)	8 fl. oz.	30	5.0
(Hain) savory soup, dip & recipe mix, no salt added	6 fl. oz.	50	9.0
(Ultra Slim Fast) creamy	6 fl. oz.	45	7.0
Oriental (Lipton) Cup-a-Soup, lite	6 fl. oz.	45	5.8
Shrimp flavor (Campbell's) Cup-a-Ramen, with vegetables, low fat	8 fl. oz.	230	45.0
Tomato:			
(Estee) instant	6 fl. oz	40	5.0
(Lipton) Cup-a-Soup, creamy & herbs, lite	6 fl. oz.	66	14.1
(Ultra Slim Fast) creamy	6 fl. oz.	60	10.0
Vegetable (Hain) savory soup, no salt added	6 fl. oz.	80	13.0
SOUP STARTER:			
Beef Barley	⅛ of pkg.	80	15.0
Chicken noodle	⅛ of pkg.	70	15.0
Chicken & rice	⅛ of pkg.	70	15.0
SOUR CREAM (See **CREAM**, Sour)			
SOURSOP, raw (USDA):			
Whole	1 lb. (weighed with skin & seeds)	200	50.3
Flesh only	4 oz.	74	18.5
SOUSE (USDA)	1 oz.	51	.3

Food	Measure	Cals.	Carbs.
SOUTHERN COMFORT:			
80 proof	1 fl. oz.	79	3.4
100 proof	1 fl. oz.	95	3.5
SOYBEAN:			
(USDA):			
Young seeds:			
Raw	1 lb. (weighed in pod)	322	31.7
Boiled, drained	4 oz.	134	11.5
Canned:			
Solids & liq.	4 oz.	85	7.1
Drained solids	4 oz.	117	8.4
Mature seeds:			
Raw	1 lb.	1828	152.0
Raw	1 cup (7.4 oz.)	846	70.4
Cooked	4 oz.	147	12.2
Oil roasted:			
(Soy Ahoy) regular, or garlic	1 oz.	152	4.8
(Soytown)	1 oz.	152	4.8
SOYBEAN CURD OR TOFU			
(USDA):			
Regular	4 oz.	82	2.7
Cake	4.2-oz. cake	86	2.9
SOYBEAN FLOUR (See **FLOUR**)			
SOYBEAN GRITS, high fat (USDA)	1 cup (4.9 oz.)	524	46.0
SOYBEAN MILK (USDA):			
Fluid	4 oz.	37	1.5
Powder	1 oz.	122	7.9
SOYBEAN PROTEIN (USDA)	1 oz.	91	4.3
SOYBEAN PROTEINATE (USDA)	1 oz.	88	2.2
SOYBEAN SPROUT (See **BEAN SPROUT**)			
SOY SAUCE (See **SAUCE**, Soy)			

Food	Measure	Cals.	Carbs.
SPAGHETTI (See also **PASTA, DRY OR FRESH, REFRIGERATED** or **NOODLE**). Plain spaghetti products are essentially the same in calorie value and carbohydrate content on the same weight basis. The longer the cooking, the more water is absorbed and this affects the nutritive and caloric value:			
Dry (Pritikin) whole wheat	1 oz.	110	18.0
Cooked dry (USDA):			
8—10 minutes, "Al Dente"	1 cup (5.1 oz.)	216	43.9
14—20 minutes, tender	1 cup (4.9 oz.)	155	32.2
Canned, regular pack:			
(Chef Boyardee) & meatballs	7½-oz. serving	170	36.0
(Franco-American):			
With meatballs in tomato sauce, *SpaghettiOs*	7⅜-oz. can	220	25.0
With meatballs, in tomato sauce	7⅜-oz. can	220	28.0
With sliced franks in tomato sauce, *SpaghettiOs*	7⅜-oz. can	220	26.0
In tomato & cheese sauce, *SpaghettiOs*	7⅜-oz. can	170	33.0
In tomato sauce with cheese	7⅜-oz. can	180	36.0
(Hormel) *Short Orders:*			
& beef	7½-oz. can	260	25.0
& meatballs	7½-oz. can	210	26.0
(Top Shelf):			
With meat sauce	10-oz. serving	260	37.0
Spaghettini	1 serving	240	35.0
(Ultra Slim Fast) with beef & mushroom sauce	12-oz. serving	370	49.0
Canned, dietetic:			
(Estee) & meatballs	7½-oz. serving	240	19.0
(Featherweight) & meatballs	7½-oz. serving	200	28.0
Frozen:			
(Armour) *Dining Lite*, with beef	9-oz. meal	220	25.0
(Banquet):			
Casserole, with meat sauce	8-oz. meal	270	35.0
Dinner, & meatballs	10-oz. meal	290	44.0

Food	Measure	Cals.	Carbs.
(Healthy Choice) with meat sauce	10-oz. meal	280	42.0
(Kid Cuisine)	9¼-oz. meal	310	43.0
(Le Menu) healthy style, with beef sauce & mushroom	9-oz. meal	280	45.0
(Morton) & meatballs	10-oz. dinner	200	39.0
(Stouffer's):			
Regular:			
With meatballs	12⅝-oz. meal	380	42.0
With meat sauce	12⅞-oz. meal	370	49.0
Lean Cuisine, with beef & mushroom sauce	11½-oz. meal	280	38.0
(Swanson):			
Regular, & meatballs	12½-oz. meal	390	46.0
Homestyle Recipe, with Italian style meatballs	13-oz. meal	490	60.0
(Weight Watchers) with meat sauce	10½-oz. meal	280	34.0

SPAGHETTI SAUCE (See PASTA SAUCE)

SPAGHETTI SAUCE MIX: (See **PASTA SAUCE MIX**)

Food	Measure	Cals.	Carbs.
SPAM, luncheon meat (Hormel):			
Regular, smoke flavored or with cheese chunks	1-oz. serving	85	0.0
Deviled	1 T.	35	0.0

SPANISH MACKEREL (See also **MACKEREL**, raw (USDA):

Food	Measure	Cals.	Carbs.
Whole	1 lb. (weighed whole)	490	0.0
Meat only	4 oz.	201	0.0

SPARKLING COOLER, CITRUS, *La Croix,* 3½% alcohol

Food	Measure	Cals.	Carbs.
	12 fl. oz.	215	30.0
SPECIAL K, cereal (Kellogg's)	1 cup (1 oz.)	110	20.0

SPICES (See individual spice names)

SPINACH:
Raw (USDA):

Food	Measure	Cals.	Carbs.
Untrimmed	1 lb. (weighed with large stems & roots)	85	14.0
Trimmed or packaged	1 lb.	118	19.5
Trimmed, whole leaves	1 cup (1.2 oz.)	9	1.4
Trimmed, chopped	1 cup (1.8 oz.)	14	2.2
Boiled (USDA) whole leaves, drained	1 cup (5.5 oz.)	36	5.6
Canned, regular pack: (USDA):			
Solids & liq.	½ cup (4.1 oz.)	21	3.5
Drained solids	½ cup	27	4.0
(Allen's) chopped, solids & liq.	½ cup	25	4.0
(Larsen) *Freshlike,* cut	½ cup (4.3 oz.)	25	4.0
(S&W) Premium Northwest	½ cup	25	3.0
(Town House) whole leaf	½ cup	28	3.0
Canned, dietetic or low calorie: (USDA) low sodium:			
Solids & liq.	4 oz.	24	3.9
Drained solids	4 oz.	29	4.5
(Allen's) low sodium, solids & liq.	½ cup	25	4.0
(Del Monte) no salt added, solids & liq.	½ cup	25	4.0
(Larsen) *Fresh-Lite,* cut, no salt added	½ cup (4.3 oz.)	20	4.0
Frozen:			
(Bel-Air)	3.3 oz.	20	3.0
(Birds Eye):			
Chopped or leaf	⅓ of pkg. (3.3 oz.)	28	3.4
Creamed	⅓ of pkg. (3 oz.)	60	4.9
& water chestnuts with selected seasonings	⅓ of 10-oz. pkg.	32	5.0
(Budget Gourmet) au gratin	6-oz. serving	150	9.0
(Green Giant):			
Creamed	3.3 oz.	70	8.0
Cut or leaf, in butter sauce	5 oz.	40	6.0
Harvest Fresh	4½ oz.	25	4.0
(McKenzie) chopped or cut	⅓ of pkg.	25	3.0
(Stouffer's) creamed	½ of 9-oz. pkg.	190	8.0

Food	Measure	Cals.	Carbs.
SPINACH, NEW ZEALAND			
(USDA):			
Raw	1 lb.	86	14.1
Boiled, drained	4 oz.	15	2.4
SPINACH PUREE, canned			
(Larsen) no salt added	½ cup (4.3 oz.)	22	3.5
SPLEEN, raw (USDA):			
Beef & calf	4 oz.	118	0.0
Hog	4 oz.	121	0.0
Lamb	4 oz.	130	0.0
SPLIT PEA (See **PEA, MATURE SEED**, dry)			
SPORTS DRINK:			
Canned:			
(All Sport)			
Fruit punch	8 fl. oz.	80	22.0
Grape or lemon-lime	8 fl. oz.	70	20.0
Orange, caffeine-free	8 fl. oz	70	19.0
(Gatorade):			
Regular, any flavor	8 fl. oz.	50	14.0
Light, lemon-lime	8 fl. oz.	25	7.0
(Knudsen & Sons) lemon,			
Isotonic Sports Beverage	8 fl. oz.	60	21.0
(Pro-formance) fruit punch,			
grape, lemon or orange	8 fl. oz.	99	26.0
(Shasta) *Body Works,*			
orange, caffeine-free	8 fl. oz.	60	15.0
Mix:			
(Tiger's Milk):			
Breakfast Booster	2 T.	70	14.0
Energy Booster	3 heaping T.	120	28.0
Protein Booster, Dutch			
chocolate or vanilla			
orange creme	3 heaping T.	90	12.0
(Weider):			
Carbo Energizer, orange	4 scoops	230	58.0
90 Plus, vanilla, sugar free	2 scoops	100	1.0

SQUAB, pigeon, raw (USDA):

Food	Measure	Cals.	Carbs.
Dressed	1 lb. (weighed with feet, inedible viscera & bones)	569	0.0
Meat & skin	4 oz.	333	0.0
Meat only	4 oz.	161	0.0
Light meat only, without skin	4 oz.	142	0.0
Giblets	1 oz.	44	.3

SQUASH, SUMMER:
Fresh (USDA):
Crookneck & straightneck, yellow:

Whole	1 lb. (weighed untrimmed)	89	19.1
Boiled, drained:			
Diced	½ cup (3.6 oz.)	15	3.2
Slices	½ cup (3.1 oz.)	13	2.7

Scallop, white & pale green:

Whole	1 lb. (weighed untrimmed)	93	22.7
Boiled, drained, mashed	½ cup (4.2 oz.)	19	4.5

Zucchini & cocazelle, green:

Whole	1 lb. (weighed untrimmed)	73	15.5
Boiled, drained slices	½ cup (2.7 oz.)	9	1.9
Canned (Progresso) zucchini, Italian style	½ cup	50	8.0

Frozen:
(Birds Eye):

Regular	⅓ of 10-oz. pkg.	22	3.9
Zucchini	⅓ of 10-oz. pkg.	19	3.3

(Larsen):

Yellow crookneck	3.3 oz.	18	4.0
Zucchini	3.3-oz.	16	3.0

(McKenzie):

Crookneck	⅓ of pkg. (3.3 oz.)	20	4.0
Zucchini	3.3 oz.	18	3.0
(Ore-Ida) zucchini, breaded	3 oz.	150	15.0

(Southland):

Crookneck	⅕ of 16-oz. pkg.	15	4.0
Zucchini	⅕ of 16-oz. pkg.	15	3.0

SQUASH, WINTER:
Fresh (USDA):

Food	Measure	Cals.	Carbs.
Acorn:			
Whole	1 lb. (weighed with skin & seeds)	152	38.6
Baked, flesh only, mashed	½ cup (3.6 oz.)	56	14.3
Boiled, mashed	½ cup (4.1 oz.)	39	9.7
Butternut:			
Whole	1 lb. (weighed with skin & seeds)	171	44.4
Baked, flesh only	4 oz.	77	19.8
Boiled, flesh only	4 oz.	46	11.8
Hubbard:			
Whole	1 lb. (weighed with skin & seeds)	117	28.1
Baked, flesh only	4 oz.	57	13.3
Boiled, flesh only, diced	½ cup (4.2 oz.)	35	8.1
Boiled, flesh only, mashed	½ cup (4.3 oz.)	37	8.4
Frozen:			
(USDA) heated	½ cup (4.2 oz.)	46	11.0
(Birds Eye)	⅓ of pkg. (3.3 oz.)	43	9.2
(Southland) butternut	⅕ of 20-oz. pkg.	45	11.0
SQUASH PUREE, canned (Larsen) no salt added	½ cup (4.5 oz.)	35	7.5
SQUASH SEEDS, dry (USDA):			
In hull	4 oz.	464	12.6
Hulled	1 oz.	157	4.3
SQUID, raw (USDA) meat only	4 oz.	95	1.7
STARCH (See **CORNSTARCH**)			
STEAK UMM	2-oz. serving	180	0.0
STEW (See individual listings such as **BEEF STEW**)			
STIR FRY ENTREE MIX, frozen			
(Green Giant) *Create A Meal:*			
Lo-mein	1¼ cups	320	32.0
Sweet & sour	1¼ cups	290	28.0
Szechuan	1¼ cups	320	21.0

Food	Measure	Cals.	Carbs.
Teriyaki	1¼ cups	240	18.1
Vegetable almond	1⅓ cup	320	23.0
STOMACH, PORK, scalded (USDA)	4 oz.	172	0.0
STRAINED FOOD (See **BABY FOOD**)			
STRAWBERRY:			
Fresh (USDA):			
Whole	1 lb. (weighed with caps & stems)	161	36.6
Whole, capped	1 cup (5.1 oz.)	53	2.1
Canned (USDA) unsweetened or low calorie, water pack, solids & liq.	4 oz.	25	6.4
Frozen (Birds Eye):			
Halves:			
Regular	⅓ of 16-oz. pkg.	164	34.9
Quick thaw in lite syrup	½ of 10-oz. pkg.	68	15.8
Whole:			
Regular	¼ of 16-oz. pkg.	89	21.4
In lite syrup	¼ of 16-oz. pkg.	61	14.4
Quick thaw	1.2 of 10-oz. pkg.	125	30.1
*STRAWBERRY DRINK, mix (Funny Face)	8 fl. oz.	88	22.0
STRAWBERRY FRUIT JUICE, canned (Smucker's)	8 fl. oz.	120	30.0
STRAWBERRY-GUAVA JUICE, canned (Knudsen & Sons)	8 fl. oz.	105	26.0
STRAWBERRY JELLY:			
Sweetened (Smucker's)	1 T. (.7 oz.)	53	13.5
Dietetic:			
(Diet Delight)	1 T. (.6 oz.)	12	3.0
(Estee)	1 T.	18	4.8
(Featherweight)	1 T.	16	4.0
STRAWBERRY NECTAR, canned (Libby's)	6 fl. oz.	60	14.0

Food	Measure	Cals.	Carbs.
STRAWBERRY PRESERVE OR JAM:			
Sweetened:			
(Smucker's)	1 T. (.7 oz.)	53	13.5
(Welch's)	1 T.	52	13.5
Dietetic or low calorie:			
(Estee)	1 T. (.6 oz.)	6	0.0
(Featherweight) calorie reduced	1 T.	16	4.0
(Louis Sherry) wild	1 T. (.6 oz.)	6	0.0
(S&W) *Nutradiet*, red label	1 T.	12	3.0
STUFFING, FROZEN (Green Giant) *Stuffing Originals*:			
Chicken	½ cup	170	21.0
Cornbread	½ cup	170	25.0
Mushroom	½ cup	150	19.0
Wild rice	½ cup	160	21.0
STUFFING MIX:			
Apple & raisin (Pepperidge Farm)	1 oz.	110	21.0
*Beef, *Stove Top*	½ cup	181	21.5
*Chicken:			
(Bell's)	½ cup	224	25.0
(Betty Crocker)	⅓ of pkg.	180	21.0
(Pepperidge Farm)	1 oz.	110	20.0
Stove Top	½ cup	178	20.2
*(Town House)	½ cup	180	20.0
Cornbread:			
(Pepperidge Farm)	1 oz.	110	22.0
Stove Top	½ cup	174	21.6
(Town House)	½ cup	170	20.0
Cube (Pepperidge Farm)	1 oz.	110	22.0
*Herb (Betty Crocker) seasoned	⅙ of pkg.	190	22.0
*New England style, *Stove Top*	½ cup	180	20.8
*Pork, *Stove Top*	½ cup	176	20.3
*Premium blend (Bell's)	½ cup	180	24.0
*Ready mix (Bell's)	½ cup	224	25.0
*San Francisco style, *Stove Top*	½ cup	175	19.9
Turkey, *Stove Top*	½ cup	177	20.7
White bread (Mrs. Cubbison's)	1 oz.	101	20.5
Wild rice & mushroom (Pepperidge Farm)	1 oz.	130	17.0

Food	Measure	Cals.	Carbs.
STURGEON (USDA)			
Raw:			
Section	1 lb. (weighed with skin & bones)	362	0.0
Meat only	4 oz.	107	0.0
Smoked	4 oz.	169	0.0
Steamed	4 oz.	181	0.0
SUBWAY **RESTAURANTS:**			
Salad:			
BMT:			
Regular	1 serving	635	14.0
Small	1 serving	360	12.0
Cold Cut combo:			
Regular	1 serving	506	14.0
Small	1 serving	305	12.0
Ham & cheese:			
Regular	1 serving	296	12.0
Small	1 serving	200	11.0
Italian, spicy:			
Regular	1 serving	696	14.0
Small	1 serving	369	12.0
Roast beef:			
Regular	1 serving	340	15.0
Small	1 serving	222	13.0
Seafood & crab:			
Regular	1 serving	639	29.0
Small	1 serving	371	18.0
Seafood & lobster:			
Regular	1 serving	597	26.0
Small	1 serving	351	18.0
Subway club:			
Regular	1 serving	346	14.0
Small	1 serving	225	12.0
Tuna:			
Regular	1 serving	756	12.0
Small	1 serving	430	12.0
Turkey breast:			
Regular	1 serving	297	14.0
Small	1 serving	201	12.0
Veggies & cheese	1 regular order	188	12.0
Salad dressing:			
Regular:			
Blue cheese	2-oz. serving	322	14.0
French	2-oz. serving	264	20.0

Food	Measure	Cals.	Carbs.
Italian, creamy	2-oz. serving	256	5.0
Thousand Island	2-oz. serving	252	10.0
Dietetic, Italian, lite	2-oz. serving	23	4.0
Sub:			
BMT	6-inch sandwich	491	41.0
Cold cut combo	6-inch sandwich	427	41.0
Ham & cheese	6-inch sandwich	322	41.0
Italian, spicy	6-inch sandwich	491	41.0
Meatball	6-inch sandwich	458	48.0
Roast beef	6-inch sandwich	345	42.0
Seafood & crab	6-inch sandwich	493	47.0
Seafood & lobster	6-inch sandwich	472	47.0
Steak & cheese	6-inch sandwich	383	42.0
Subway club	6-inch sandwich	346	42.0
Tuna	6-inch sandwich	552	41.0
Turkey breast	6-inch sandwich	322	41.0
Veggies & cheese	6-inch sandwich	268	41.0
SUCCOTASH:			
Canned, solids & liq.:			
(Comstock):			
Cream style	½ cup (4.4 oz.)	110	20.0
Whole kernel	½ cup (4.4 oz.)	80	15.0
(Larsen) *Freshlike*	½ cup (4.5 oz.)	80	18.0
(S&W) country style	½ cup	80	16.0
Frozen (Bel-Air)	⅓ of 10-oz. pkg.	100	19.0
SUCKER, CARP (USDA) raw:			
Whole	1 lb. (weighed whole)	196	0.0
Meat only	4 oz.	126	0.0
SUCKER, including **WHITE MULLET** (USDA) raw:			
Whole	1 lb. (weighed whole)	203	0.0
Meat only	4 oz.	118	0.0
SUET, raw (USDA)	1 oz.	242	0.0
SUGAR, beet or cane (there are no differences in calories and carbohydrates among brands) (USDA):			
Brown:			

Food	Measure	Cals.	Carbs.
Regular	1 lb.	1692	437.3
Brownulated	1 cup (5.4 oz.)	567	146.5
Firm-packed	1 cup (7.5 oz.)	791	204.4
Firm-packed	1 T. (.5 oz.)	48	12.5
Confectioner's:			
Unsifted	1 cup (4.3 oz.)	474	122.4
Unsifted	1 T. (8 grams)	30	7.7
Sifted	1 cup (3.4 oz.)	366	94.5
Sifted	1 T. (6 grams)	23	5.9
Stirred	1 cup (4.2 oz.)	462	119.4
Stirred	1 T. (8 grams)	29	7.5
Granulated	1 lb.	1746	451.3
Granulated	1 cup (6.9 oz.)	751	194.0
Granulated	1 T. (.4 oz.)	46	11.9
Granulated	1 lump (1⅛" × ¾" × ⅜", 6 grams)	23	6.0
Maple	1 lb.	1579	408.0
Maple	1¾" × 1¼" × ½" piece (1.2 oz.)	104	27.0
SUGAR APPLE, raw (USDA):			
Whole	1 lb. (weighed with skin & seeds)	192	48.4
Flesh only	4 oz.	107	26.9
SUGAR PUFFS, cereal (Malt-O-Meal)	⅞ cup (1 oz.)	109	24.7
SUGAR SUBSTITUTE:			
(Estee) fructose	1 tsp.	12	3.0
(Equal) aspartame	1 pkg.	4	<1.0
(NutraSweet) aspartame	1 tsp.	2	<1.0
Spoon for Spoon	1 tsp.	2	1.0
Sprinkle Sweet (Pillsbury)	1 tsp.	2	.5
Sweet 'N Low:			
Brown	1 tsp.	20	10.0
Granulated	1-gram packet	14	.9
Liquid	1 drop	0	0.0
Sweet'n It (Estee) liquid	6 drops	0	0.0
*Sweet *10* (Pillsbury)	⅛ tsp.	0	0.0
(Weight Watchers) *Sweet'ner*	1-gram packet	4	1.0
SUKIYAKI DINNER, canned:			
(Chun King) stir fry	6-oz. serving	257	9.6
(La Choy)	⅜ cup	210	9.0

Food	Measure	Cals.	Carbs.
SUNFLAKES MULTI-GRAIN, cereal (Ralston Purina)	1 cup (1 oz.)	100	24.0
SUNFLOWER SEED:			
(USDA):			
In hulls	4 oz. (weighed in hull)	343	12.2
Hulled	1 oz.	159	5.6
(Fisher):			
In hull, roasted, salted	1 oz.	86	3.0
Hulled, roasted:			
Dry, salted	1 oz.	164	5.6
Oil, salted	1 oz.	167	5.6
(Party Pride) dry roasted	1 oz.	190	3.0
(Planters):			
Dry roasted	1 oz.	160	5.0
Unsalted	1 oz.	170	5.0
SUNFLOWER SEED FLOUR, (See **FLOUR**)			
SUNSHINE PUNCH DRINK, canned (Johanna Farms) *Ssips*	8.45-fl.-oz. container	130	32.0
SUNTOPS (Dole)	1 bar	40	9.0
SURIMI (See **CRAB, IMITATION**)			
SUZY Q's (Hostess)			
Banana	1 piece	240	38.0
Chocolate	1 piece	250	37.0
SWAMP CABBAGE (USDA):			
Raw, whole	1 lb. (weighed untrimmed)	107	19.8
Boiled, trimmed, drained	4 oz.	24	4.4
SWEETBREADS (USDA):			
Beef:			
Raw	1 lb.	939	0.0
Braised	4 oz.	363	0.0
Calf:			
Raw	1 lb.	426	0.0

Food	Measure	Cals.	Carbs.
Braised	4 oz.	363	0.0
Hog (See **PANCREAS**)			
Lamb:			
Raw	1 lb.	426	0.0
Braised	4 oz.	198	0.0
SWEET POTATO (See also **YAM**):			
Baked (USDA) peeled after baking	5" × 2" potato (3.9 oz.)	155	35.8
Candied, home recipe (USDA)	3½" × 2¼" piece (6.2 oz.)	294	59.8
Canned:			
(USDA):			
In syrup	4-oz. serving	129	31.2
Vacuum or solid pack	½ cup (3.8 oz.)	118	27.1
(Joan of Arc):			
Mashed	½ cup (4 oz.)	90	24.0
Whole:			
Candied	½ cup (5.2 oz.)	240	60.0
Heavy syrup	½ cup (4.5 oz.)	130	34.0
Light syrup	½ cup (4 oz.)	110	28.0
In pineapple-orange sauce	½ cup (5 oz.)	210	54.0
(Trappey's) *Sugary Sam:*			
Cut, in light syrup	½ cup (4.3 oz.)	110	25.0
Mashed	½ cup (4.3 oz.)	100	25.0
Whole, in heavy syrup	½ cup (4.3 oz.)	130	30.0
Frozen (Mrs. Paul's) candied:			
Regular	4-oz. serving	170	42.0
N' apples	4-oz. serving	160	38.0
SWEET POTATO PIE (USDA) home recipe	⅙ of 9" pie (5.4 oz.)	324	36.0
SWEET N' SOUR COCKTAIL MIX, liquid (Holland House)	1 fl. oz.	31	8.0
SWEET & SOUR PORK (See **PORK**)			
SWEET SUCCESS (Nestlé):			
Bar, chewy	1 bar	120	18.0

Food	Measure	Cals.	Carbs.
Canned, chocolate mocha, creamy milk chocolate & dark chocolate & dark chocolate fudge	10 fl. oz.	200	32.0
*Mix:			
Chocolate raspberry truffle or dark chocolate fudge	8 fl. oz.	180	23.0
Rich chocolate almond	8 fl. oz.	180	24.0
SWISS STEAK, frozen:			
(Budget Gourmet)	11.2-oz. meal	450	40.0
(Swanson) 4-compartment dinner	10-oz. dinner	350	37.0
SWORDFISH (USDA):			
Raw, meat only	1 lb.	535	0.0
Broiled, with butter or margarine	3" × 3" × ½" steak (4.4 oz.)	218	0.0
Canned, solids & liq.	4 oz.	116	0.0
Frozen (Captain's Choice)	3-oz. steak	132	0.0
SYRUP (See also **TOPPING**):			
Regular:			
Apricot (Smucker's)	1 T. (.6 oz.)	50	13.0
Blackberry (Smucker's)	1 T. (.6 oz.)	50	13.0
Blueberry (Smucker's)	1 T.	50	13.0
Boysenberry	1 T.	50	13.0
Chocolate or chocolate-flavored:			
(Hershey's)	1 T. (.7 oz.)	40	8.5
(Nestlé) *Quik*	1 oz.	80	18.0
Cane (USDA)	1 T. (.7 oz.)	55	14.0
Corn, *Karo*, dark or light	1 T. (.7 oz.)	58	14.5
Maple:			
(USDA)	1 T. (.7 oz.)	50	13.0
(Home Brands)	1 T. (.7 oz.)	55	13.0
Karo, imitation	1 T.	57	14.2
Pancake or waffle:			
(Aunt Jemima)	1 T. (.7 oz.)	53	13.1
Golden Griddle	1 T. (.7 oz.)	55	14.2
Karo	1 T. (.7 oz.)	60	14.9
Mrs. Butterworth's	1 T. (.7 oz.)	55	7.5
Strawberry (Smucker's)	1 T.	50	13.0
Dietetic or low calorie:			
Blueberry:			
(Estee) breakfast	1 T. (.5 oz.)	12	3.0
(Featherweight)	1 T.	16	4.0

Food	Measure	Cals.	Carbs.
Chocolate or chocolate-flavored:			
(Estee) *Choco-Syp*	1 T.	20	5.0
(Diet Delight)	1 T. (.6 oz.)	8	2.0
(No-Cal)	1 T.	6	0.0
Coffee (No-Cal)	1 T.	6	1.2
Cola (No-Cal)	1 T.	0	Tr.
Maple:			
(Cary's)	1 T.	6	2.0
(S&W) *Nutradiet*, imitation	1 T.	12	3.0
Pancake or waffle:			
(Aunt Jemima)	1 T. (.6 oz.)	29	7.3
(Diet Delight)	1 T. (.6 oz.)	6	4.0
(Estee)	1 T.	8	1.0
Log Cabin	1 T. (.7 oz.)	34	9.1
(Mrs. Butterworth's)	1 T.	30	7.5
(Weight Watchers)	1 T. (.6 oz.)	25	6.0

T

Food	Measure	Cals.	Carbs.
TABOULI MIX:			
(Casbah)	1 oz.	90	20.0
*(Near East)	⅔ cup	120	23.0
TACO:			
*(Ortega)	1 oz.	54	.9
*Mix:			
*(Durkee)	½ cup	321	3.7
(French's)	1¼-oz. pkg.	120	24.0
(McCormick)	1¼-oz. pkg.	123	23.7
(Old El Paso)	1 pkg.	100	20.7
Shell:			
(Gebhardt)	1 shell (.4 oz.)	30	4.0
(Lawry's)	1 shell	50	8.0
(Old El Paso):			
Regular	1 shell	55	6.0
Mini	1 shell	23	2.3
Super	1 shell	100	11.0
(Rosarita)	1 shell (.4 oz.)	45	6.0

Food	Measure	Cals.	Carbs.
TACO BELL RESTAURANTS:			
Burrito:			
Bean:			
Green sauce	6¾-oz. serving	351	52.9
Red sauce	6¾-oz. serving	357	54.5
Beef:			
Green sauce	6¾-oz. serving	398	37.7
Red sauce	6¾-oz. serving	403	39.1
Supreme:			
Regular:			
Green sauce	8½-oz. serving	407	45.2
Red sauce	8½-oz. serving	413	46.6
Double beef:			
Green sauce	9-oz. serving	451	40.3
Red sauce	9-oz. serving	456	41.7
Cinnamon crispas	1.7-oz. serving	259	27.5
Enchirito:			
Green sauce	7½-oz. serving	371	28.0
Red sauce	7½-oz. serving	382	30.9
Fajita:			
Chicken	4¾-oz. serving	225	19.8
Steak	4¾-oz. serving	234	19.5
Guacamole	¾-oz. serving	34	2.9
Meximelt	3¾-oz. serving	266	18.7
Nachos:			
Regular	3¾-oz. serving	345	37.5
Bellgrande	10.1-oz. serving	648	60.6
Pepper, jalapeño	3½-oz. serving	20	4.0
Pico De Gallo, relish	1-oz. serving	8	1.1
Pintos & cheese:			
Green sauce	4½-oz. serving	184	17.5
Red sauce	4½-oz. serving	190	18.9
Pizza, Mexican	7.9-oz. serving	575	39.7
Ranch dressing	2.6-oz. serving	235	1.5
Salsa	.3-oz. serving	18	3.6
Sour cream	¾-oz. serving	46	.9
Taco:			
Regular	2¾-oz. serving	183	10.6
Bellgrande	5¾-oz. serving	355	17.6
Light	6-oz. serving	410	18.1
Platter, light	1 serving	1062	97.0
Soft:			
Regular	3¼-oz. serving	338	17.9
Supreme	4.4-oz. serving	275	19.1
Super combo	5-oz. serving	286	20.9
Taco salad:			
With shell	18.7-oz. serving	502	26.3

Food	Measure	Cals.	Carbs.
With salsa:			
Regular	21-oz. serving	941	63.1
Without shell	18.7-oz. serving	520	30.0
Taco sauce:			
Regular	.4-oz. packet	2	.4
Hot	.4-oz. packet	2	.3
Tostada:			
Green sauce	5½-oz. serving	237	25.1
Red sauce	5½-oz. serving	243	26.6
TACO JOHN'S:			
Burrito:			
Bean	5-oz. serving	197	37.0
Beef	5-oz. serving	303	25.0
Chicken:			
Regular	5-oz. serving	227	19.0
With green chili	12¼-oz. serving	344	29.0
Combo	5-oz. serving	250	31.0
Smothered:			
With green chili	12¼-oz. serving	367	40.0
With Texas chili	12¼-oz. serving	455	47.0
Super:			
Regular	8¼-oz. serving	389	51.0
With chicken	8¼-oz. serving	366	40.0
Chimichanga:			
Regular	12-oz. serving	464	67.0
With chicken	12-oz. serving	441	55.0
Mexican rice	1 serving	567	93.9
Nachos:			
Regular	5-oz. serving	468	45.0
Super	11¼-oz. serving	669	60.0
Potato Ole, large	6-oz. serving	414	96.0
Taco:			
Regular	4¼-oz. serving	178	15.0
With chicken	4¼-oz. serving	140	12.0
Softshell:			
Regular	5-oz. serving	224	23.0
With chicken	5-oz. serving	180	20.0
Taco Bravo:			
Regular	6¾-oz. serving	319	42.0
Super	8-oz. serving	361	43.0
Taco burger	6-oz. serving	275	29.0
Taco salad:			
Regular:			
Without dressing	6-oz. serving	229	30.0
With dressing	8-oz. serving	359	35.0
Chicken:			

Food	Measure	Cals.	Carbs.
Without dressing	12¼-oz. serving	377	56.0
With dressing	14¼-oz. serving	507	61.0
Super:			
Without dressing	12¼-oz. serving	428	59.0
With dressing	14¼-oz. serving	558	65.0
TAMALE:			
Canned:			
(Hormel) beef:			
Regular	1 tamale	70	4.0
Hot & Spicy	1 tamale	70	4.5
Short Orders	7½-oz. can	270	17.0
(Old El Paso), with chili gravy	1 tamale	95	8.0
(Pride of Mexico) beef	2-oz. tamale	115	7.5
Frozen (Patio)	13-oz. dinner	470	58.0
TAMARIND, fresh (USDA):			
Whole	1 lb. (weighed with peel, membrane & seeds) ½ cup (4.4 oz.)	104	24.6
Juice	½ cup (4.4 oz.)	51	12.0
TANG:			
Canned, *Fruit Box*:			
Cherry or strawberry	8.45-fl. oz. container	121	31.5
Grape	8.45-fl. oz. container	131	33.7
Mixed fruit	8.45-fl. oz. container	137	36.0
Orange, tropical	8.45-fl. oz. container	147	37.2
*Mix:			
Regular	6 fl. oz.	86	22.0
Dietetic	6 fl. oz.	5	Tr.
TANGELO, fresh (USDA):			
Whole	1 lb. (weighed with peel, membrane & seeds)	104	24.6
Juice	½ cup (4.4 oz.)	51	12.0

Food	Measure	Cals.	Carbs.
TANGERINE OR MANDARIN ORANGE:			
Fresh (USDA):			
Whole	1 lb. (weighed with peel, membrane & seeds)	154	38.9
Whole	4.1-oz. tangerine (2⅜" dia.)	39	10.0
Sections (without membranes)	1 cup (6.8 oz.)	89	22.4
Canned, regular pack:			
(Dole)	½ cup (4.4 oz.)	70	19.0
(S&W) in heavy syrup	½ cup	76	20.0
(Town House)	5½-oz.	100	25.0
Canned, dietetic or low calorie, solids & liq.:			
(Diet Delight) juice pack	½ cup (4.3 oz.)	50	13.0
(S&W) *Nutradiet*	½ cup	28	7.0
*TANGERINE JUICE, frozen (Minute Maid)	6 fl. oz.	91	21.9
TAPIOCA, dry, *Minute,* quick cooking	1 T. (.3 oz.)	32	7.9
TAQUITO, frozen, shredded (Van de Kamp's) beef	8-oz. serving	490	45.0
TARO, raw (USDA):			
Tubers, whole	1 lb. (weighed with skin)	373	90.3
Tubers, skin removed	4 oz.	111	26.9
Leaves & stems	1 lb.	181	33.6
TARRAGON (French's)	1 tsp. (1.4 grams)	5	.7
TAUTUG OR BLACKFISH, raw (USDA):			
Whole	1 lb. (weighed whole)	149	0.0
Meat only	4 oz.	101	0.0
TCBY all flavors:			
Regular, 96% fat free:			
Regular	8.2 oz.	267	47.0
Giant	31.6 oz.	1027	182.0

Food	Measure	Cals.	Carbs.
Kiddie	3.2 oz.	104	18.0
Large	10½ oz.	342	60.0
Small	5.9 oz.	192	34.0
Super	15.2 oz.	494	87.0
Fat free:			
Regular	8.2 oz.	226	47.0
Giant	31.6 oz.	869	182.0
Kiddie	3.2 oz.	88	18.0
Large	10½ oz.	289	60.0
Small	5.9 oz.	162	34.0
Super	15.2 oz.	418	87.0
Fat free, sugar free:			
Regular	8.2 oz.	164	37.0
Giant	31.6 oz.	632	142.0
Kiddie	3.2 oz.	64	18.0
Large	10½ oz.	210	47.0
Small	5.9 oz.	118	27.0
Super	15.2 oz.	304	68.0

*TEA:
Bag:
  (Celestial Seasonings):
    After dinner:

Food	Measure	Cals.	Carbs.
Amaretto Nights or *Cinnamon Vienna*	1 cup	<3	.3
Bavarian Chocolate Orange	1 cup	7	1.6
Caffeine free	1 cup	4	.8
Fruit & tea	1 cup	<3	1.0
Herb:			
Almond Sunset, Cinnamon Rose or *Cranberry Cove*	1 cup	3	<2.0
Emperor's Choice, Lemon Zinger or *Raspberry Patch*	1 cup	4	<2.0
Mandarin Orange Spice or *Orange Zinger*	1 cup	5	<2.0
Roastaroma	1 cup	11	2.0
Premium black tea	1 cup	3	.4
(Lipton):			
Plain or flavored	1 cup	2	Tr.
Herbal:			
Almond pleasure, dessert mint, gentle orange or cinnamon apple	1 cup	2	0.0

Food	Measure	Cals.	Carbs.
Quietly chamomile or toasty spice	1 cup	4	Tr.
(Sahadi):			
Herbal	6 fl. oz.	2	0.0
Spearmint	6 fl. oz.	4	Tr.
Instant (Lipton) 100% tea or lemon flavored	8 fl. oz.	2	0.0
TEA, ICED:			
Canned:			
Regular:			
(Arizona) peach or raspberry flavored	8 fl. oz.	95	25.0
(Johanna Farms) *Ssips* container	8.45 fl. oz.	100	26.0
(Lipton) lemon & sugar flavored	6 fl. oz.	70	18.0
(Mistic):			
Lemon flavored	8 fl. oz.	90	24.0
Peach flavored	8 fl. oz.	100	30.0
(Shasta)	6 fl. oz.	61	16.5
(Snapple):			
Lemon or orange flavored	8 fl. oz.	110	27.0
Peach flavored	8 fl. oz.	110	9.0
Dietetic:			
(Arizona) low calorie, sugar free	8 fl. oz.	40	0.0
(Lipton) lemon flavored	8 fl. oz.	3	0.0
(Snapple) lemon or raspberry flavored	8 fl. oz.	4	<1.0
*Mix:			
Regular:			
Country Time, sugar & lemon flavored	8 fl. oz.	121	30.2
(Lipton)	8 fl. oz.	60	16.0
(Nestea) lemon & sugar flavored	8 fl. oz.	93	12.0
Decaffeinated (Lipton) sugar & lemon flavored	8 fl. oz.	80	20
Dietetic:			
Crystal Light	8 fl. oz.	2	.2
(Lipton) lemon flavored	8 fl. oz.	2	0.0
(Nestea) light	8 fl. oz.	5	1.3
TEAM, cereal (Nabisco)	1 cup (1 oz.)	110	24.0

Food	Measure	Cals.	Carbs.
TEENAGE MUTANT NINJA TURTLES, cereal (Ralston Purina)	1 cup (1-oz.)	110	26.0
TEQUILA SUNRISE COCKTAIL (Mr. Boston) 12% alcohol	3 fl. oz.	120	14.4
TERIYAKI, frozen:			
(Armour) *Dining Lite,* beef	9-oz. meal	270	36.0
(Chun King) beef	13-oz. entree	379	68.0
(La Choy) Fresh & Light, with rice & vegetables	10-oz. meal	240	39.9
(Stouffer's) beef, with rice & vegetables	9¾-oz. meal	290	33.0
TERIYAKI BASTE & GLAZE (Kikkoman)	1 T. (.8 oz.)	28	6.0
TERIYAKI MARINADE & SAUCE (La Choy)	1 oz.	30	5.0
***TEXTURED VEGETABLE PROTEIN,** Morningstar Farms:*			
Breakfast link	1 link	73	1.3
Breakfast patties	1 patty (1.3 oz.)	100	3.5
Breakfast strips	1 strip (.3 oz.)	37	.6
Grillers	1 patty (2.3 oz.)	190	6.0
THURINGER:			
(Eckrich):			
Sliced	1-oz. slice	90	1.0
Smoky Tangy	1-oz. serving	80	1.0
(Hormel):			
Packaged, sliced	1 slice	80	0.0
Whole:			
Regular or tangy, chub	1 oz.	90	0.0
Beefy	1-oz. serving	100	0.0
Old Smokehouse	1-oz. serving	90	1.0
(Louis Rich) turkey	1-oz. slice	50	Tr.
(Ohse):			
Regular	1 oz.	75	2.0
Beef	1 oz.	80	1.0
(Oscar Mayer):			
Regular	.8-oz. slice	71	.3
Beef	.8-oz. slice	69	.1

Food	Measure	Cals.	Carbs.
THYME (French's)	1 tsp.	5	1.0
TOASTED WHEAT AND RAISINS, cereal (Nabisco)	1 oz.	100	23.0
TOASTER CAKE OR PASTRY:			
Pop-Tarts (Kellogg's):			
Regular:			
Blueberry or cherry	1.8-oz. pastry	200	37.0
Brown sugar cinnamon	1¾-oz. pastry	210	33.0
Strawberry	1.8-oz. pastry	200	37.0
Frosted:			
Blueberry or strawberry	1 pastry	190	35.0
Brown sugar cinnamon	1 pastry	210	34.0
Cherry chocolate fudge	1 pastry	200	36.0
Chocolate-vanilla creme	1 pastry	210	37.0
Concord grape, dutch apple or raspberry	1 pastry	210	36.0
Toaster Tarts (Pepperidge Farm):			
Apple cinnamon	1 piece	170	25.0
Cheese	1 piece	190	22.0
Strawberry	1 piece	190	28.0
Toastettes (Nabisco):			
Regular, any flavor	1 pastry	200	36.0
Frosted:			
Brown sugar cinnamon or strawberry	1 pastry	190	35.0
Fudge	1 pastry	190	34.0
Toast-R-Cake (Thomas'):			
Blueberry	1 piece	100	17.0
Bran	1 piece	103	17.6
Corn	1 piece	120	19.2
TOASTY O's, cereal (Malt-O-Meal)	1¼ cups (1 oz.)	107	20.3
TOFU (See **SOYBEAN CURD**)			
TOFUTTI:			
Frozen:			
Regular:			
Chocolate	4 fl. oz.	180	18.0
Maple walnut	4 fl. oz.	230	20.0
Vanilla	4 fl. oz.	200	21.0
Vanilla almond bark	4 fl. oz.	210	21.0
Wildberry supreme	4 fl. oz.	210	22.0

Food	Measure	Cals.	Carbs.
Cuties:			
Chocolate	1 piece	140	21.0
Vanilla	1 piece	130	21.0
Lite Lite, chocolate-vanilla	4 fl. oz.	90	20.0
Love Drops	4 fl. oz.	230	26.0
Soft serve:			
Regular	4 fl. oz.	190	20.0
Lite	4 fl. oz.	90	20.0
TOMATO:			
Fresh (USDA):			
Green:			
Whole, untrimmed	1 lb. (weighed with core & stem end)	99	21.1
Trimmed, unpeeled	4 oz.	27	5.8
Ripe:			
Whole:			
Eaten with skin	1 lb.	100	21.3
Peeled	1 lb. (weighed with skin, stem ends & hard core)	88	18.8
Peeled	1 med. (2" × 2½", 5.3 oz.)	33	7.0
Peeled	1 small (1¾" × 2½", 3.9 oz.)	24	5.2
Sliced, peeled	½ cup (3.2 oz.)	20	4.2
Boiled (USDA)	½ cup (4.3 oz.)	31	6.7
Canned, regular pack, solids & liq.:			
(Contadina):			
Sliced, baby	½ cup (4.2 oz.)	50	10.0
Pear shape	½ cup (4.2 oz.)	25	6.0
Stewed	½ cup (4.3 oz.)	35	9.0
Whole, peeled	½ cup (4.2 oz.)	25	5.0
(Del Monte):			
Stewed	4 oz.	35	8.0
Wedges	½ cup (4 oz.)	30	8.0
Whole, peeled	½ cup (4 oz.)	25	5.0
(Hunt's):			
Crushed	½ cup	40	9.0
Cut, peeled	4-oz. serving	20	5.0
Pear shaped, Italian	4-oz. serving	20	5.0
Stewed, regular	4-oz. serving	35	8.0

Food	Measure	Cals.	Carbs.
Whole	4-oz. serving	20	5.0
(La Victoria) green, whole	1 T.	4	1.0
(S & W):			
Aspic, supreme	½ cup	60	16.0
Diced, in rich puree	½ cup	35	8.0
Sliced	½ cup	35	9.0
Whole, peeled	½ cup	25	6.0
(Town House):			
Stewed	½ cup	35	9.0
Whole	½ cup	25	6.0
Canned, dietetic pack, solids & liq.:			
(Diet Delight) whole, peeled	½ cup (4.3 oz.)	25	5.0
(Furman's) crushed	½ cup	72	13.1
(Hunt's) no added salt:			
Stewed	4-oz. serving	35	8.0
Whole	4-oz. serving	20	5.0

TOMATO, PICKLED

Food	Measure	Cals.	Carbs.
(Claussen) green	1 piece (1 oz.)	6	1.1

TOMATO & PEPPER, HOT CHILI:

Food	Measure	Cals.	Carbs.
(Old El Paso), Jalapeño	¼ cup	13	2.5
(Ortega) Jalapeño	1 oz.	10	2.6

TOMATO JUICE, CANNED:
Regular pack:

Food	Measure	Cals.	Carbs.
(Ardmore Farms)	6 fl. oz.	36	7.8
(Campbell's)	6 fl. oz.	40	8.0
(Hunt's)	6 fl. oz.	30	7.0
(Knudsen & Sons) organic)	8 fl. oz.	50	10.0
(S & W) California	6 fl. oz.	35	8.0
(Town House)	6 fl. oz.	35	8.0
Dietetic pack:			
(Diet Delight)	6 fl. oz.	35	7.0
(Hunt's) no added salt	6 fl. oz.	30	8.0
(S & W) *Nutradiet*	6 fl. oz.	35	8.0

TOMATO PASTE, canned:
Regular pack:

Food	Measure	Cals.	Carbs.
(Contadina):			
Regular	6 oz.	150	35.0
Italian:			
Plain	6 oz.	210	36.0
With mushroom	6 oz.	180	36.0

Food	Measure	Cals.	Carbs.
(Hunt's):			
Regular	2 oz.	45	11.0
Garlic	2 oz.	60	11.0
Italian style	2 oz.	50	11.0
(Town House)	6 oz.	150	35.0
Dietetic (Hunt's) low sodium	2 oz.	45	11.0
TOMATO PUREE, canned:			
Regular (Hunt's)	½ cup (4.2 oz.)	45	10.0
Dietetic (Featherweight) low sodium	1 cup	90	20.0
TOMATO SAUCE (See also **PASTA SAUCE** or **SAUCE**)			
Fresh, refrigerated (Contadina):			
Light	4 oz.	40	7.2
Marinara	4 oz.	53	6.4
Plum tomatoes, with basil	4 oz.	53	7.5
Canned:			
(Contadina):			
Regular	½ cup (4.4 oz.)	45	9.0
Italian style	½ cup (4.4 oz.)	40	8.0
(Furman's)	½ cup	58	9.8
(Hunt's):			
Regular or with bits	4 oz.	30	7.0
With garlic	4 oz.	70	10.0
Herb	4 oz.	70	12.0
Italian	4 oz.	60	10.0
With mushrooms	4 oz.	25	6.0
With onions	4 oz.	40	9.0
Special	4 oz.	35	8.0
(Town House)	4 oz.	40	9.0
TOMATO, SUN-DRIED, (Bella Sun Luci) in oil with herbs	1 oz.	90	9.0
TOMCOD, ATLANTIC, raw (USDA):			
Whole	1 lb. (weighed whole)	136	0.0
Meat only	4 oz.	87	0.0
TOM COLLINS (Mr. Boston) 12½% alcohol	3 fl. oz.	111	10.8

Food	Measure	Cals.	Carbs.
*TOM COLLINS MIX			
(Bar-Tender's)	6 fl. oz.	177	18.0
TONGUE (USDA):			
Beef, medium fat:			
Raw, untrimmed	1 lb.	714	1.4
Braised	4 oz.	277	.5
Calf:			
Raw, untrimmed	1 lb.	454	3.1
Braised	4 oz.	181	1.1
Hog:			
Raw, untrimmed	1 lb.	741	1.7
Braised	4 oz.	287	.6
Lamb:			
Raw, untrimmed	1 lb.	659	1.7
Braised	4 oz.	288	.6
Sheep:			
Raw, untrimmed	1 lb.	877	7.9
Braised	4 oz.	366	2.7
TONGUE, CANNED:			
(USDA):			
Pickled	1 oz.	76	Tr.
Potted or deviled	1 oz.	82	.2
(Hormel) cured	1 oz.	63	0.0
TONIC WATER (See **SOFT DRINK**, quinine or tonic)			
TOOTIE FRUITIES, cereal			
(Malt-O-Meal)	1 cup (1-oz.)	113	24.7
TOPPING:			
Regular:			
Butterscotch (Smucker's)	1 T. (.7 oz.)	70	16.5
Caramel (Smucker's) hot	1 T.	75	14.0
Chocolate:			
(Hershey's) fudge	1 T.	50	9.0
(Smucker's):			
Regular	1 T.	65	13.5
Fudge:			
Regular	1 T.	65	15.5
Hot	1 T.	55	9.0
Milk	1 T.	70	15.5
Marshmallow (Smucker's)	1 T.	60	14.5
Nut (Planters)	½ oz.	90	4.5

Food	Measure	Cals.	Carbs.
Peanut butter caramel			
(Smucker's)	1 T.	75	14.5
Pecans in syrup (Smucker's)	1 T.	65	14.0
Pineapple (Smucker's)	1 T. (.7 oz.)	65	16.0
Strawberry (Smucker's)	1 T.	60	15.0
Walnuts in syrup (Smucker's)	1 T.	65	13.5
Dietetic, chocolate (Smucker's)	1 T. (.6 oz.)	35	9.5

TOPPING, WHIPPED:
Regular:
Cool Whip (Birds Eye):

Dairy	1 T.	16	1.2
Non-dairy	1 T.	13	1.0
Dover Farms, dairy	1 T. (.2 oz.)	17	1.2
(Johanna Farms) aerosol	1 T. (3 grams)	8	*1.0
Dietetic (Featherweight)	1 T.	3	.5

*Mix:

Regular, *Dream Whip*	1 T. (.2 oz.)	9	.9
Dietetic (Estee)	1 T.	4	Tr.

TORTELLINI:
Fresh, refrigerated (See
**PASTA, DRY
OR FRESH,
REFRIGERATED**)

Canned (Chef Boyardee) meat, microwave main meal	10½-oz. serving	220	50.0

Frozen:

(Armour) *Classics Lite,* with meat	10-oz. dinner	250	8.0
(Budget Gourmet) cheese, side dish	5½-oz. serving	200	25.0

(Buitoni):
Cheese filled:

Regular	2.6-oz. serving	222	29.8
Tricolor	2.6-oz. serving	221	29.7
Verdi	2.6-oz. serving	220	29.8

Meat filled:

Plain	2.4-oz. serving	212	21.9
Entree	2.5-oz. serving	223	32.4

(Green Giant):

Cheese, marinara, One Serving	5½-oz. pkg.	260	37.0
Provencale, microwave Garden Gourmet	9½-oz. pkg.	210	36.0

(Le Menu) cheese, healthy
style:

Food	Measure	Cals.	Carbs.
Dinner	10-oz. dinner	230	35.0
Entree	8-oz. entree	250	34.0
(Stouffer's):			
Cheese:			
Alfredo sauce	8⅞-oz. meal	600	32.0
Tomato sauce	9⅝-oz. meal	360	37.0
Vinaigrette	6⅞-oz. meal	400	24.0
Veal, in Alfredo sauce	8⅝-oz. meal	500	32.0
(Weight Watchers)	9-oz. meal	310	50.0
TORTILLA (Old El Paso):			
Corn	1 piece	60	10.0
Flour	1 piece	150	27.0
TOSTADA SHELL:			
(Old El Paso)	1 shell (.4 oz.)	55	6.0
(Ortega)	1 shell (.4 oz.)	50	6.0
TOTAL, cereal (General Mills):			
Regular	1 cup (1 oz.)	110	22.0
Corn	1 cup (1 oz.)	110	24.0
Raisin bran	1 cup (1.5-oz.)	140	33.0
TOWEL GOURD, raw (USDA):			
Unpared	1 lb. (weighed with skin)	69	15.8
Pared	4 oz.	20	4.6
TRICOLOR PASTA (See **PASTA, DRY OR FRESH, REFRIGERATED**)			
TRIPE:			
Beef (USDA):			
Commercial	4 oz.	113	0.0
Pickled	4 oz.	70	0.0
Canned (Libby's)	¼ of 24-oz. can	290	1.1
TRIPLE SEC LIQUEUR (Mr. Boston)	1 fl. oz.	79	8.5

Food	Measure	Cals.	Carbs.
TRIX, cereal (General Mills)	1 cup (1 oz.)	110	25.0
TROPICAL CITRUS DRINK, chilled or *frozen (Five Alive)	6 fl. oz.	85	21.3
TROPICAL FRUIT JUICE, canned (Juicy Juice)	8.45-fl.-oz. container	150	36.0
TROPICAL LIME COOLER, canned (Knudsen & Sons)	8 fl. oz.	130	32.0
TROPICAL PASSION JUICE, canned (Knudsen & Sons)	8 fl. oz.	80	20.0
*TROPIC QUENCHER DRINK, mix, dietetic, *Crystal Light*	8 fl. oz.	3	Tr.
TROUT (USDA):			
Brook, fresh:			
Whole	1 lb. (weighed whole)	224	0.0
Meat only	4 oz.	115	0.0
Lake (See **LAKE TROUT**)			
Rainbow:			
Fresh, meat with skin	4 oz.	221	0.0
Canned	4 oz.	237	0.0
TUNA:			
Raw (USDA) meat only:			
Bluefin	4 oz.	164	0.0
Yellowfin	4 oz.	151	0.0
Canned in oil:			
(Bumble Bee):			
Chunk, light, solids & liq.	½ of 6½-oz. can	265	0.0
Solid, white, solids & liq.	½ cup (3.5 oz.)	285	0.0
(Carnation) solids & liq.	6½-oz. can	427	0.0
(Progresso) light, solid	⅓ cup	150	*1.0
(Sea Trader) chunk, light	3¼ oz.	230	0.0
(Star Kist) solid, white, solids & liq.	7-oz. serving	503	0.0
(S&W) light, chunk, fancy	2 oz.	140	0.0
Canned in water:			
(Breast O'Chicken)	6½-oz. can	211	0.0
(Bumble Bee):			
Chunk, light, solids & liq.	½ cup	117	0.0

Food	Measure	Cals.	Carbs.
Solid, white, solids & liq.	½ cup	126	0.0
(Sea Trader):			
Chunk, light	3¼ oz.	110	0.0
White albacore	2 oz.	100	0.0
(Star Kist) light	7-oz. can	220	0.0

*TUNA HELPER
(General Mills):

Au gratin	⅕ of pkg.	280	30.0
Cheesy noodles 'n tuna	⅕ of pkg.	250	28.0
Creamy mushroom	⅕ of pkg.	220	28.0
Creamy noodles 'n tuna	⅕ of pkg.	300	30.0
Pot pie	⅙ of pkg.	420	31.0
Tetrazzini	⅕ of pkg.	240	27.0

TUNA NOODLE CASSEROLE:

Canned, *Dinty Moore* (Hormel)	10-oz. can	240	28.0
Frozen:			
(Stouffer's)	10-oz. meal	280	33.0
(Weight Watchers)	9-oz. meal	230	27.0

TUNA PIE, frozen

(Banquet)	7-oz. pie	540	44.0

TUNA SALAD:

Home recipe, (USDA) made with tuna, celery, mayonnaise, pickle, onion and egg	4-oz. serving	193	4.0
Canned (Carnation)	¼ of 7½-oz. can	100	3.3

TURBOT, GREENLAND
(USDA) raw:

Whole	1 lb. (weighed whole)	344	0.0
Meat only	4 oz.	166	0.0

TURKEY:
Raw (USDA):

Ready-to-cook	1 lb. (weighed with bones)	722	0.0
Dark meat	4 oz.	145	0.0
Light meat	4 oz.	132	0.0
Skin only	4 oz.	459	0.0
Raw, ground (Perdue)	4 oz.	160	0.0

Food	Measure	Cals.	Carbs.
Barbecued (Louis Rich) breast, half	1 oz.	40	0.0
Roasted (USDA):			
Flesh, skin & giblets	From 13½-lb. raw, ready-to-cook turkey	9678	0.0
Flesh & skin	From 13½-lb. raw, ready-to cook turkey	7872	0.0
Flesh & skin	4 oz.	253	0.0
Meat only:			
Chopped	1 cup (5 oz.)	268	0.0
Diced	4 oz.	200	0.0
Light	1 slice (4" × 2" × ¼", 3 oz.)	75	0.0
Dark	1 slice (2½" × 1⅝" × ¼", .7 oz.)	43	0.0
Skin only	1 oz.	128	0.0
Giblets, simmered (USDA)	2 oz.	132	.9
Gizzard (USDA):			
Raw	4 oz.	178	1.2
Simmered	4 oz.	222	12.
Canned (Swanson) chunk	2½-oz. serving	120	0.0
Packaged:			
(Carl Buddig) smoked:			
Regular	1 oz.	50	Tr.
Ham or salami	1 oz.	40	Tr.
Hebrew National, breast	1 oz.	37	*1.0
(Hormel) breast:			
Regular	1 slice	30	0.0
Smoked	1 slice	25	0.0
(Louis Rich):			
Turkey bologna	1-oz. slice	60	1.0
Turkey breast:			
Oven roasted	1-oz. slice	30	0.0
Smoked	.7-oz. slice	25	0.0
Turkey cotto salami	1-oz. slice	50	Tr.
Turkey ham:			
Chopped	1-oz. slice	45	Tr.
Cured	1-oz. slice	35	Tr.
Turkey pastrami	1-oz. slice	35	Tr.
(Ohse):			
Oven cooked or smoked breast	1 oz.	30	1.0
Turkey bologna	1 oz.	70	2.0
Turkey salami	1 oz.	50	1.0

Food	Measure	Cals.	Carbs.
(Oscar Mayer) breast, smoked	¾-oz. slice	19	.2
Smoked (Louis Rich):			
Breast	1 oz.	35	0.0
Drumsticks	1 oz. (without bone)	40	Tr.
Wing drumettes	1 oz. (without bone)	45	Tr.
TURKEY, POTTED (USDA)	1 oz.	70	0.0
TURKEY DINNER OR ENTREE:			
Canned:			
(Hormel):			
Dinty Moore, with dressing & gravy	10-oz. serving	290	33.0
Health Selections, & vegetables, microwave cup	7¼-oz. serving	220	35.0
(Libby's) *Diner,* with dressing & gravy, microwave cup	7-oz. serving	170	15.0
Frozen:			
(Armour) *Dinner Classics,* & dressing	11½-oz. dinner	320	34.0
(Banquet)	10½-oz. dinner	390	35.0
(Budget Gourmet) glazed, *Light and Healthy*	9-oz. meal	260	38.0
(Freezer Queen) sliced:			
Cook-in-Pouch, with gravy	5-oz. serving	70	6.0
Family Supper, with gravy	7-oz. serving	110	8.0
Single-serve, with dressing & gravy	9-oz. serving	230	32.0
(Healthy Choice):			
Breast, roasted, with mushrooms in gravy	8½-oz. meal	200	26.0
With vegetables, homestyle	9½-oz. meal	230	28.0
(Le Menu):			
Regular	10½-oz. dinner	300	38.0
Healthy style:			
Dinner:			
Divan	10-oz. dinner	260	23.0
Sliced	10-oz. dinner	210	21.0
Entree:			
Glazed	8¼-oz. entree	260	18.0
Traditional	8-oz. entree	250	19.0
(Morton)	10-oz. meal	226	28.0

Food	Measure	Cals.	Carbs.
(Stouffer's):			
Regular:			
Casserole with gravy & dressing	9¾-oz. meal	360	29.0
Tetrazzini	10-oz. meal	380	28.0
Lean Cuisine:			
Breast, sliced, in mushroom sauce	8-oz. meal	240	20.0
Dijon	9½-oz. meal	270	22.0
(Swanson):			
Regular	11½-oz. dinner	350	42.0
Homestyle Recipe, with dressing & potatoes	9-oz. entree	290	30.0
Hungry Man	17-oz. dinner	550	61.0
(Ultra Slim Fast):			
Glazed, with dressing	10½-oz. serving	340	49.0
Medallions, in herb sauce	12-oz. serving	280	33.0
(Weight Watchers) *Smart Ones*, medallion roasted	8½-oz. meal	200	35.0
TURKEY NUGGETS, frozen:			
(Empire Kosher)	¼ of 12-oz. pkg.	255	14.0
Purdue Done It	1 piece	54	3.0
TURKEY PATTY, frozen			
(Empire Kosher)	¼ of 12-oz. pkg.	188	12.0
TURKEY PIE, frozen			
(Banquet):			
Regular	7-oz. pie	370	39.0
Supreme microwave	7-oz. pie	470	45.0
(Empire Kosher)	8-oz. pie	491	50.0
(Morton)	7-oz. pie	420	27.0
(Stouffer's)	10-oz. pie	540	35.0
(Swanson):			
Regular	7-oz. pie	440	44.0
Hungry Man	16-oz. pie	650	65.0
TURKEY SALAD, canned			
(Carnation)	¼ of 7½-oz. can	110	31.1
TURKEY SPREAD, canned:			
(Libby's) *Spreadables*	1.9 oz.	100	6.0
(Underwood) chunky, light	2.1 oz.	75	2.0
TURNIP (USDA):			
Fresh:			

Food	Measure	Cals.	Carbs.
Without tops	1 lb. (weighed with skins)	117	25.7
Pared, diced	½ cup (2.4 oz.)	20	4.4
Pared, slices	½ cup (2.3 oz.)	19	4.2
Boiled, drained:			
Diced	½ cup (2.8 oz.)	18	3.8
Mashed	½ cup (4 oz.)	26	5.6
TURNIP GREENS, leaves & stems:			
Fresh (USDA):	1 lb. (weighed untrimmed)	107	19.0
Boiled (USDA):			
In small amount water, short time, drained	½ cup (2.5 oz.)	14	2.6
In large amount water, long time, drained	½ cup (2.5 oz.)	14	2.4
Canned:			
(USDA) solids & liq.	½ cup (4.1 oz.)	21	3.7
(Allen's) chopped, with diced turnips	½ cup	20	1.0
(Stokely-Van Camp) chopped	½ cup (4.1 oz.)	23	3.5
(Sunshine) solids & liq.:			
Chopped	½ cup (4.1 oz.)	19	2.5
& diced turnips	½ cup (4.1 oz.)	21	3.2
Frozen:			
(Bel-Air) chopped	3.3-oz.	20	4.0
(Birds Eye):			
Chopped	⅓ of 10-oz. pkg.	20	3.0
Chopped, with sliced turnips	⅓ of 10-oz. pkg.	20	3.0
(Frosty Acres)	3.3-oz. serving	20	4.0
TURNIP ROOT, frozen (McKenzie) diced	1 oz.	4	1.0
TURNOVER:			
Frozen (Pepperidge Farm):			
Apple	1 turnover	300	34.0
Blueberry	1 turnover	310	32.0
Cherry	1 turnover	310	22.0
Peach	1 turnover	310	34.0
Raspberry	1 turnover	310	36.0
Refrigerated (Pillsbury)	1 turnover	170	23.0
TURTLE, GREEN (USDA):			
Raw:			

Food	Measure	Cals.	Carbs.
In shell	1 lb. (weighed in shell)	97	0.0
Meat only	4 oz.	101	0.0
Canned	4 oz.	120	0.0
TWINKIES (Hostess):			
Banana	1 piece	150	26.0
Golden, cream filled:			
Regular	1 piece	150	27.0
Light	1 piece	110	21.0
Strawberry, Fruit n' Cream	1 piece	140	27.0

U

Food	Measure	Cals.	Carbs.
ULTRA DIET QUICK			
(TKI Foods):			
Bar	1.2-oz. piece	130	17.0
*Mix:			
Dutch chocolate:			
Lowfat milk	8 fl. oz.	200	37.0
Water	8 fl. oz.	220	40.0
Strawberry	8 fl. oz.	100	19.0
Vanilla	8 fl. oz.	100	19.0
ULTRA SLIM FAST:			
Canned, French vanilla	12 fl. oz.	220	38.0
*Mix:			
Regular:			
Cafe mocha	8 fl. oz.	200	38.0
French vanilla	8 fl. oz.	190	36.0
Plus:			
Chocolate fantasy	12 fl. oz.	250	50.0
Piña colada	8 fl. oz.	190	38.0
Mix with fruit juice	8 fl. oz.	200	43.0

Food	Measure	Cals.	Carbs.

V

V-8 JUICE (See **VEGETABLE JUICE COCKTAIL**)

Food	Measure	Cals.	Carbs.
VANDERMINT, liqueur	1 fl. oz.	90	10.2
VANILLA EXTRACT (Virginia Dare) pure, 35% alcohol	1 tsp.	10	DNA
VEAL, medium fat (USDA):			
Chuck:			
Raw	1 lb. (weighed with bone)	628	0.0
Braised, lean & fat	4 oz.	266	0.0
Flank:			
Raw	1 lb. (weighed with bone)	1410	0.0
Stewed, lean & fat	4 oz.	442	0.0
Foreshank:			
Raw	1 lb. (weighed with bone)	368	0.0
Stewed, lean & fat	4 oz.	245	0.0
Loin:			
Raw	1 lb. (weighed with bone)	681	0.0
Broiled, medium done, chop, lean & fat	4 oz.	265	0.0
Plate:			
Raw	1 lb. (weighed with bone)	828	0.0
Stewed, lean & fat	4 oz.	344	0.0
Rib:			
Raw, lean & fat	1 lb. (weighed with bone)	723	0.0
Roasted, medium done, lean & fat	4 oz.	305	0.0

Food	Measure	Cals.	Carbs.
Round & rump:			
Raw	1 lb. (weighed with bone)	573	0.0
Broiled, steak or cutlet, lean & fat	4 oz. (weighed with bone)	245	0.0
VEAL DINNER, frozen:			
(Armour) *Dinner Classics,* parmigiana	11¼-oz. meal	400	34.0
(Banquet) parmigiana:			
Cookin' Bags	4-oz. meal	230	20.0
Family Entree, patties	¼ of 2-lb. pkg.	370	33.0
(Le Menu) parmigiana	11½-oz. dinner	390	36.0
(Morton) parmigiana	10-oz. dinner	260	35.0
(Stouffer's) with pasta Alfredo, homestyle	9¼-oz. meal	350	26.0
(Swanson) parmigiana:			
Regular, 4-compartment	12¾-oz. dinner	430	42.0
Homestyle Recipe	10-oz. entree	330	33.0
Hungry Man	18¼-oz. dinner	590	57.0
(Weight Watchers) *Ultimate 200*	8.2-oz. meal	150	5.0
VEAL STEAK, frozen (Hormel):			
Regular	4-oz. serving	130	2.0
Breaded	4-oz. serving	240	13.0
VEGETABLE (See specific variety such as **CAULIFLOWER; SQUASH;** etc.)			
VEGETABLE, MIXED:			
Canned, regular pack:			
(Chun King) chow mein, drained	½ of 8-oz. can	32	6.3
(La Choy) drained:			
Chinese	⅓ of 14-oz. can	12	2.0
Chop suey	½ cup (4.7 oz.)	9	2.0
(Pathmark)	½ cup	35	8.0
(Town House)	½ cup	45	7.0
(Veg-all) solids & liq.	½ cup	35	8.0
Canned, dietetic pack:			
(Featherweight) low sodium	½ cup (4 oz.)	40	8.0
(Larsen) *Fresh-Lite,* no added salt	½ cup	35	8.0

Food	Measure	Cals.	Carbs.
(Pathmark) no salt added	½ cup	35	7.0
Frozen:			
(Bel-Air):			
Regular	3.3 oz.	65	13.0
Chinese	3.3 oz.	30	6.0
Hawaiian	3.3 oz.	50	14.0
Japanese	3.3 oz.	35	8.0
Winter mix	3.3 oz.	40	5.0
(Birds Eye):			
Regular:			
Broccoli, cauliflower & carrot in butter sauce	⅓ of 10-oz. pkg.	51	5.7
Broccoli, cauliflower & carrot in cheese sauce	⅓ of 10-oz. pkg.	72	7.9
Broccoli, cauliflower & red pepper	⅓ of 10-oz. pkg.	31	4.7
Carrot, pea & onion, deluxe	⅓ of 10-oz. pkg.	52	10.0
Medley, in butter sauce	⅓ of 10-oz. pkg.	62	9.7
Mixed	⅓ of 10-oz. pkg.	68	13.3
Mixed, with onion sauce	⅓ of 8-oz. pkg.	103	11.7
Pea & potato in cream sauce	⅓ of 8-oz. pkg.	164	15.6
Farm Fresh:			
Broccoli, carrot & water chestnut	⅕ of 16-oz. pkg.	36	6.5
Broccoli, cauliflower & carrot strips	⅕ of 16-oz. pkg.	30	5.3
Broccoli, corn & red pepper	⅕ of 16-oz. pkg.	58	10.9
Broccoli, green bean, onion & red pepper	⅕ of 16-oz. pkg.	31	5.4
Brussels sprout, cauliflower & carrot	⅕ of 16-oz. pkg.	38	6.5
Cauliflower, green bean & carrot	⅕ of 16-oz. pkg.	42	8.1
Green bean, corn, carrot & pearl onion	⅕ of 16-oz. pkg.	49	10.1
Green bean, cauliflower & carrot	⅕ of 16-oz. pkg.	32	6.1
Pea, carrot & pearl onion	⅕ of 16-oz. pkg.	59	10.7
International:			
Bavarian style beans & spaetzle	⅓ of 10-oz. pkg.	112	11.5

Food	Measure	Cals.	Carbs.
Chinese style	⅓ of 10-oz. pkg.	85	8.4
Far Eastern style	⅓ of 10-oz. pkg.	84	8.4
Italian style	⅓ of 10-oz. pkg.	114	11.4
Japanese style	⅓ of 10-oz. pkg.	102	10.4
Mexican style	⅓ of 10-oz. pkg.	133	16.1
New England style	⅓ of 10-oz. pkg.	129	14.2
San Francisco style	⅓ of 10-oz. pkg.	99	10.9
Stir Fry:			
Chinese style	⅓ of 10-oz. pkg.	36	6.9
Japanese style	⅓ of 10-oz. pkg.	32	5.9
(Green Giant):			
Regular:			
Broccoli, carrot fanfare	½ cup	25	5.0
Broccoli, cauliflower & carrot in cheese sauce	½ cup	60	8.0
Broccoli, cauliflower supreme	½ cup	20	4.0
Cauliflower, green bean festival	½ cup	16	3.0
Corn, broccoli bounty	½ cup	60	11.0
Mixed, butter sauce	½ cup	80	12.0
Mixed, polybag	½ cup	50	10.0
Pea, pea pod & water chestnut in butter sauce	½ cup	80	10.0
Pea & cauliflower medley	½ cup	40	7.0
Harvest Fresh	½ cup	60	13.0
Harvest Get Togethers:			
Broccoli-cauliflower medley	½ cup	60	10.0
Broccoli fanfare	½ cup	80	14.2
Cauliflower-carrot bonanza	½ cup	60	7.0
Chinese style	½ cup	60	7.0
Japanese style	½ cup	45	8.0
(Frosty Acres):			
Regular	3.3-oz. serving	65	13.0
Dutch style	3.2-oz. serving	30	5.0
Italian	3.2-oz. serving	40	8.0
Oriental	3.2-oz. serving	25	5.0
Rancho Fiesta	3.2-oz. serving	60	13.0
Soup mix	3-oz. serving	45	11.0
Stew	3-oz. serving	42	10.0
Swiss mix	3-oz. serving	25	5.0
(La Choy) stir fry	4-oz. serving	40	7.9

Food	Measure	Cals.	Carbs.
(Larsen):			
Regular	3.3-oz. serving	70	13.0
California or Italian blend	3.3-oz. serving	30	6.0
Chuckwagon blend	3.3-oz. serving	70	16.0
Midwestern blend	3.3-oz. serving	40	8.0
Oriental or winter blend	3.3-oz. serving	25	5.0
Scandinavian blend	3.3-oz. serving	45	9.0
For soup or stew	3.3-oz. serving	50	11.0
Wisconsin blend	3.3-oz. serving	50	12.0
(Ore-Ida) medley, breaded	3 oz.	160	17.0
VEGETABLE BOUILLON:			
(Herb-Ox):			
Cube	1 cube	6	.6
Packet	1 packet	12	2.2
(Knorr)	1 packet	16	.9
(Wyler's) instant	1 tsp.	6	1.0
VEGETABLE DINNER OR ENTREE, frozen:			
(Budget Gourmet) *Light and Healthy*:			
Chinese, & chicken	10-oz. meal	280	47.0
Italian, & chicken	10¼-oz. meal	310	50.0
(Stouffer's) *Lean Cuisine*, & pasta mornay with ham	9⅜-oz. meal	280	29.0
VEGETABLE FAT (See **FAT, COOKING**)			
VEGETABLE JUICE COCKTAIL:			
Regular:			
(Knudsen & Sons) *Very Veggie,* regular, organic or spicy	6 fl. oz.	30	6.0
(Mott's)	6 fl. oz.	30	7.0
(Smucker's) hearty or hot & spicy	6 fl. oz.	43	9.7
(V-8) regular, light & tangy, picante mild or spicy hot	6 fl. oz.	35	8.0
Dietetic:			
(Knudsen & Sons) *Very Veggie,* low sodium	6 fl. oz.	30	6.0
(V-8) no salt added	6 fl. oz.	35	8.0

Food	Measure	Cals.	Carbs.
VEGETABLE POT PIE,			
frozen:			
(Banquet):			
& Beef	7 oz.	510	39.0
& Chicken	7 oz.	550	39.0
(Morton):			
With beef	7 oz.	430	27.0
With chicken	7 oz.	320	32.0
With turkey	7 oz.	300	29.0
"VEGETARIAN FOODS":			
Canned or dry:			
Chicken, fried (Loma Linda)			
with gravy	1½-oz. piece	70	2.0
*Chicken, supreme (Loma			
Linda)	¼ cup	50	4.0
Chili (Worthington)	½ cup (4.9 oz.)	177	13.2
Choplet (Worthington)	1 choplet		
	(1.6 oz.)	50	1.7
Dinner cuts (Loma Linda)			
drained:			
Regular	1 piece (1.8 oz.)	55	2.0
No salt added	1 piece (1.8 oz.)	55	2.0
Dinner loaf (Loma Linda)	¼ cup (.6 oz.)	50	4.0
Franks, big (Loma Linda)	1.8-oz. frank	100	4.0
Franks, sizzle (Loma Linda)	1.2-oz. frank	85	1.5
FriChik (Worthington)	1 piece (1.6 oz.)	75	2.5
Granburger (Worthington)	1 oz.	96	5.8
Linkettes (Loma Linda)	1.3-oz. link	75	2.5
Little links (Loma Linda)			
drained	.8-oz. link	40	1.0
Non-Meatballs	1 meatball		
(Worthington)	(.6 oz.)	32	1.9
Numete (Worthington)	½" slice (2.4 oz.)	145	7.1
Nuteena (Loma Linda)	½" slice (2.4 oz.)	160	5.0
*Ocean platter (Loma Linda)	¼ cup	50	5.0
*Patty mix (Loma Linda)	¼ cup	50	4.0
Peanuts & soya (USDA)	4 oz.	269	15.2
Prime Stakes	1 slice	171	7.8
Proteena (Loma Linda)	½" slice	144	6.5
Protose (Worthington)	½" slice	140	5.0
Redi-burger (Loma Linda)	½" slice (2.4 oz.)	130	5.0
Sandwich spread			
(Loma Linda)	1 T. (.5 oz.)	23	1.3
Savorex (Loma Linda)	1 tsp.	16	1.0

Food	Measure	Cals.	Carbs.
*Savory dinner loaf (Loma Linda)	1 slice (¼ cup dry)	110	4.0
Skallops (Worthington) drained	½ cup (3 oz.)	89	3.0
Soyagen (Loma Linda):			
All purpose or no sucrose	½ cup	65	7.0
Carob	½ cup	70	8.0
Soyameat (Worthington):			
Beef, sliced	1 slice (1 oz.)	44	2.6
Chicken, diced	1 oz.	40	1.4
Soyamel, any kind (Worthington)	1 oz.	120	12.2
Stew pack (Loma Linda) drained	2 oz.	70	4.0
Super Links (Worthington)	1 link (1.9 oz.)	110	3.7
Swiss steak with gravy (Loma Linda)	1 steak (2¾ oz.)	140	8.0
Taystee cuts (Loma Linda)	1 cut (1.3 oz.)	35	1.0
Tender bits (Loma Linda) drained	1 piece	20	1.0
Tender rounds (Loma Linda)	1-oz. piece	20	1.2
Vege-burger (Loma Linda):			
Regular	½ cup	110	4.0
No salt added	½ cup	140	4.0
Vegelona (Loma Linda)	½" slice (2.4 oz.)	100	6.0
Vega-links (Worthington)	1 link (1.1 oz.)	55	2.8
Veg-scallops (Loma Linda)	1 piece (.5 oz.)	12	.3
Vita-Burger (Loma Linda)	1 T. (¼ oz.)	23	2.3
Wheat protein (USDA)	4 oz.	170	10.8
Worthington 209	1 slice (1.1 oz.)	58	2.2
Frozen:			
Beef pie (Worthington)	8-oz. pie	278	41.8
Bologna (Loma Linda)	1 oz.	75	2.5
Bolono (Worthington)	¾-oz. slice	23	1.0
Chicken (Loma Linda)	1-oz. slice	46	2.1
Chicken, fried (Loma Linda)	2 oz. serving	180	2.0
Chicken pie (Worthington)	8-oz. pie	346	37.5
Chic-Ketts (Worthington)	1 oz.	53	2.2
Chik-Nuggets (Loma Linda)	1 piece (.6 oz.)	45	3.4
Chik-Patties (Loma Linda)	1 patty (3 oz.)	226	15.0
Corn dogs (Loma Linda)	1 piece (2.6 oz.)	250	7.0
Corned beef, sliced (Worthington)	1 slice (.5 oz.)	32	1.9
Fillets (Worthington)	1½-oz. piece	90	4.6
FriPats (Worthington)	1 patty	204	5.2

Food	Measure	Cals.	Carbs.
Griddle steak (Loma Linda)	1 piece (2 oz.)	190	5.0
Meatballs (Loma Linda)	1 meatball (.3 oz.)	63	.8
Meatless salami (Worthington)	¾-oz. slice	44	1.2
Ocean fillet (Loma Linda)	1 piece (2 oz.)	160	5.0
Olive loaf (Loma Linda)	1 slice (1 oz.)	59	2.7
Prosage (Worthington):			
Links	1 link	60	1.5
Patty	1.3-oz. piece	96	2.8
Roll	⅜" slice (1.2 oz.)	86	2.0
Roast beef (Loma Linda)	1 oz.	53	2.6
Salami (Loma Linda)	1 slice (1 oz.)	49	2.8
Sizzle burger (Loma Linda)	1 burger (2.5 oz.)	210	13.0
Smoked beef, slices (Worthington)	1 slice	14	1.1
Stakelets (Worthington)	3-oz. piece	164	9.4
Tuno (Worthington)	2-oz. serving	81	3.4
Turkey (Loma Linda)	1 slice (1 oz.)	47	2.3
Wahm roll (Worthington)	1 slice (.8 oz.)	36	1.9
VENISON (USDA) raw, lean, meat only	4 oz.	143	0.0
VERMICELLI (See **PASTA, DRY OR FRESH, REFRIGERATED**)			
VERMOUTH:			
Dry & extra dry (Lejon; Noilly Pratt)	1 fl. oz.	33	1.0
Sweet (Lejon; Taylor)	1 fl. oz.	45	3.8
VICHY WATER (Schweppes)	Any quantity	0	0.0
VINEGAR:			
Balsamic (Luigi Vitelli)	1 T. (.5 oz.)	5	2.0
Cider:			
(USDA)	1 T. (.5 oz.)	2	.9
(USDA)	½ cup (4.2 oz.)	17	7.1
(Town House)	1 T.	0	0.0
(White House) Apple	1 T.	2	1.0
Distilled:			
(USDA)	1 T. (.5 oz.)	2	.8
(USDA)	½ cup (4.2 oz.)	14	6.0

Food	Measure	Cals.	Carbs.
Red, red with garlic or white wine (Regina)	1 T. (.5 oz.)	Tr.	Tr.
VINESPINACH OR BASELLA (USDA) raw	4 oz.	22	3.9
VODKA, unflavored (See **DISTILLED LIQUOR**)			

W

Food	Measure	Cals.	Carbs.
WAFFLE:			
Home recipe (USDA)	7" waffle (2.6 oz.)	209	28.1
Frozen:			
(Aunt Jemima) jumbo	1 waffle	86	14.5
(Downyflake):			
Regular:			
Regular	1 waffle	60	10.0
Hot-N-Buttery	1 waffle	90	13.5
Jumbo	1 waffle	85	15.0
Blueberry	1 waffle	90	16.0
Buttermilk	1 waffle	85	15.0
(Eggo):			
Regular	1 waffle	120	16.0
Apple cinnamon	1 waffle	130	18.0
Blueberry	1 waffle	130	18.0
Buttermilk	1 waffle	120	16.0
Home style	1 waffle	120	16.0
(Roman Meal):			
Regular	1 waffle	140	16.5
Golden Delight	1 waffle	131	15.1
WAFFLE BREAKFAST, frozen (Swanson) *Great Starts*:			
Regular, with bacon	2.2-oz. meal	230	19.0
Belgian:			
& sausage	2.85-oz. meal	280	21.0
& strawberries with sausage	3½-oz. meal	210	31.0

Food	Measure	Cals.	Carbs.
WAFFLE MIX (See also **PANCAKE & WAFFLE MIX**) (USDA):			
Complete mix:			
Dry	1 oz.	130	18.5
*Prepared with water	2.6-oz. waffle	229	30.2
Incomplete mix:			
Dry	1 oz.	101	21.5
*Prepared with egg & milk	2.6-oz. waffle	206	27.2
*Prepared with egg & milk	7.1-oz. waffle (9" × 9" × ⅝", 1⅛ cups)	550	72.4
WAFFLE SYRUP (See **SYRUP**)			
WALNUT:			
(USDA):			
Black, in shell, whole	1 lb. (weighed in shell)	627	14.8
Black, shelled, whole	4 oz. (weighed whole)	712	16.8
Black, chopped	½ cup (2.1 oz.)	377	8.9
English or Persian, whole	1 lb. (weighed in shell)	1327	32.2
English or Persian, shelled, whole	4 oz.	738	17.9
English or Persian, halves	½ cup (1.8 oz.)	356	6.5
(California) halves & pieces	½ cup (1.8 oz.)	356	6.5
(Fisher):			
Black	½ cup (2.1 oz.)	374	8.8
English	½ cup (2.1 oz.)	389	9.5
WATER CHESTNUT, CHINESE:			
Raw (USDA):			
Whole	1 lb. (weighed unpeeled)	272	66.5
Peeled	4 oz.	90	21.5
Canned:			
(Chun King) drained:			
Sliced	½ of 8-oz. can	89	21.5
Whole	½ of 8-oz. can	85	22.9
(La Choy) drained, sliced	½ of 8-oz. can	32	7.8
WATERCRESS, raw (USDA):			
Untrimmed	½ lb. (weighed untrimmed)	40	6.2

Food	Measure	Cals.	Carbs.
Trimmed	½ cup (.6 oz.)	3	.5
WATERMELON, fresh (USDA):			
Whole	1 lb. (weighed with rind)	54	13.4
Wedge	4" × 8" wedge (2 lb. weighed with rind)	111	27.3
Diced	½ cup	21	5.1
WAX GOURD, raw (USDA):			
Whole	1 lb. (weighed with skin & cavity contents)	41	9.4
Flesh only	4 oz.	15	3.4
WEAKFISH (USDA):			
Raw, whole	1 lb. (weighed whole)	263	0.0
Broiled, meat only	4 oz.	236	0.0
WELSH RAREBIT:			
Home recipe	1 cup (8.2 oz.)	415	14.6
Canned (Snow's)	½ cup	170	10.0
Frozen (Stouffer's)	5-oz. serving	270	8.0
WENDY'S:			
Bacon, breakfast	1 strip	55	Tr.
Breakfast sandwich:			
Regular	1 serving	370	33.0
With bacon	1 serving	430	33.0
With sausage	1 serving	570	33.0
Buns:			
Kaiser	1 bun	180	32.0
Multi-grain	1 bun	140	25.0
White	1 bun	140	26.0
Cheeseburger:			
Double	1 serving	620	26.0
Jr.:			
Regular	4.4-oz. serving	310	34.0
Bacon	5½-oz. serving	410	34.0
Swiss deluxe	5.8-oz. serving	360	35.0
Kids Meal	4.1-oz. serving	320	33.0
Chicken nuggets, crispy:			
6 pieces	1 serving	310	14.0
9 pieces	1 serving	465	21.0

Food	Measure	Cals.	Carbs.
20 pieces	1 serving	1023	46.0
Chicken sandwich:			
Breast, on white bun	1 serving	340	30.0
Club	7.2-oz. serving	505	43.0
Fried	6.9-oz. serving	440	43.0
Grilled	6.2-oz. serving	340	32.0
Chicken sandwich on multi-grain bun	1 sandwich	320	31.0
Chili:			
Regular	8 oz.	210	21.0
Large	12 oz.	310	32.0
Condiments:			
Bacon	½ strip	30	Tr.
Cheese, American	1 slice	70	Tr.
Ketchup	1 tsp.	6	1.0
Mayonnaise	1 T.	100	Tr.
Mustard	1 tsp.	4	Tr.
Onion rings	.3-oz. piece	4	Tr.
Pickle, dill	4 slices	1	Tr.
Relish	.3-oz. serving	14	3.0
Tomato	1 slice	2	Tr.
Cookie, chocolate chip	2¼-oz. serving	275	40.0
Danish:			
Apple	1 piece	360	53.0
Cheese	1 piece	430	52.0
Cinnamon raisin	1 piece	430	52.0
Drinks:			
Coffee	6 fl. oz.	2	Tr.
Cola:			
Regular	12 fl. oz.	110	29.0
Dietetic	12 fl. oz.	Tr.	Tr.
Fruit flavored drink	12 fl. oz.	110	28.0
Hot chocolate	6 fl. oz.	100	17.0
Milk:			
Regular	8 fl. oz.	150	11.0
Chocolate	8 fl. oz.	210	26.0
Non-cola	12 fl. oz.	100	26.0
Orange juice	6 fl. oz.	80	17.0
Egg, scrambled	1 order	190	7.0
Fish sandwich, fillet	6-oz. serving	460	42.0
Frosty dairy dessert:			
Small	12 fl. oz.	400	59.0
Medium	16 fl. oz.	533	78.7
Large	20 fl. oz.	680	98.3
Hamburger:			
Regular:			
Plain	4.4-oz. serving	340	30.0

Food	Measure	Cals.	Carbs.
With everything	1 serving	420	35.0
Quarter-pound, on white bun	1 serving	350	26.0
Big Classic on kaiser bun:			
Regular	1 serving	470	36.0
Double	1 serving	680	36.0
Double, on white bun	1 serving	560	26.0
Kids Meal	3.7-oz. serving	260	33.0
Omelet:			
Ham & cheese	1 omelet	290	7.0
Ham, cheese & mushroom	1 omelet	290	7.0
Ham, cheese, onion & green pepper	1 omelet	280	7.0
Mushroom, onion & green pepper	1 omelet	210	7.0
Potato:			
Baked, hot stuffed:			
Plain	1 potato	310	71.0
Bacon & cheese	1 potato	540	78.0
Broccoli & cheese	1 potato	470	80.0
Cheese	1 potato	570	78.0
Chili & cheese	1 potato	620	83.0
Sour cream & chives	1 potato	460	53.0
Stroganoff & sour cream	1 potato	490	60.0
French fries	regular order	260	33.0
Home fries	1 order	360	37.0
Salad:			
Caesar, side order	1 serving	160	18.0
Chef's:			
Regular	9.1-oz. serving	130	8.0
Take out	1 serving	180	10.0
Chicken, grilled	1 serving	200	9.0
Garden:			
Regular	8-oz. serving	70	9.0
Deluxe	1 serving	110	9.0
Take out	1 serving	102	9.0
Pasta:			
Regular	¼ cup	130	18.0
Deli	¼ cup	35	6.0
Potato, red skins	¼ cup	110	6.0
Side	1 serving	60	6.0
Taco	17.3-oz. serving	530	55.0
3-bean, deluxe	¼ cup	60	13.0
Salad bar, *Garden Spot:*			
Alfalfa sprouts	2 oz.	20	2.0
Bacon bits	⅛ oz.	10	Tr.
Blueberries, fresh	1 T.	8	2.0
Breadstick	1 piece	20	2.0

Food	Measure	Cals.	Carbs.
Broccoli	½ cup	14	2.0
Cantaloupe	1 piece	9	2.0
Carrot	¼ cup	12	3.0
Cauliflower	½ cup	14	3.0
Cheese:			
American, imitation	1 oz.	90	1.0
Cheddar, imitation	1 oz.	90	1.0
Cottage	½ cup	110	3.0
Mozzarella, imitation	1 oz.	90	Tr.
Swiss, imitation	1 oz.	80	Tr.
Chow mein noodles	¼ cup	60	6.0
Coleslaw	½ cup	90	3.0
Cracker, saltine	1 piece	11	2.0
Crouton	1 piece	2	.2
Cucumber	1 piece	<1	Tr.
Eggs	1 T.	14	Tr.
Mushroom	¼ cup	6	Tr.
Onions, red	1 slice	2	Tr.
Orange, fresh	1 piece	5	1.4
Pasta salad	½ cup	134	17.0
Peas, green	½ cup	60	9.0
Peaches, in syrup	1 piece	8	2.0
Peppers:			
Banana or mild			
pepperoncini	1 T.	18	4.0
Bell	¼ cup	4	1.0
Jalapeño	1 T.	9	2.0
Pineapple chunks in juice	½ cup	70	20.0
Sunflower seeds & raisins	¼ cup	180	12.0
Tomato	1 oz.	6	1.0
Turkey ham	¼ cup	46	1.0
Watermelon, fresh	1 piece (1 oz.)	1	Tr.
Salad dressing:			
Regular:			
Blue cheese	2 T. (1 ladle)	170	Tr.
French, red	2 T.	130	9.0
Italian, golden	2 T.	45	3.0
Oil	2 T.	130	Tr.
Ranch	2 T.	90	1.0
1000 Island	2 T.	130	3.0
Dietetic:			
Bacon & tomato	2 T.	45	2.0
Cucumber, creamy	2 T.	50	2.0
Italian	2 T.	40	2.0
Wine vinegar	2 T.	2	Tr.
Sauce:			
Alfredo	2 oz.	35	5.0

Food	Measure	Cals.	Carbs.
Barbecue	1 oz.	50	11.0
Cheese	2 oz.	39	5.0
Honey	.5 oz.	45	12.0
Mustard, sweet	1 oz.	50	9.0
Picante	2 oz.	18	4.0
Sweet & sour	1 oz.	45	11.0
Taco	1 oz.	16	3.0
Sausage	1 patty	200	Tr.
Steak sandwich, country fried	5.1-oz. serving	440	45.0
Toast:			
Regular, with margarine	1 slice	125	17.5
French	1 slice	200	22.5
WESTERN DINNER, frozen:			
(Banquet)	11-oz. dinner	630	40.0
(Morton)	10-oz. dinner	290	29.0
(Swanson):			
Regular, 4-compartment dinner	11½-oz. dinner	430	43.0
Hungry Man	17¾-oz. dinner	820	73.0
WHEAT GERM:			
(USDA)	1 oz.	103	13.2
(Elam's) raw	1 T. (.3 oz.)	28	3.2
(Kretschmer)	1 oz.	110	13.0
WHEAT GERM CEREAL (Kretschmer):			
Regular	¼ cup (1 oz.)	110	13.0
Brown sugar & honey	¼ cup (1 oz.)	110	17.0
WHEAT HEARTS, cereal (General Mills)	1 oz. dry	110	21.0
WHEATIES, cereal (General Mills)	1 cup (1 oz.)	100	23.0
WHEAT PUFF, cereal (Post)	⅞ cup	104	26.0
WHEAT, ROLLED (USDA):			
Uncooked	1 cup (3.1 oz.)	296	66.3
Cooked	1 cup (7.7 oz.)	163	36.7

WHEAT, SHREDDED, cereal
(See **SHREDDED WHEAT**)

Food	Measure	Cals.	Carbs.
WHEAT, WHOLE GRAIN			
(USDA) hard red spring	1 oz.	94	19.6
WHEAT, WHOLE-MEAL,			
cereal (USDA):			
Dry	1 oz.	96	20.5
Cooked	4 oz.	51	10.7
WHEY (USDA):			
Dry	1 oz.	99	20.8
Fluid	1 cup (8.6 oz.)	63	12.4
WHIPPED TOPPING (See **TOPPING, WHIPPED**)			
WHISKEY (See **DISTILLED LIQUOR**)			
WHISKEY SOUR COCKTAIL:			
(Mr. Boston) 12½% alcohol	3 fl. oz.	120	14.4
*Mix (Bar-Tender's)	3½ fl. oz.	177	18.0
WHITE CASTLE:			
Breakfast sandwich:			
Sausage	1.7-oz. serving	196	13.0
Sausage & egg	3.4-oz. serving	322	16.0
Bun	.8-oz. bun	74	13.9
Cheeseburger	2.3-oz. serving	200	15.5
Chicken sandwich	2¼-oz. sandwich	186	20.5
Fish sandwich without tartar sauce	2.1-oz. serving	155	20.9
French fries	3.4-oz. serving	301	37.7
Hamburger	1 burger	161	15.4
Onion chips	1 serving	329	38.8
Onion rings	1 serving	245	26.6
WHITEFISH, LAKE (USDA):			
Raw, meat only	4 oz.	176	0.0
Baked, stuffed, home recipe, with bacon, butter, onion, celery & breadcrumbs	4 oz.	244	6.6
Smoked	4 oz.	176	0.0
WHOPPER (See **BURGER KING**)			

Food	Measure	Cals.	Carbs.
WIENER (See **FRANKFURTER**)			
WILD BERRY DRINK, canned (Hi-C)	6 fl. oz.	92	22.5
WINE (See individual listings)			
WINE, COOKING (Regina):			
Burgundy or sauterne	¼ cup	2	Tr.
Sherry	¼ cup	20	5.0
WINE COOLER (Bartles & Jaymes):			
Regular:			
Berry	6 fl. oz.	110	16.0
Cherry, black	6 fl. oz.	104	16.1
Peach	6 fl. oz.	107	16.5
Premium	6 fl. oz.	99	14.0
Sangria, red	6 fl. oz.	107	14.5
Strawberry	6 fl. oz.	110	16.0
Tropical	6 fl. oz.	115	18.5
Light:			
Berry	6 fl. oz.	75	16.0
Premium	6 fl. oz.	67	12.0
Tropical	6 fl. oz.	76	16.5
WONTON WRAPPER (Nasoya)	1 piece	18	3.6

Y

Food	Measure	Cals.	Carbs.
YAM (USDA):			
Raw:			
Whole	1 lb. (weighed with skin)	394	90.5
Flesh only	4 oz.	115	26.3
Canned & frozen (See **SWEET POTATO**)			

Food	Measure	Cals.	Carbs.
YAM BEAN, raw (USDA):			
Unpared tuber	1 lb. (weighed unpared)	225	52.2
Pared tuber	4 oz.	62	14.5
YEAST:			
Baker's:			
Compressed:			
(USDA)	1 oz.	24	3.1
(Fleischmann's)	1 cube	15	2.0
Dry:			
(USDA)	1 oz.	80	11.0
(USDA)	7-gram pkg.	20	2.7
(Fleischmann's)	1 packet	20	3.0
YOGURT: (See also *TCBY*)			
Regular:			
Plain:			
(Bison)	8-oz. container	160	16.8
(Borden) *Lite-Line*	8-oz. container	140	18.0
(Dannon):			
Lowfat	8-oz. container	140	16.0
Nonfat	8-oz. container	110	16.0
(Friendship)	8-oz. container	150	17.0
(Johanna Farms) sundae style	8-oz. container	150	17.0
(La Yogurt)	6-oz. container	140	12.0
(Lucerne):			
Gourmet	6-oz. container	130	12.0
Lowfat	8-oz. container	160	17.0
Nonfat	8-oz. container	130	18.0
(Mountain High)	8-oz. container	200	16.0
(Weight Watchers) nonfat	8 oz.	90	13.0
(Whitney's)	6-oz. container	150	13.0
Yoplait, regular	6-oz. container	130	13.0
Apple:			
(Dannon) Dutch, Fruit-on-the-Bottom	8-oz. container	240	43.0
(Lucerne) spice, lowfat	8-oz. container	260	46.0
(Sweet'n Low) Dutch	8-oz. container	150	33.0
Apple-cinnamon, *Yoplait, Breakfast Yogurt*	6-oz. container	220	38.0
Apricot (Lucerne) lowfat	8-oz. container	260	46.0
Apricot-pineapple (Lucerne) lowfat	8-oz. container	260	46.0
Banana (Dannon) Fruit-on-the-Bottom	8-oz. container	240	43.0

Food	Measure	Cals.	Carbs.
Berry:			
(Whitney's) wild	6-oz. container	200	33.0
Yoplait:			
Breakfast Yogurt	6-oz. container	200	39.0
Custard Style	6-oz. container	180	32.0
Blackberry (Lucerne)	8-oz. container	260	46.0
Blueberry:			
(Breyers) lowfat	8-oz. container	250	48.0
(Dannon):			
Fresh Flavors	8-oz. container	200	34.0
Fruit-on-the-Bottom	4.4-oz. container	130	23.0
Fruit-on-the-Bottom	8-oz. container	240	43.0
Light, nonfat	8-oz. container	100	19.0
(Lucerne):			
Gourmet	6-oz. container	190	32.0
Lowfat	8-oz. container	260	46.0
Nonfat	8-oz. container	180	10.0
(Mountain High)	8-oz. container	220	31.0
(TCBY):			
Regular	8 oz.	220	42.0
Light, nonfat	8 oz.	100	17.0
(Weight Watchers)			
Ultimate 90	8 oz.	90	13.0
(Whitney's)	6-oz. container	200	33.0
Yoplait:			
Regular	6-oz. container	180	32.0
Custard Style	6-oz. container	180	30.0
Light	6-oz. container	90	14.0
Boysenberry:			
(Dannon) Fruit-on-the-			
Bottom	8-oz. container	240	43.0
(Lucerne) lowfat	8-oz. container	260	46.0
(Whitney's)	6-oz. container	200	33.0
Yoplait	6-oz. container	180	32.0
Caramel pecan (Lucerne)	8-oz. serving	260	46.0
Cherries jubilee (Weight			
Watchers) *Ultimate 90*	8 oz.	90	13.0
Cherry:			
(Breyers) black, lowfat	8-oz. container	260	49.0
(Dannon) Fruit-on-the-			
Bottom	8-oz. container	240	43.0
(Sweet'n Low)	8-oz. container	150	33.0
(TCBY) light	8-oz.	100	17.0
(Whitney's)	6-oz. container	200	33.0
Yoplait:			
Breakfast Yogurt, with			
almonds	6-oz. container	200	38.0

Food	Measure	Cals.	Carbs.
Custard Style	6-oz. container	180	30.0
Cherry-vanilla:			
(Borden) *Lite-Line,* Swiss style	8-oz. container	240	45.0
(TCBY)	8 oz.	220	42.0
Coffee:			
(Dannon) Fresh Flavors	8-oz. container	200	34.0
(Friendship)	8-oz. container	210	35.0
(Johanna Farms) sundae style	8-oz. container	220	17.0
(Whitney's)	6-oz. container	200	28.0
Cranberry-raspberry (Weight Watchers) *Ultimate 90*	8 oz.	90	13.0
Exotic fruit (Dannon) Fruit-on-the-Bottom	8-oz. container	240	43.0
Lemon:			
(Dannon) Fresh Flavors	8-oz. container	200	34.0
(Johanna Farms) sundae style	8-oz. container	220	17.0
(Lucerne) lowfat	8-oz. container	260	46.0
(Weight Watchers) *Ultimate 90*	1 cup	90	13.0
(Whitney's)	6-oz container	200	28.0
Yoplait:			
Regular	6-oz. container	190	32.0
Custard Style	6-oz. container	180	30.0
Lime (Lucerne) lowfat	1 cup	260	46.0
Mixed Berries (Dannon):			
Extra Smooth	4.4-oz. container	130	24.0
Fruit-on-the-Bottom	4.4-oz. container	130	23.0
Fruit-on-the-Bottom	8-oz. container	240	43.0
Peach:			
(Borden) *Lite-Line*	8-oz. container	230	42.0
(Breyers)	8-oz. container	270	46.0
(Dannon) Fruit-on-the-Bottom	8-oz. container	240	43.0
(Lucerne):			
Gourmet	6-oz. container	190	32.0
Lowfat	8-oz. container	260	46.0
Nonfat	8-oz. container	180	34.0
(TCBY)	8 oz.	220	36.0
(Weight Watchers) *Ultimate 90*	8 oz.	90	13.0
(Whitney's)	6-oz. container	200	33.0
Yoplait	6-oz. container	190	32.0
Pina colada:			

Food	Measure	Cals.	Carbs.
(Dannon) Fruit-on-the-Bottom	8-oz. container	240	43.0
(Lucerne) lowfat	1 cup	260	46.0
Yoplait	6-oz. container	190	32.0
Pineapple:			
(Breyers)	8-oz. container	270	45.0
(Light n' Lively)	8-oz. container	240	48.0
Yoplait	6-oz. container	190	32.0
Pineapple-grapefruit (Lucerne)	8-oz. container	260	46.0
Raspberry:			
(Breyers) red	8-oz. container	260	44.0
(Dannon):			
Extra Smooth	4.4-oz. container	130	24.0
Fresh Flavors	8-oz. container	200	34.0
Fruit-on-the-Bottom	4.4-oz. container	130	23.0
Fruit-on-the-Bottom	8-oz. container	240	43.0
(Light n' Lively) red	8-oz. container	230	43.0
(Lucerne):			
Regular or red	8-oz. container	260	46.0
Gourmet, red	6-oz. container	190	32.0
(Meadow-Gold) sundae style	8-oz. container	250	42.0
(TCBY)	8 oz.	220	42.0
(Weight Watchers) *Ultimate 90*	8 oz.	90	13.0
(Whitney's)	6-oz. container	200	33.0
Yoplait:			
Regular	6-oz. container	190	32.0
Custard Style	6-oz. container	180	30.0
Light	6-oz. container	90	14.0
Strawberry:			
(Borden) *Lite-Line*	8-oz. container	240	46.0
(Breyers)	8-oz. container	270	46.0
(Dannon):			
Extra Smooth	4.4-oz. container	130	24.0
Fresh Flavors	8-oz. container	200	34.0
Fruit-on-the-Bottom	4.4-oz. container	130	23.0
Fruit-on-the-Bottom	8-oz. container	240	43.0
(TCBY)	8 oz.	220	43.0
(Weight Watchers) *Ultimate 90*	8 oz.	90	13.0
(Whitney's)	6-oz. container	200	33.0
Yoplait:			
Regular	6-oz. container	190	32.0
Breakfast Yogurt, with almonds	6-oz. container	200	38.0

Food	Measure	Cals.	Carbs.
Custard Style	6-oz. container	180	30.0
Light	6-oz. container	90	14.0
Strawberry-banana:			
(Dannon):			
Fresh Flavors	8-oz. container	200	34.0
Fruit-on-the-Bottom	4.4-oz. container	130	23.0
Fruit-on-the-Bottom	8-oz. container	240	43.0
(Light n' Lively)	8-oz. container	260	52.0
(Sweet'n Low)	8-oz. container	190	33.0
(Weight Watchers)			
Ultimate 90	8 oz.	90	13.0
(Whitney's)	6-oz. container	200	33.0
Yoplait:			
Breakfast Yogurt	6-oz. container	240	43.0
Custard Style	6-oz. container	180	30.0
Strawberry colada (Colombo)	8-oz. container	230	36.0
Tropical, *Yoplait, Breakfast*			
Yogurt	6-oz. container	230	41.0
Tropical fruit (Sweet n' Low)	8-oz. container	150	33.0
Vanilla:			
(Breyers)	8-oz. container	230	31.0
(Dannon):			
Fresh Flavors	4.4-oz. container	110	20.0
Fresh Flavors	8-oz. container	220	34.0
(Lucerne) lowfat	1 cup	260	46.0
(Weight Watchers)			
Ultimate 90	8 oz.	90	13.0
(Whitney's)	6-oz. container	200	28.0
Yoplait, Custard Style	6-oz. container	180	30.0
Wild berries (Whitney's)	6-oz. container	200	33.0
Frozen, hard:			
Almond praline (Edy's			
Inspirations)	½ cup	130	22.0
Apple pie (Ben & Jerry's)	4 oz.	170	32.0
Banana split (Colombo)			
gourmet, lowfat, Sundae			
Style	3 oz.	100	20.0
Banana-strawberry:			
(Ben & Jerry's)	½ cup	160	32.0
(Häagen-Dazs)	½ cup	170	27.0
Blueberry (Ben & Jerry's)	½ cup	160	32.0
Boysenberry-vanilla (Edy's			
Inspirations)	½ cup	110	19.0
Brownie nut blast (Häagen-			
Dazs) Exträs	½ cup	220	29.0
Cafe mocha (Baskin-			
Robbins) *Trulyfree*	1 serving	70	16.0

Food	Measure	Cals.	Carbs.
Cappuccino coffee (Colombo) gourmet	3 oz.	120	19.0
Caramel fudge sundae (Colombo) lowfat	3 oz.	100	21.0
Caramel pecan chunk (Colombo) gourmet	3 oz.	120	19.0
Cheesecake, wild raspberry (Colombo) gourmet	3 oz.	100	18.0
Cherry:			
(Ben & Jerry's) *Cherry Garcia*	½ cup	170	31.0
(Sealtest) black, free	½ cup	110	24.0
Cherry almond chunk (Colombo) gourmet	3 oz.	110	17.0
Cherry-vanilla swirl:			
(Dannon) light, nonfat	4 oz.	90	21.0
(Edy's Inspirations) black, nonfat	½ cup	90	19.0
Chocolate:			
(Breyers)	½ cup	120	24.0
(Dannon):			
Light, nonfat	4 oz.	80	19.0
Pure Indulgence	3 oz.	130	24.0
(Edy's Inspirations):			
Regular	½ cup	110	18.0
nonfat	½ cup	90	18.0
(Häagen-Dazs)	3 oz.	130	21.0
(Sealtest) *Free*, nonfat	½ cup	110	24.0
Chocolate fudge brownie (Ben & Jerry's)	½ cup	190	35.0
Chocolate nut (Dannon) *Pure Indulgence,* chunky	4 oz.	190	24.0
Chocolate peanut butter twist sundae (Colombo)	3 oz.	110	18.0
Chocolate raspberry swirl (Ben & Jerry's)	½ cup	200	40.0
Citrus heights (Edy's Inspirations)	½ cup	120	21.0
Coconut (Baskin-Robbins) nonfat:			
Large	9 oz.	180	45.0
Medium	7 oz.	140	35.0
Small	5 oz.	100	25.0
Coffee (Häagen-Dazs)	½ cup	180	28.0
Coffee almond fudge (Ben & Jerry's)	½ cup	200	30.0
Cookies & cream:			

Food	Measure	Cals.	Carbs.
(Dannon) *Pure Indulgence*	4 oz.	180	18.0
(Edy's Inspirations)	½ cup	130	22.0
Dream (Colombo) gourmet	3 oz.	90	16.0
English toffee crunch (Ben & Jerry's)	½ cup	190	32.0
Heath bar crunch:			
(Colombo) gourmet	3 oz.	130	19.0
(Dannon) *Pure Indulgence*	4 oz.	170	25.0
(Edy's Inspirations)	½ cup	130	20.0
Marble fudge (Edy's Inspirations)	½ cup	120	20.0
Mocha Swiss almond (Colombo) gourmet	3 oz.	120	17.0
Orango tango (Häagen-Dazs) Exträas	½ cup	130	26.0
Orange-vanilla swirl (Edy's Inspirations)	½ cup	110	19.0
Peach:			
(Breyers)	½ cup	110	22.0
(Dannon) light, nonfat	4 oz.	80	19.0
(Edy's Inspirations)	½ cup	110	19.0
(Häagen-Dazs)	½ cup	170	26.0
Peanut butter cup (Colombo) gourmet	3 oz.	140	16.0
Praline Pandemonium (Häagen-Dazs) Exträas	4 oz.	240	33.0
Raspberry:			
(Dannon) red, light, nonfat	4 oz.	90	21.0
(Edy's Inspirations):			
Regular	½ cup	110	19.0
Nonfat	½ cup	90	20.0
(Sealtest) Free, nonfat	½ cup	100	23.0
Raspberry rendezvous (Häagen-Dazs) Exträas	½ cup	130	26.0
Raspberry-vanilla swirl (Edy's Inspirations)	½ cup	110	19.0
Strawberry:			
(Breyer's)	½ cup	110	22.0
(Dannon) light, nonfat	4 oz.	80	19.0
(Edy's Inspirations):			
Regular	½ cup	110	18.0
Nonfat	½ cup	90	20.0
(Häagen-Dazs)	3 oz.	120	21.0
(Sealtest) Free, nonfat	½ cup	100	22.0
Strawberry cheesecake craze (Häagen-Dazs) Exträas	4 oz.	210	31.0

Food	Measure	Cals.	Carbs.
Strawberry passion			
(Colombo) gourmet	3 oz.	100	18.0
Vanilla:			
(Baskin-Robbins) lowfat:			
Large	9 oz.	270	54.0
Medium	7 oz.	211	42.0
Small	5 oz.	150	30.0
(Breyers)	½ cup	120	23.0
(Dannon):			
Light, nonfat	3 oz.	80	20.0
Pure Indulgence	3 oz.	130	25.0
(Edy's Inspirations):			
Regular	½ cup	110	19.0
Nonfat	½ cup	90	18.0
(Häagen-Dazs)	½ cup	170	26.0
Vanilla-almond crunch			
(Häagen-Dazs)	3 oz.	150	22.0
Frozen, soft-serve:			
(Bresler's) all flavors:			
Gourmet	1 oz.	29	5.5
Lite	1 oz.	27	6.0
(Dannon):			
Blueberry, butter pecan, cappuccino, cheesecake, lemon meringue, peach, piña colada, raspberry, strawberry or strawberry banana	½ cup	100	18.0
Chocolate	½ cup	120	23.0
Red raspberry, nonfat	½ cup	90	21.0
(Häagen-Dazs):			
Regular:			
Chocolate	1 oz.	30	4.0
Coffee or vanilla	1 oz.	28	4.0
Raspberry	1 oz.	30	5.0
Nonfat:			
Chocolate	1 oz.	30	6.0
Strawberry	1 oz.	25	5.0
YOGURT BAR, frozen			
(Dole) *Fruit & Yogurt*:			
Cherry	1 bar	80	17.0
Strawberry	1 bar	70	17.0
(Häagen-Dazs):			
Cherry chocolate fudge	1 bar	230	28.0
Peach	1 bar	100	19.0
Piña colada	1 bar	100	21.0

Food	Measure	Cals.	Carbs.
Raspberry & vanilla	1 bar	100	19.0
Tropical orange passion	1 bar	100	21.0
YOGURT DESSERT, frozen (Sara Lee) *Free & Light*	¹⁄₁₀ of pkg.	120	26.0
YOGURT SHAKE, frozen (Weight Watchers) *Sweet Celebrations*, chocolate	7½ fl. oz.	220	44.0

Z

ZINFANDEL WINE (Louis M. Martini):			
Red, 12½% alcohol	3 fl. oz.	64	Tr.
White, 11% alcohol	3 fl. oz.	55	1.5
ZINGERS (Dolly Madison):			
Devil's food or white	1¼-oz. piece	140	23.0
Raspberry	1¼-oz. piece	130	20.0
ZITI, dry (see **PASTA, DRY OR FRESH, REFRIGERATED**)			
ZWEIBACK:			
(USDA)	1 oz.	120	21.1
(Gerber)	7-gram piece	30	5.1
(Nabisco)	1 piece	30	5.0

NUTRITION GUIDES BY ED BLONZ, PH.D.

❏ YOUR PERSONAL NUTRITIONIST: FIBER AND FAT COUNTER

Here is the only guide to fiber that also includes calorie and fat-gram counts. Nutrition expert Dr. Ed Blonz tells you everything you have to know about the remarkable gifts of fiber. How much you need to keep healthy, and how to easily include the right amount in your daily diet.   (184874—$3.99)

❏ YOUR PERSONAL NUTRITIONIST: ANTIOXIDANT COUNTER

Antioxidant vitamins, found in certain nutrient-rich foods, help your body guard against health threats you can't control—like air pollution, water pollution, a deteriorating ozone, and food additives. Nutrition expert Dr. Ed Blonz supplies the fat, calorie, and antioxidant vitamin contents of over 3,000 common and brand-name foods.

(184882—$3.99)

❏ YOUR PERSONAL NUTRITIONIST: CALCIUM AND OTHER MINERALS COUNTER

Most Americans—especially women—just don't include enough calcium and other minerals in their daily diet. These essential nutrients offer the best protection from brittle bones, anemia, and fatigue. Nutrition expert Dr. Ed Blonz supplies the fat, calorie, and mineral contents of over 3,000 common and popular brand-name foods.

(188802—$3.99)

❏ YOUR PERSONAL NUTRITIONIST: FOOD ADDITIVES

To help you make wise choices about the foods you buy, nutrition expert Dr. Ed Blonz brings you the facts about more than 300 natural and artificial chemical additives that are used in bakery items, canned foods, boxed foods, dairy, and meat products.

(188810—$3.99)